Living with Cancer

Living with Cancer:

A Practical Guide

Dave Visel

Rutgers University Press
New Brunswick, New Jersey, and London

Library of Congress Cataloging-in-Publication Data

Visel, Dave, 1938–
    Living with cancer : a practical guide / Dave Visel.
        p. cm.
    Includes bibliographical references and index.
    ISBN–13: 978–0–8135–3819–8 (hardcover : alk. paper)
    ISBN–13: 978–0–8135–3820–4 (pbk. : alk. paper)
    1. Cancer—Popular works. 2. Cancer—Treatment—Popular works.
3. Cancer—Psychological aspects. 4. Cancer—Patients—Family
relationships 1. Title.
    RC263.V57 2006
    616.99'4—dc22   2005020074

A British Cataloging-in-Publication record for this book is available from the
British Library

Manufactured in the United States of America

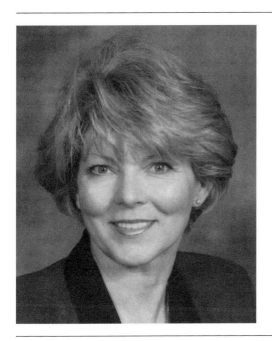

The reason for this book

Lymphoma patient,
my lady,
mother of Scott and Amy,
Kate and Drew's granny

. . . and in these better
times, project advisor and
content supervisor

Karen

Cancer also teaches us about ourselves.

Contents

Foreword

As a medical oncologist and palliative care specialist in a large cancer center, I care for individuals whose lives have been affected by serious chronic illness and work to develop more effective strategies for eliminating cancer and the suffering it causes. Because I try to offer my patients encouragement as well as treatment, I am always on the lookout for tools that will help them navigate through difficult issues that may arise. *Living with Cancer* is one such tool.

Dave Visel has not written this book from the perspective of a health-care professional or science writer. He does not work in a field related to health products, pharmaceuticals, or health information. Dave is a man whose wife, Karen, was diagnosed with cancer. He did not know what to do about her diagnosis or how to do it, but he knew he needed to learn everything about cancer—the disease itself, science, heath-care professionals, health-care systems, humanity, friendship, love, and personal coping. The result is a gift for the rest of us, a useful "What do I do now and how do I do it?" guide for all of us who have been affected by cancer or acknowledge that we are at risk for being affected by it. This book represents something that I have long wished I could give not only to my patients and their families but also to my own family, friends, and neighbors. It is not a book with all the answers, but it provides a solid foundation upon which one can build an understanding of what might be needed to deal with cancer.

> This book represents something that I have long wished I could give not only to my patients and their families but also to my own family, friends, and neighbors.

Why do I want to give this book to my family, friends, and neighbors rather than to just my patients and their families? The reason is simple—because virtually everyone I know has some reason to wish that they could understand cancer better. This is not particularly surprising, as more than 1.3 million Americans are diagnosed with invasive (and thus risky) cancer each year. About 560,000 persons die of cancer each year; however, there are also more than ten million cancer survivors among us. As our populations grow older and live longer, cancer will touch each of our lives in some way.

Cancer has touched my personal life. I was eleven years old when my mother was diagnosed with breast cancer. She underwent surgery, radiation therapy, and chemotherapy. It was hard and scary for all of us, but she survived. Two years later, she had another breast cancer, and her treatment was again successful. She currently lives with chronic lymphocytic leukemia and advanced lung cancer. In the interim, her mother died of stomach cancer, her father died of a brain tumor, and her youngest brother died of pancreatic cancer. Within sight of my own home, I have one neighbor with advanced pancreatic cancer, two neighbors whose parents died of cancer within the past year, and one neighbor whose sister is receiving treatment of advanced breast cancer. My daughter's elementary-school teacher is helping her mother deal with lung cancer; the unavoidable disruption in her personal life impacts her colleagues and our children. It is not that we live near power lines or a chemical plant or necessarily did anything wrong. This is simply the reality of our world today. At some point in our lives, we will all face the unwelcome task of understanding and navigating the confusing world of cancer.

Living with Cancer is a book that I want to have and want others to have, but it is not a book I could have written. Even health-care professionals, many of whom are gifted communicators and educators, cannot reproduce the perspective of a layperson who learned about cancer by trial and error and is willing to openly share his or her experiences. Moreover, professional organizations such as the American Cancer Society and American Society of Clinical Oncologists are well suited for providing terrific up-to-date information on a variety of cancer topics but not personal, day-to-day, how-to-live-through-cancer information of the sort in this book. Specifically, this book has a conversational style that makes it readable. Also, Dave's extensive consultations with reputable medical professionals, lawyers, philanthropists, and counselors make the information provided here credible. No physician or professional organization is going to agree with or vouch for every page of this book, however. To achieve that kind of consensus would change the nature of the book.

It is unfortunate that the typical person who comes face-to-face with the need to understand cancer is overwhelmed by the myriad of available Internet resources, as well as advice (and occasional misinformation) from friends, neighbors, and even health-care professionals. Although all the factual information in this book is attainable through other means, no other book provides this kind of comprehensive format with information and personal advice framed in a reassuring manner.

The book is not just about cancer. It is also about solving problems, finding meaning and hope in our lives even when faced with difficult circumstances, and striving to live as long and as well as possible. This book will inspire you as well as inform you.

Michael J. Fisch, MD, MPH
Medical Director, Community Clinical Oncology Program Research Base
Associate Professor, Sections of General Oncology and Palliative Care
The University of Texas, MD Anderson Cancer Center

Preface

Returning home after a wonderful winter holiday, my wife took what she thought was persistent flu to our family doctor. "Karen," he told her, "I don't like those swollen lymph glands in your neck. I think you need to be checked for lymphoma."

When she told me, I presumed that lymphoma was worse than flu. I had no idea how much worse.

The Los Angeles basin in which we live houses the largest metropolitan area in the world, more than a thousand square miles of sprawl. Within it are some of the nation's best-known cancer-treatment centers. Though we were both frightened by her lymphoma, we figured that the medical establishment would put an orderly process in place for us that would lead to treatment.

That's exactly what happened. One referral led to another, a trail we followed without understanding—or question.

Our story begins in January 2000. A month later, a friend who had lost his wife to cancer about a year earlier asked us several pointed questions about Karen's diagnosis, the selection of her medical team, and our general understanding of what was happening and why. I realize now that our answers revealed our poor support of the doctors who were trying to save Karen's life.

The following Monday, our widowed friend, LJ, piled me into his car for a visit to one of the treatment centers his wife had used. In the car, he began a gentle explanation of what a cancer patient should know and do to optimize the work of an oncology team. He talked about resources such as cancer nonprofits, government agencies, patient-support groups, reference books, survivor hot lines, and Internet sites that might help us. He explained that some medical components of success, such as second opinions and optional testing, were our responsibility as much as the medical team's. Perhaps most important, he helped me understand why I had to become an effective partner for my cancer-patient wife, and what that entailed.

By then we were pulling into the parking lot of the USC/Norris Comprehensive Cancer Center, where he had arranged for me to meet several key members of the staff. This was my first introduction to world-class oncology, its facilities, and its amazing scientist-physicians.

Years have passed. There have been surprising and very fortunate turns—beyond anything we could have predicted. It may interest you to know that, despite the outstanding credentials of thousands of local doctors, despite the presence of some of the world's most sophisticated cancer-research facilities, the lead oncologist on Karen's team is 1,500 miles away. A department head at USC Norris suggested the referral, which put Karen into the hands of the world's leading authority on her particular form of the disease. You may end up in a similar circumstance. This is a small part of a complex issue that you will learn more about as you read on.

My training as a reporter and researcher caused me to presume that I would find a book to help Karen and me deal with all the complexities of cancer. Two years later, I realized that, despite mountains of literature, videos, Web sites, there was no such collected guidance. As my lady's condition began to improve, it became clear that I needed to impart the lessons she and I had learned from thousands of sources to as many new cancer patients as possible. I needed to pay forward the quiet talk that LJ had with me in his car those years ago, and all the tutelage that followed.

Living with Cancer is not a medical book. It is about how normal everyday people like you and me *live* with cancer. It is a listing of tips and tactics that my wife and I have collected, offered to you from the point of view of those who've been down this trail ahead of both you and me, edited and reviewed by experts in the fields involved. It is about understanding your cancer, sure. It's also about how to be the most successful patient possible, which is much different. Homelife, work, personal relationships, career, children, negotiations with health and life insurers, payments of vast sums for things that you don't have vast sums for, possible physical handicaps, tax matters, legal assistance—all these change, too.

Cancer will strike more than 1.3 million other Americans besides you this year. That does not count the million-plus cases of skin cancers that are generally considered nonthreatening, though people die of them, too, on occasion. Close to ten million Americans are now classified as "cancer survivors." An industry and huge pieces of governmental machinery have clanked into place to help you. The leaps in technology are breathtaking. Estimates of the annual expenditure in all areas of this enterprise run as high as $170 billion a year, and climbing.

Imagine that you are walking down a peaceful street, minding your own business. You come to a windowless building that's a thousand stories high and goes on for as far down the block as you can see. Strangers run out of the bushes. Grab you. Push you through the door. Inside is frenetic chaos. The size, the noise, smells, confusion, bright lights, armies of scurrying people are beyond imagining. The one thing you desperately need and can't find is a receptionist.

Hi, there! Can I help you?

Acknowledgments

Special thanks to Daniel J. Lieber, MD, Oncology/Hematology, the Angeles Clinic and Research Institute and the USC School of Medicine, who served as medical editor to this book.

Several hundred others helped and deserve to be thanked. Some contributed anonymously or in passing. Of the remainder, a core group of seventy is organized so that you can appreciate both the givers and the areas of expertise they brought to this gift of knowledge and encouragement to you.

The *Living with Cancer* Team

Contributors to the outlook, the background, the insight, and providers of expertise and criticism, with affection and gratitude:

Dana Anderson, Jr., Esq.	Attorney
Kenneth Anderson, MD	Oncologist, research scientist
Rick Anderson	Cancer survivor, innovator
Rachel Beller, RN	Oncology nutritionist
Vergil Best	Christian minister
Richard Bloch	Author, cancer survivor, philanthropist
Joy Braunlich	EAP worklife coordinator
Melanie Buhrman	Internet marketing expert
Dwight Carlson, MD	Father of an AML patient, psychiatrist, author
Roy Chitwood	CEO, Max Sacks International
Roger Cicala, MD	Pain man, author
Jim Cypher	Mentor, literary agent
Robert Drew	Spouse/partner of cancer patient
Ed English	Advisor, succumbed to cancer
Nancy Fawzy, RN, PhD	Psychosocial patient-care innovator
Michael Fisch, MD	Medical Director, Community Clinical Oncology Program Research Base
Preston Gable, MD	Oncology/hematology; cdr., USN
Otis Glasscock	Advisor, great tenor, succumbed to cancer
Mitch Golant, PhD	Vice president, Research and Development, Wellness Community
Scott Goodwin	HR consultant
Peggy Guziak	Spouse/partner of cancer patient, HR expert

Jo Hanson	Advisor, succumbed to cancer
Tom Hanson	Spouse/partner of cancer patient, pharmacist
Carolita Hart, CSC	Advisor; Archdioceses of Los Angeles
Phil Hodges	HR expert, author
Ruth Ip	Financial officer, cheerleader
Safy Jacob	Intercessor, pharmacist
Glen and Julie Johnson	Family counselors
Sue Kaled, RN	Psychosocial patient-care specialist
Song Kang, MD	Radiation oncology; lt. cdr., USN
Dale and Maxine Kaufman	A model partner/patient team
Michael Keating, MD	Oncologist, research scientist
Nancy Kolanz, RN	Oncology nurse
Jim Lack	CEO, RCA Media
Susan Lerner	Clinical protocol administrator
Jim Lester	Hospital CEO, health industry leader
Gwynn Lewis	Christian missionary
Judy Lindberg-McFarland	Founder, Lindberg Nutrition
Letty McGowan	Facilitator extraordinary
Brenda McNamara	Cancer survivor, educator
Mike McNamara, Esq.	Spouse/partner of cancer patient
Robert Mayer, MD	Oncologist
Arnold Nagely, DVM	Veterinarian, CEO
Judy Nagely	Educator
Bobbe Needham	Extraordinary editor
Jim Nentwig	Spouse/partner, hospital trustee, patron
Nelly Northcross, RN	Oncology nursing supervisor
Deirdre O'Reilly-Marblestone, Esq.	Staff counsel, Patient Advocate Foundation
Richard Pavlick, Esq	Engineer, attorney
Lawrence Piro, MD	Oncologist, research scientist, CEO
David Pulsifer	CEO, BD Healthcare Consulting
Vangie Rich	Executive director, Bloch Cancer Foundation
Glenn Ridgway	Group health insurance expert
Howard Rosenberg	Father's Day Council, cancer survivor
Liz Safly	Harry S. Truman Library
Ahmad Sakr, PhD	Islam theologian
Barbara Schwerin, Esq,	Disability-rights attorney
Nancy Siever	Bereavement counselor
Steven Silver	Rabbi
June Simmons	CEO, Partners in Care Foundation
Joshua Smith	Navy journalist
Benjamin Spock, MD	Pediatrician, author
L.J. Stogsdill	Spouse/partner of cancer patient, mentor
Jim Tamkin, MD	Endocrinologist, cancer patient
Claire Tehan	CEO, Trinity Care Hospice
Karen Visel	Cancer survivor, author's conscience

Catherine Walden	Executive director, American Amputee Foundation
Derek White	Cancer survivor, retail executive
Deane Wolcott, MD	Psychiatrist, hospital services innovator
Audra Wolfe, PhD	Science editor, Rutgers University Press
Linda Yarger, MLS	Medical librarian
Joe Zanetta, Esq.	Hospital economics authority

Quick Starts

Dear cancer patient:

You, or someone who matters to you, is under attack. This book is your survival guide. This section is intended to help you make the most of all the information that follows, quickly and efficiently.

You need only one chapter, the first, to get oriented. Following it, you will see many areas of interest. It is absolutely fine either to continue reading chapter by chapter, or to skip about in whatever sequence seems best to you. For example, if finances are today's biggest worry, go right to "Supporting Resources," Part IV.

Rather than treat this as a traditional book, think of it as a bag of tips and tactics or a box of tools held between two covers to keep things off the floor. There is information here that you need right now, and other stuff that may leave you scratching your head. Please don't be distracted if the first topics you come across aren't what concern you most. Move on. If, for example, there is no possible way for you, a cancer patient, to take advantage of the recommendation that you find a supporting partner to go to treatments with, don't conclude that all is lost and close the book. A partner will make it better. Perhaps one will come along later. Knowing that you need one will help you stay on the lookout. Okay. We're done with that subject. Go on to the next. Learn about leads to advanced treatment centers, effective ways to negotiate with your health-insurance provider, finding survivors of your kind of cancer to talk to, how to break the news to your boss and your kids, the tax implications of this thing, whether or not you're going to lose your hair or end up a drug addict.

One area is particularly sensitive to a few readers—the references to spirituality. Eighty-seven percent of cancer patients want this information. If you are part of the other 13 percent, don't conclude that *Living with Cancer* is a sneaky way to involve you in the God thing, or to "convert" you from one faith to another. Just move on.

To relatives and friends:

When a loved one is diagnosed with cancer, close friends and relatives feel a great need to know all the details and what they can do to help. It's not gonna happen.

You're not going to get whole, candid insight because, in the beginning, nobody has much more than the rudimentary facts, which he or she may or may not understand or even have gotten right. Moreover, the patient may or may not be inclined to divulge these details, or much of anything else, to you.

You're not going to learn what you can do to help, either, because that won't be evident to the shocked patient, at least for some time. So be the supporting, caring friend that's really needed. Read on. Learn how to provide the help your loved one may not even know how to ask you for.

To the oncology team:

When you're looking at a cancer patient, you're thinking about diagnosis and treatment. What do you suppose your typical patient thinks about, looking at you? There are family worries and the contemplation of disfigurement or death. Patients must also actively struggle with the financial challenges and the impersonal conduct of health insurers and government "welfare" agencies. Patients have to deal with a plethora of problems at work, some of them grossly unfair. All of it handed to people who feel lousy anyway, and very insecure.

Living with Cancer leaves the technical side of surviving the disease to you, and recommends that cancer patients do, too. There is really quite enough to deal with, being a patient. You learned about some of this in medical school, but it was mostly psych related. There's much more.

If you've never been exposed to the canons of today's real cancer patient, take a look at the Contents. Maybe sample a chapter or two in "Team Building" and "Supporting Resource," Parts III and IV, or read about the patient's treatment issues discussed later in the book. These are the further dimensions of those vessels of disease now leafing through back issues of *Good Housekeeping* in your waiting room. These concerns impact the decisions your patients make and their chances for survival.

To the family's established physicians, pharmacists, therapists, counselors, and other caregivers:

Your patient's episode with cancer will go better with you in the loop to make direct, regular, and meaningful contributions. With your busy schedule over very long hours, that's hard, of course. Particularly because you will probably have to take the initiative at least some of the time to be certain that the communications line stays open.

Even though cancer has distracted your patient, even though it hasn't occurred to the cancer patient to keep you informed, please give time to the case.

There are short sections about each of you later in *Living with Cancer,* with reasons why the patient should continue to actively solicit your expertise. But during the cancer-fighting experience, most patients lose the focus necessary to do everything that might be good for them. Please recognize the patient's need for your active interest. Keep in touch. It reinforces the traditional, core value that is the very basis of family medicine.

To students of cancer care:

The literature you reviewed before opening *Living with Cancer* dealt with cancer care from other points of view. The material coming from the oncology community and the pharmaceutical houses spent its energies on scientific cause and effect. You may have also read about psychoanalytical issues pertaining to the patient and the patient's loved ones and family members. In addition to commentaries on science, there are excellent discussions focused on theological issues available, and some truly well-told first-person narratives by cancer survivors.

Now you come to a new perspective. This is a handbook for those who have recently been diagnosed that aims to give the patient general directions learned from the been-there-done-that school of hard knocks.

Living with Cancer's benefit for you should be an understanding of how the clinical, spiritual, and psychological aspects of feeling miserable and scared tie together with the insurance, tax, family, financial, and work issues and the impositions of social engineers.

One wonderful outcome could be that some of these data will help you design better policies or services, or in some other way lighten the load that so many vested interests have placed on these wounded people.

I Introduction

Setting the Stage

1 Now What?

The diagnosis is cancer.
Unbelievable.
Scary.

Irritating.
Looks expensive,
Demanding, disruptive.

There's so much to figure out.
Now what?

"Now what?" is not a simple question. It will take this whole book to answer. But even after your first few minutes in these pages, you'll have more confidence in what you're doing. More to the point, you'll be going in the right direction.

Maybe not the one you had in mind. Be open to that.

You'll get help finding all the resources you may need for recovery, including some you haven't thought about yet. This breadth and depth will become increasingly important as you learn more ways to defeat this very complicated disease.

The illness will impact the rest of your life too. Your job, your family, your finances. By deciding to survive this disease, you have a bigger project to manage than you realize right now. But *Living with Cancer* offers chapters on every area where you may need help.

Forget What You Think You Know

Just about everyone has impressions of cancer based on the experiences of people they have known who suffered from it. These recollections may give you insights into your own predicament—or you may be completely misled.

Misled is more likely. Cancer treatments have radically changed and improved from what they were like even a few years ago. Things that have the same names are much different, more effective, more comfortable to go through, less damaging to our lives and our appearance than you may believe.

People's attitudes regarding cancer have changed too. In years past, polite society didn't discuss the effects of cancer for many reasons, often having to do with someone's impending death. The unstated usually had a more frightening visage than the problem would have if it had been explained.

People were also silent because the colon, rectum, men's prostate, and women's breasts—sites of large numbers of cancers—were not referred to in mixed company. We still observe this convention. As a result, mysteries and myths persist.

As difficult as it may be for you, set aside these ideas and beliefs for the moment. Whether these concepts of yours are true or false doesn't matter. Erase the blackboard and go back to your seat. We're starting class over, together.

Telling People That You Have Cancer

Let's be clear: For many, many reasons, you need to announce your condition. Keeping cancer a secret is a very bad idea. That leaves us with how and when, which deserves some thought.

A reminder: Conditions like a broken bone, or even a bad appendix— which are serious—are in a different league. With those sorts of things, your doc is absolutely confident of the proper treatment and of your recovery. By contrast, with cancer, medical science offers hope, but no assurances. People start giving you statistics of probability: "We're 65 percent sure . . . "; "In 80 percent of the cases . . . " These are great gambling odds, but not promises of recovery.

The seriousness of cancer changes the impact of your announcement. You need a little perspective, and a plan, to avoid potholes in the road just ahead.

The perspective is this: Your very serious health condition is going to upset everyone who loves you and, a second group, those who count on you. Your loved ones will be upset because they love you and they hurt for you. Your announcement needs to deftly serve each one, particularly your frightened children, your spouse, and aging parents.

You have a professional relationship with others who count on you at work. Though some or all of these acquaintances may also love you, those who think of you as a team member will also quickly consider what they have to lose if your sickness progresses. If you happen to play a role that could impact the wealth of others, your cancer announcement is going to rivet their attention too. Shareholders, employees, and a former spouse whom you support are in this category. Before you make any disclosure to these people, see Chapter 12, "The Patient's Workplace."

You have probably formulated a sufficient plan in your head, just by having read the last few paragraphs. But let's broadly touch on a few planning principles for you to consider.

- Keep the description of the disease, and what your medical team expects to do about it, short, direct, and simple. ("I have lung cancer. X-rays show a tumor that has to come out. After that, I'm told to expect both radiation and chemotherapy. Looks like I could be in treatment and then recovery for several months.")
- Don't speculate. ("I'm not certain when all this is going to start or how long it will take. We have some tests first and then I'm going to get second opinions. I should know more in a week or so.")
- Be positive. ("Everyone I work with on this is optimistic. It certainly is serious, but I'm told there are far more effective procedures now than ever before, and some terrific new drugs.")

- Be yourself. This time, above all times, calls for absolute, complete honesty. The fear and sickness are real and earned. Be candid with your medical team and your "care unit," the team of family and friends that surrounds you. This probity is an important tool for fighting your cancer—and for keeping from going absolutely nuts while you're at it.
- Be prepared for awkward comments and questions. People you think you know well will say things to you that are jaw-droppers. Others will find that they can't complete a sentence in your presence, or they get teary eyed talking to you. Keep a pleasant expression. Don't rush to reply. Your pause may be as good as an answer. Don't be offended. With practice, and honesty, you will find ways to give these encounters the grace and dignity they need.

Planning what you say, how and when you say it, and what you will do then is an intensely personal business. There is no prototype plan to use as a guide. Think about what you want to do. Bounce ideas off your doc or a nurse. Get your spouse or a close friend to help you put together a plan for telling everyone else.

Sample Jaw-Dropper:

"Gee, you look really good . . . for a guy with cancer."

A Quick Backgrounder

Your personal success will largely come from ignoring the big picture and the "facts" that "everybody knows." You'll learn here to focus instead on managing your disease and to minimize the damage it might do to the rest of your life.

But we'll begin with a quick look at the big picture anyway. "Cancer" is actually a family of diseases, more than two hundred. Some say thousands. The courses for treatment of them vary, as do success rates. About ten million people in the United States are living with one or more of them at any given time, of whom more than half a million will succumb this year. Cancer is the nation's second-greatest killer, after heart disease.

Cancer has been of formal interest to medical practitioners for some 3,500 years. But the majority of the advances against it are less than 25 years old. This process is accelerating at a breathtaking rate. More has been learned about cancer in the last three years than in the entire preceding course of human history.

You are one of about 1.3 million men, women, and children who will be diagnosed with cancer this year in the United States. This large number may be because the incidence of cancer is greater now than in the past, as some claim. Or it may be that the improved methods of early detection, the ever-growing population of the United States, and our generally greater health consciousness have caused this "epidemic."

None of this is going to make you feel any better about having your disease. But it will help you understand why your treatment world is shaped and flavored as it is. Though the consolation is minimal, you may also come to believe that this is a much better time than any other to have been afflicted with cancer.

When you first hear, "I'm terribly sorry to tell you . . . ," a shock wave rapidly builds behind the words. You feel like you've been hit by a ton of bricks. You fall into a deep, dark, cold, lonely place you never expected to be. It is a bleak region that holds nothing but questions and fears. It's as if a giant tsunami wave came out of nowhere and left you breathless and blinded. Totally helpless. This is what I call no-man's-land.

If you or your loved one is sucked under by that wave right now, please know that soon, out of the confusion, darkness, and fear, sanity will reappear. Yes, you or your loved one has cancer. Yes, the situation is bad. But you are not alone. There are lifeguards on duty. All sorts of help are on the way. Hang in there. Millions of Americans—like me—have taken the awful plunge ahead of you, and made it back to shore.

James A. Tamkin, MD, endocrinologist, cancer patient

Preview of Next Medical Things to Do

This thing that has happened to you is sort of like being hit by a truck in a hospital parking lot. You didn't need the experience, but since it happened, at least help is handy.

Now that it's happened, you want to get on with treatment. Before you do, you need a plan and priorities. Otherwise, it's almost a certain bet that you will make costly, maybe painful mistakes.

Cancer is not like a cut finger or a broken bone. There's no bleeding to stop, no dangling limb to cast. And it is a much more elusive problem to understand. Your medical team has to pinpoint which of this large number of similar diseases it will be dealing with. Beyond that, your specific cancer probably belongs to a subtype. Your doctors know that the best treatment for one form of cancer may actually make another, maybe closely related form more aggressive. So getting the proper diagnosis is the most important next thing to do, by far.

Because of the complex nature of cancer, this exact naming of what you have may require the concurrence of several medical specialties, after multiple tests and possibly surgical procedures. Attend to this part of the situation as quickly as possible, but if it takes days or even weeks, so be it. Until your panel of experts agrees on everything that needs to be known, disastrous—even fatal—decisions are distinct possibilities.

The Power of "We"

It will help to have someone share this experience with you from this point on. Ideally, this person has made a commitment to be constantly at your side during treatments and evaluations, though a group of friends can also serve this need. A spouse, a parent, an adult child, or another close relative would all be good choices, so long as the person is caring and alert. A close friend is a next alternative, followed by a professional caregiver. This strong suggestion is the point of Chapter 3. Part VII of this book, "Relationships," also contributes information you may need to consider. After you have decided on a partner, that person should read Chapter 9.

But I Was Planning To . . .

No plan, nothing that happened before your cancer diagnosis, takes priority over the cancer-based activities now crowding into your life, except maybe your children's needs if you are a parent. That new job, the school, the trip, the marriage—the life you had—has changed. Subordinate everything to the care you need. Later, as your diagnosis and treatment programs progress, you will learn how and when you can relax this strict discipline a little. Until then, play it safe, focus, and learn.

A New Place

It's all right if you find the hurried, antiseptic world of medicine unsettling. Despite the flowers and friendly smiles, this is a place full of sick people and those trying to fix them up. Science and strange apparatus dominate the environment. People with needles and things to peer into your ears or down your throat seem to be everywhere.

The saving grace is that they are nice people with magnificent, encyclopedic knowledge of your health needs and with awesome energy. They care a great deal about you. You will learn to forgive their strangeness and marvel at the deftness and grace with which they help their patients through good and bad times alike.

Settle In

You need to become one with them. First, you must learn the details of your particular illness. It isn't just cancer. It's some particular kind of cell that originated in some specific place in your body, and it has developed into something or other for which certain remedies are to be applied, which you should know how to describe. The help you need for this part of living with cancer starts in Chapter 4. Another part is the learning of what these tests, lotions, potions, doping, scraping, zapping, and cutting are all about. See Chapter 5. Nobody is expected to become as conversant with the technical terms as your medical team is. But you will benefit by learning a bit about cancer-treatment terminology. Chapter 6 expounds on why that is so.

Team Building

People don't beat cancer. Teams of people do.

As you read this, you may be sick, lonely, worried, and overburdened. And now, you are thinking, here's even more I have to do.

No. The main points of these few paragraphs on team building are these: First, teams, rather than individuals, are the norm in every aspect of cancer fighting. Second, teams will naturally form around you to help fight your cancer. Recognize and encourage them.

Since your diagnosis, a lot of people have already come into your life specifically to help you fight cancer. More will join them. Others—support groups, legal aides, helpers with finances and certain services you suddenly discover you need, and people to pray with—stand ready for you or your partner to request. For much more, see "Team Building" and "Supporting Resources," Parts III and IV.

Workplace Issues, Including Your Professional Standing

You can be fired for having cancer. You can lose your professional standing. People will tell you that there are laws that protect a person with a critical illness from job discrimination. It is true that many such laws exist. It is not true that a person receives much protection as a result, with notable exceptions.

This situation and the measures a person can take for protection are one focus of Chapter 12, "The Patient's Workplace." Until you have digested it and decided which parts are most helpful in your situation, it is suggested that you not disclose your diagnosis to anyone you know professionally. Just wait a day or two. There is a great deal to lose and not much upside until you have taken the time to put a positive plan of action in place.

Your Big Guns

A great many people and resources will be coming to help you with this cancer. There are fabulous medical treatment complexes, sophisticated health insurers, federal, state, and local government support, private-sector help—which should include a cancer-care group, your employer, and your place of worship. You are supported by multiple billion-dollar research and development projects with new pharmaceuticals, equipment, and techniques. This generating and spending of resources exceeds the gross national product of all but a handful of nations. And all this is available to help you.

More personally, you have a medical team that has more capabilities than any team anywhere in the world had a generation ago. In 1980, the queen's crown jewels couldn't have bought the sophisticated care you will receive.

Everything associated with your cancer treatment is *big*. Don't shy away from the army sent to your rescue. Accept the attention. Be comforted.

You may live in a rural place and see no more than one doctor or a few. Or you may find yourself at a clinic that uses armies of doctors and nurses to treat hundreds of cancer patients a day. No matter. The behind-the-scenes support of your healing team and the science they use can be pretty much the same.

Some of the equipment is StarTrek spooky. The medicines do weird and wonderful things and are priced accordingly. Individual pills may cost more than a hundred dollars. Some shots and intravenous medications cost thousands each. Forty minutes in a body scanner may top a thousand dollars.

You're worth it. You can afford it. The "how" will be answered in "Supporting Resources," Part IV, so move forward with confidence.

Your Personal Resources

The bad news is that we live in a country without cradle-to-grave medical care. This makes the process of selecting from the myriad of medical options, and then paying the bills, very complex. The good news is that all of the world that has adopted the socialized approach to medicine sends its best and brightest citizens to the United States when cancer becomes life-threatening. Now that you have major health-care needs, someone may bemoan your lack of free doctors and medicines. Don't take it to heart. No system is perfect. But ours in the United States is by far the most likely to meet your health needs.

"Supporting Resources," Part IV, can simplify the issues somewhat. It provides help negotiating with the third parties that fund the most expensive cancer procedures. It opens windows on programs that have been created for the poor and the elderly. It gives some insight into the charitable efforts of public and private institutions that may be new to you. It comments on some of their strengths and limitations. More important—at least to some—you will learn how to join support groups that help patients and their partners with specific problems. These groups are made up of experts who know exactly where you're coming from, have been there, done that, got the T-shirt. Though this help is priceless, it is also free. See Chapter 19.

Financial Survival

A Siamese twin comes joined at the chest to every major treatment decision you make. Its name is Payforitby. You dare not try to separate this twin. Decision and Payforitby share one heart. Unless you plan to pay cash for your cancer-treatment program, Payforitby has to be addressed at each step, from this moment forward.

Yes, I am going to have an MRI. I will Payforitby ——.

I will have the biopsy surgery at ——. I will Payforitby ——.

My medications, my chemo, my radiation, my recovery arrangements, my plastic and reconstruction surgeries? I will Payforitby —— .

"You must make arrangements for all the financial support, beforehand. It has to be specific, signed, sealed, and delivered. Get careless, and there's a chance of a nasty surprise," advises George Russell, CPA, advisor, and veteran of many wars over cancer care finance. "We're talking about a mistake that could cost tens of thousands of dollars."

There are plenty of creative ways to get things paid for. Some of the best require you to obtain approval before beginning the procedure.

You may find huge gaps in the health protection you thought you had. For example, "comprehensive" health-insurance and health-maintenance plans often specifically exclude transplants, prosthetic devices, and some advanced medicines. They may exclude expensive support items, such as home-care supplies and things like wigs. You may get them covered. But only if Payforitby is taken care of up front. Part IV, "Supporting Resources," is in place to help.

Some Notable Things about Being Very Ill

By the time a person is diagnosed, there are usually symptoms. But often the worst is yet to come. Cancer and its treatments have terrible reputations. In general, both the effects of the disease and the perturbations of treatments are much less threatening today. So it is particularly disturbing to the oncology community to see that, out of fear and ignorance, some people never seriously attempt to receive treatment. They forget: Dying is worse.

Part V, "The Illness," gives you a patient's view of the experiences current cancer patients go through. It explains all the basic types of cancer treatments. Chemotherapy gets an introduction in Chapter 27 and then the whole of Chapter 33. The first is on what the experience is and how it works. The second is evidence submitted in defense of a treatment that has a really, really bad rep—not always deserved. It offers every special tip for reducing the problems associated with chemo that a large assortment of chemo veterans and nurses could come up with.

Nutrition and physical fitness are examined in Chapter 28. It includes programs that prepare the body for certain treatments and ways to recover more quickly through exercise and diet. There is also a discussion of "cures" claimed through nutrition and food supplementation. The controversy is heartbreaking because of the schism between opposite opinions and because of the finality of decisions patients sometimes make. As with all medical issues, you don't get the answer here. You get tools, references, and the confidence to pursue a wise path.

Modern Doctoring's Limits

After advising you on matters concerning your illness, your medical teams will, as best they can, help with your insurance claims. They will also coordinate with your pharmacist. They may give you referrals to other necessary medical services and therapies. Do not expect more from your doctors. Legal and social practices have changed from the probably mythical day when a physician had an encyclopedic grasp of all manner of topics outside the strict and narrow bounds of clinical services. It is unfair for you to expect your doctors to counsel you on matters such as your finances, your problems at work, your new relationships with all kinds of people, and the host of other nonmedical things going on in your life.

A closely related point: While many people expect a book on living with cancer to be written by a doctor, medical care is only one part of this journey. The broad view of living with cancer needs to be taken from the patient's perspective, not the doctor's. Any of many gifted physicians who also happen to be good reporters could have written *Living with Cancer*. But it is the reporting, the eclectic drudgery of the ink-stained wretch, that has value—not the mastery of medicine. (As an aside, a pediatrician named Benjamin Spock provided both the inspiration and the editorial concept for *Living with Cancer*.)

Core Concept: You Are the Patient

The most important part of being a patient with a potentially fatal disease is following orders. Once you have picked your team and have a program underway, you must listen and obey.

If you are like most adults, you have become accustomed to making illness bend a bit to suit the other things going on in your life. Got a cold? Wait a day before treatment and see if it goes away. Hurt? Headache? We all play through pain when we have to. Take an aspirin and soldier on.

These are lifestyle habits that are absolutely suitable to noncritical illnesses.

Don't confuse then and now. Play the role of patient with every care. If the doctor says come back in six weeks, first, come back, and second, do it in exactly six weeks. If something comes along to make it difficult or inconvenient to follow your doctor's orders, explain the problem to the doctor. Listen to the reply. Be prepared to subordinate everything else to your role as patient.

Forget the Hospital Soaps

You may imagine that living with cancer will involve hospital environments like the ones on daytime TV. There you are in a bed, tubes and wires everywhere, surrounded by gizmos and monitors. Wrong. Most of your treatments are likely to be provided on an outpatient basis. Your medical personnel may be as good-looking as the TV actors, but, sadly, you don't get the hand-holding. They will tend to work with you in teams rather than as individuals, and then you have to go home at the end of the day and complain to somebody else.

Except for the warm-fuzzy ministration you never got, this is a good thing. There are extraordinarily wealthy cancer patients in this world who can afford to buy whole hospitals if they choose to. Even they receive outpatient team medicine. It is the best, most effective means of fighting cancer at most stages.

How to Use This Book

There is a secret to successful eating at a wedding-reception buffet: Don't load up on salad. If you can get away with it, do a reconnaissance walk around the table, taking careful note of where the best stuff is. Then put a courtesy leaf of lettuce on your plate, saving plenty of room for the strawberries, roast beef, and dessert.

To this point, the intent of this book has been to provide an overview of a table with many entrees and a large, empty plate on which to heap the topics of most pressing concern. Nobody consumes all of what's here in one sitting or even several. You have to go at it in stages. Even then, there are things one is apt to forget.

Here's the recommended drill.

Get a yellow highlighter, some of those 1 1/2″ × 2″ Post-it Notes, and a mechanical pencil—pencil so you can erase, mechanical because the point stays reasonably sharp. You won't run out of lead in the midst of an important note to yourself.

Every time you open this book, have these supplies handy. Highlight the things that are most important to you or that you want to ask somebody about. Use Post-Its for tabbing pages and for notes where you can't find room to write on the page. Use some of the blank area in the front or back as your personal topical index and treatment-notes sections.

Don't treat this book like some little collector's item perched daintily on a shelf. Carry it around. Write in it. Paste and tape in stuff. Keep taking what you need from it, whenever and however that works best for you.

www.aboutmycancer.com

Aboutmycancer is a supporting Web site created to give you a place to look for updates of information that constantly changes. The latest phone numbers and addresses of the resources in the back of this book are good examples. You may also find important links to supporting Web sites.

Aboutmycancer also has a direct private channel to the author, Dave Visel. Its purpose is to collect comments, suggestions, updates, and any other information you think may enrich the service of this project to others struggling with cancer.

Each individual must become an active participant in the choices to be made.

Richard Klausner, MD, Director, National Cancer Institute, 1995–2001

Your Expectations

As time passes and events unfold, you will learn how to take maximum advantage of what is known about your cancer and apply it rigorously to your unique circumstances. This is the shortest path to a remission, when there is one. When there isn't, this gives cancer the longest and toughest obstacle course to complete before it can harm you. It also buys time for the promising new developments constantly being introduced.

It is a process for living with cancer.

II Orientation

Some Preliminary Introductions and Suggestions

2 Personal Decisions

The decision to take action against cancer—or not to take it—has implications and consequences to understand.

You Da Man

Cancer has a way of focusing lives. Youngsters grow up. Workers suit up. Fighters step up. The timid curl up. Some people give up. The one thing that you as a cancer patient cannot do is assign the disease and its consequences to someone else. In the parlance of the day, you da man.

So what are you going to do?

Thoughts on Doing Nothing

You can choose to do nothing. People do it all the time. Life goes on for a while, and then things change.

You don't need to listen to another word from your oncologist. You can also make it clear to those who know about your diagnosis that the subject is taboo with you. All but the really pushy ones will respect your request. They will think you're weird and discuss you ad nauseum behind your back. But you won't hear any of it except by accident.

You will be able to continue ignoring the subject until a doctor is forced by circumstances to clarify some matters with you. Such a conversation is not apt to help you avoid impending consequences. Its objectives are to keep surprises from making your life worse than it needs to be, to reduce physical unpleasantness, and maybe to help loved ones understand a process.

There is a chance that this course of nonaction will produce a miraculous result. Your cancer could go away on its own. Vanish. For more on this long shot, see Chapter 37, "Getting 'Better.'"

Intervention

Few if any of those who look the other way after learning that cancer has entered their lives will read this far. Possibly someone who hasn't given up on the patient is still reading. A word to that friend: Convincing a person who has not taken action to change his or her mind can be difficult. Consider getting help from someone who understands this circumstance and who has successfully convinced the reticent to seek treatment in the past.

Those who do not seek treatment may be in denial or immobilized by fear. Some think they ought to die. Some are ambivalent because of cost or an anticipated physical loss. Others may be willing to risk their lives to get attention. None of these are trivial matters for the amateur psychologist to tinker with.

To find an intervention specialist:

- Talk to the patient's physician.
- Go to the Reference Center. Discuss your problem with people at one or more of the resources listed under the form of cancer involved.
- Is there an employee-assistance professional at the patient's workplace (see Chapter 12)?
- Is there an appropriate spiritual advisor?
- If a government agency such as VA or welfare is involved, talk to the patient's caseworker.
- Talk to the nurse-advocate or case nurse at the patient's health-insurance carrier or HMO (see Chapter 14).

Intervention makes most sense during the window in which the patient can be reasonably expected to enjoy a good recovery. A person planning to reason with a patient should also be prepared for the possibility that the patient's choice is not only final, but that it has merit.

Patients Decide Two Issues in Their Favor—Or in Cancer's

Doctors will do what they have to do—are duty-bound to do—unless the patient takes charge.

Those who have served in the military understand that a war game is not an amusement, nor is it sporting. When you see gaming phrases used here, think in terms of war, which is what a cancer fight is. Outcomes can be quite final. Any strategy that puts the enemy at a disadvantage is good. In this case, the patient has two matters to settle that give recovery major advantages. These issues are always present at the start of the illness. Each involves a limited-time offer. Expiration of these offers is without notice and pretty much irrevocable. If the patient doesn't grab the ball, the cancer will.

Issue One: Choose to Be Effectively Treated

You have the right to make disease-management decisions. You are actually expected to. Somebody is going to decide modes of treatment, types, tests, places, objectives that you want to shoot for—that sort of thing. You get first crack. You, your doctor, this book, and others come up with ideas and alternatives. You decide. If you demur, some parts of the matter will hang within easy reach for a while and then go away. Other parts of treatment issues won't ever go away and will eventually demand action. Once they have gone critical, these decisions will bounce from an indecisive patient to the spouse or closest family member, to the doctor in charge, or to some social worker if you are in a government-controlled program like Medicaid or the VA. Sometimes irresolution brings issues of law into play, which makes things messier still. Can you imagine being forced to be part of a mental competency hearing simply because you didn't want to make a decision? In most cases, you will avoid all this by deciding something up front. Just about anything resembling a choice will do. Change your mind later if circumstances permit.

Issue Two: Pick the Most Healthful Environment

It boils down to this. You can choose to be sick at home or at somebody else's place. You can choose the people you are going to be sick with or let strangers wipe your chin.

The needs of a patient are individual. There are times when all the high-tech gear has to be rolled in and all the caregivers are pros. But where you have a choice, pick home over the hospital and family over other caregivers. Even when you feel you might be imposing—even when you *are* imposing—you will recover better in familiar surroundings among friends and family.

Will Anyone Listen to You?

Particularly early and late in life, cancer patients have special trouble asserting themselves.

- If you are thirteen years old, it may be hard to get your mom and dad to listen to something important that you have to tell them about your illness. It may also be hard for you to listen carefully to them. Lead by example: Listen to your parents. See if they won't return the courtesy.
- If you are a seasoned citizen, how do you tell your frantic children and grandchildren that you've decided for or against an operation? Then how do you get them to stop trying to change your mind?
- If your spouse has always provided the leadership in the marriage, how do you take charge of a treatment issue now? Even if the matter is complex and directly affects both of you, such as an endangered unborn child, the cancer patient should make the final decision.

Partners and caregivers who are inclined to take charge, please note: Even the very young and the elderly will improve the conditions in which they endure their illness by taking active roles in the management of their treatments and in the selection of their support teams.

Making a Request Effectively

The person that you, the patient, need to reach may be unaccustomed to listening—to really paying attention—to you. Or the shock and sadness of the disease may have so filled their ears and stiffened their neck that getting a considerate hearing seems hopeless.

Try this, as one possibly effective strategy: (1) Make eye contact. (2) Pause. Maybe take the person's hand in yours. (3) Say something like, "This is very important to me. Please just listen." (4) Deliver your message succinctly. (5) At this point, if this is a tough case, your listener will usually object to some part of what you have just said. (6) Reply, "I'm not asking for a discussion. I am asking if [the request] is possible." (7) If yes, mission accomplished. (8) Thank the person, whose mouth is undoubtedly still open, stifled words jammed back between the ears. (9) Suggest, with a smile, that the person close their mouth. (10) Change the subject.

If the person could not stifle a no, ask why not. Just listen. Don't argue. There may be an excellent reason, or you may have a bit more negotiating to do. You have planted the seed. Give the topic a rest for now.

A second possible strategy is to give your message to a trusted friend for delivery. This may take skill and finesse on the part of your messenger. Fireworks may follow.

Sometimes a note works.

Sometimes you will need multiple tries, through multiple channels, to be heard and believed. The energy you may need for this might be hard to come by. At the point where your energy and patience are gone, play the "I've decided and I'm too sick to discuss it further" card. Close the case.

More on Control Issues

If the family is riled up over multiple issues surrounding your sickness, perhaps with multiple solutions in furious debate, think nothing of it. Your kin are a bunch of pansies compared to professional politicians.

Congress is the most notoriously chaotic body known to humanity. How is it that bitterly opposed partisans in the House and Senate manage to come to agreement on laws? The contrivance is the whip. Each side in each house picks a leader, a whip, who is allowed to establish general order and to negotiate with the other party leaders. Could that same principle work for your gang?

The Whip(s)

There is a family member—your partner in cancer therapy, your spouse, your older sister from college who can sweet-talk your dad, your son—or your doctor or your nurse who can get the attention of the rest, or of some faction. Call this person aside. Explain the whip concept. Ask for help. Make it an assignment.

When the whip operates properly, at least some laughter and kidding will blend in with some of the serious disagreements. One or more whips may also help the rest of the family grow together, be a family. Later, this process can lead to some imaginative presentations at the ceremony where the family declares victory over the patient's cancer.

This method doesn't always work, but something has to. Family ties and friendships must not be allowed to become secondary casualties of the disease.

A Personal or Family Web Site

Some may find the idea of an electronic cancer update practical, even appealing. Presuming that you have a home computer and that you use it to send and receive e-mail, your Internet provider can help with both the physical arrangements and the design ideas. A simple Web page may be low cost or even free.

Every case is different. Many times, someone close to the patient or to the patient's family may take on the chore of setting up a site and keeping it current.

3 The Idea of Patient Partnering

Allow others to give you help and companionship. Nobody should face cancer alone.

Say Hello to a New Place and Settle In

A special circumstance has been forced on you because you are a cancer patient. The rules by which you have lived must be temporarily changed. Existing practices either have to be suspended or modified for the term of this ordeal. Places have to be carved out for new parts of your life that have to do with tests, treatments, rest, and recovery. Things you enjoy and don't want to give up must go, at least for now.

The patient's first responsibility is to avoid denial. Recognize cancer as a fact and accept this need for accommodation. "De-nial" is not a river in Egypt, nor is it a useful recovery tool.

The next step is to expect and welcome help. To begin with, somebody should be with you on cancer-care visits from today on. A great deal of information is presented very quickly at these gatherings. Two sets of eyes and ears will improve understanding. Two in-sync brains will think of more issues to clarify and will suggest more creative solutions to problems. The meeting will be more fruitful. There'll be less chance you'll miss something important. You'll feel much better about what was accomplished.

There are a number of other reasons to welcome companionship. Among the most obvious is that you need physical assistance on occasion, or soon will. Besides, the whole thing's much more bearable with a friend alongside.

The Patient's Division of Tasks

It doesn't always happen, but usually there are one or more low points in the battle during which the patient feels quite ill. Cancer may cause these. So may surgery or a drug. Successful living with cancer requires planning for this contingency. A certain dividing up of tasks is needed. The patient should have things well enough organized in advance so that being on top of your game at every moment is not necessary. You need to have others appointed and in place—we'll call them partners—who can take responsibility for certain segments of this business in your name.

Making the Split

You will always want to be in charge of certain everyday tasks—toilet and personal grooming, for example. But you can give up laundry. If you are a mommy or a daddy, you may give up some of the routine nursing that is physically demanding, but not contact with your children. It's okay to have someone else fix the meals, answer the phone, maybe screen phone calls—but there are people who call you whom you want to speak with. These are the sorts of division of tasks to work on. From such planning comes a most beneficial release of pieces of your life to those who want to help you.

At work, there will be responsibilities you can allow others to help you with, and there will be other tasks that you really can't relinquish. You may already be concerned about some present situations. Partnership principles can be applied here along with other tools. (All this is examined in Chapter 12.)

Keep control of this process. Don't let anyone take charge and perhaps make arrangements without consulting with you first, either at work or in any other part of your life. People sometimes do this for the best and most caring of reasons. But the result is stressful. Point that out firmly, with thanks and an understanding smile. You have reestablished control, and the friend/relative/partner learns more about how to work with you. You also keep a valued team member instead of sending someone away feeling unappreciated.

Your Supporting Cast

Successful living with cancer seems to be quite a social business. In the course of treatment, you will meet hundreds of new people: practitioners, patients, and an assorted cast of other characters. The oncologist who ends up taking charge of your case will be memorable. After all, he or she is the quarterback on your medical team. But the person you are apt to be closest to will be your treatment partner.

Picking Your Spouse to Be Your Treatment Partner

If you are in a committed relationship, your partner in life is the logical choice to be with you during treatments. This may take some getting used to, but it is an important continuation of the relationship (see Chapter 9 for a discussion of the details).

If this person does not immediately step up to this responsibility for a career (too busy) or lifestyle reason, this reluctance can be the symptom of a serious side issue. You many need family counseling or the intercession of the psychosocial unit on your oncologist's staff to resolve it. Do not delay in addressing this. Every moment that elapses before resolution of this problem may make things worse.

That is not to imply that a couple would be wrong to have one or more outside treatment partners support the cancer patient. But there are issues in such an arrangement that should be carefully examined, including likely intimate emotional and physical exposure and how emergency treatment decisions are to be managed.

Considering a Former Spouse

Suppose there is no spouse—but there used to be. If you are divorced and you can see your way clear to considering it, give your ex a call. Talk over your medical condition and see what kinds of offers waft in your general direction. This may strike you as a long shot. Then again . . .

Other Partner Relationships

If you are a child, your parent, a guardian, or a relative will take this job. If you have adult children, one of them may be most suitable.

The role of partner most easily fits someone who is already bonded to you by love and kinship. For this person, the depth of the commitment and the intimate nature of the experience pose less problem. Other relationships can work, too. A friend or group of friends may share you. Young adult singles and the elderly who have lost their mates may find friends that easily and pleasantly slip into partner relationships. There are also professional caregivers, though this can be an expensive alternative. (Part VII, "Relationships," provides more discussion.)

When Picking a Partner Is Hard

You are unattached. No family. No friends. No workplace associates. No fraternal- or service-organization friendships. No place of worship. No psychosocial staff on your medical team.

The objective here is to locate general volunteer help for the specific needs that have materialized with this illness. Don't use the term "partner." It suggests more involvement than those you are going to contact are prepared to discuss with you. You are looking for people to help with first steps.

Here are some suggested contacts:

- Wellness Community National Headquarters: 888/793-WELL (during business hours, Washington, D.C., time); or www.thewellnesscommunity. org; e-mail: help@wellness-community.org.
- Call the local number of the charitable organization serving those with your specific cancer (breast, prostate, leukemia, lung, colorectal, etc.). It will probably have the name of your affliction in its title, for example, the Leukemia and Lymphoma Society.
- Call the American Cancer Society.

Cooties

The physical assault of implacable illness has terrified people since the dawn of time. The hand of demons was seen in it. Parents taught their children to flee from those with a "mark of the devil," the "evil eye," the "curse." Medieval religious leaders used disease as evidence of the devil or of a soiled life. Sorry to say, much more than vestiges of these outdated sentiments and prejudices remain with us today.

Do not be shocked to discover that a friend can no longer look you in the eye, or that certain children can no longer visit. Cancer phobias are very, very common.

There is also squeamishness about simply touching something unfamiliar. Again, you never know when this is going to get in the way of the hug or kiss you expected.

It is not personal. Nor, probably, is it something you can fix by laughing it off. These feelings are serious. It is best to respect their power, not demand the person do something uncomfortable. Find a meeting ground for a relationship rather than chase the person away completely, if you can.

4 The Patient's New World

Do not presume that you are who you were.

The "You Have Cancer" Moment

Some people get angry. Some people's ears burn. Eyes water. Legs weaken. Few if any find the news that they have cancer trivial. Disorientation follows. You are physically transported to a place you never expected to be, and dumped.

There is nothing wrong with being shocked, surprised, scared. Whatever you want to call it, this bit of news is riveting.

Whatever you do, deal with it. One of the great sorrows in the oncology community is that so many cancer patients who could be helped go into some form of denial. Your doctor and your medical teams are waiting, ready for you. But you must join them. Suit up and show up. Nothing can be done if you don't.

A Short To-Do-First List

There are things you can and should do immediately to fight back:

- Get a second medical opinion. Maybe a third.
- Stop using tobacco products of all kinds.
- Maintain a healthy weight. Both over- and underweight conditions are dangerous for you right now.
- Do not abuse alcohol.
- If you are addicted to any substance, tell your doctor.
- Exercise regularly.
- Follow the health-checkup recommendations of your oncologist.
- Pay attention to your diet.

Get a Second Independent Medical Diagnosis

You probably have never received more serious health news. That in itself is sufficient reason to demand time-out and a recount. The best doctors take no

Telephone 800/4-CANCER

The National Cancer Institute, one of our federal government's highest-quality public services, will give you the latest info on your specific disease and its most successful treatments.

1. Ask for a Physicians Data Query, a PDQ, for your type and stage of cancer (formerly called a Protocol Data Query).
2. Ask for open protocols for your condition. These are alternative treatments you may need to know about.
3. Call the Bloch Cancer Hotline, 800/433-0464, for a list of places nearest you to get unbiased second opinions for your specific kind and stage of cancer.

insult. They are the first to demand second opinions. The more one knows about this complex and enigmatic condition, the more one realizes how comforting it is to have broad agreement on the issues.

If the second opinion does not exactly agree with the first one, get a third. If the third finding disagrees with the other two, get a fourth. Get the picture?

At some point in this process, there may be costs beyond what you planned or can afford. Everyone who understands this situation will recommend that you go forward anyway. They understand how important this groundwork is. Everything depends on agreement about what needs to be fixed.

Every year stories appear in the press about people who made snap decisions—the woman who had her breasts removed by mistake, the lung operation for a benign cyst. Don't make a silly mistake.

Later, you may face treatment decisions. A lumpectomy or a mastectomy? Chemotherapy with nausea and hair loss or radiation that may be no more than palliative (helps you feel better; doesn't contribute to remission)? The second-opinion rule remains in effect.

Stop Using Tobacco Products

There is total, unreserved agreement among U.S. health agencies that 30 percent of all the cancer deaths this year, including 87 percent of lung-cancer deaths, can be attributed to tobacco. Tobacco use also increases the risk of cancer of the mouth, nasal cavities, larynx, pharynx, esophagus, stomach, liver, pancreas, kidney, bladder, uterine cervix, and myeloid leukemia.

Those are just the cancer risks. Tobacco also helps thin the population through heart disease, stroke, and numerous other illnesses. About 440,000 men and women will die of tobacco-related illnesses this year, 180,000 of whom will have cancer listed as the primary cause of death. The American Cancer Society, which assembled these facts, estimates that the cost of caring for those 440,000 will exceed $157.7 billion. We fight whole wars, then rebuild shattered nations, on smaller budgets.

The fact that you already have cancer is not an excuse for continuing to use tobacco products. You need to quit because:

1. Every day you don't smoke will improve you ability to breathe, which will come in handy when you need oxygen or respiration therapy.
2. If you continue to smoke, your immune system's ability to fight for you will be unnecessarily restricted. If you survive, it will take longer.
3. Pain medications may not work as well as they should.
4. Medical centers may reject you for certain treatments or delay helping you until other patients who don't use tobacco products have been served.
5. An organ transplant of any kind is out of the question, if there is a waiting list. You're probably going to be discriminated against for stem cells or bone marrow, too.
6. You are going to go out of your mind trying to find a place to smoke or chew in or near a cancer-treatment center.

Kicking the habit is hard. But cancer treatment requires it. For that reason, the tobacco-cessation programs in place at almost all cancer-treatment centers are excellent. In the end, cancer may give you this gift of health, which will shock you, it's so unexpectedly wonderful.

Maintain a Healthy Weight

If you are overweight, fat may have brought on or contributed to your cancer. Statisticians say that breast cancer is particularly apt to occur in overweight women and men. (One percent of breast cancers strike men. One in three of them die.)

In any case—too fat or too thin—weight is often an issue during a fight with cancer. Aggressive disease takes weight away that you may need. Some medications put weight on or make the patient susceptible to water retention. However body weight enters into the cancer-fighting equation for you, it is not a casual issue like getting back into a high-school-era dress size for the class reunion. Body size, fat content, and the several related aspects that nutritionists work on with you are based on highly technical issues. Follow directions. Don't freelance this one.

Do Not Abuse Alcohol

If you don't drink, cancer is not a particularly good reason to start. If you do drink, it is unlikely you will be told to stop unless a specific circumstance mitigates.

There are reasons and times not to drink. Some medications do not perform properly with alcohol or can make you nauseous if mixed with alcohol. Certain therapeutic diets require abstinence. Booze thwarts some pain medications. And sometimes people just abuse the stuff, which is never a good idea. You'll get less out of a doctor visit you don't remember.

Your oncologist will probably mention it if alcohol figures into your treatment program. A glass of wine or beer with dinner may be suggested. Or you may be warned against drinking at some point.

If there comes a time during treatment when you wonder about alcohol, ask without embarrassment. Even in hospitals run by groups that oppose drinking, your physicians, nurses, nutritionists, and even technicians and volunteers will probably give you unbiased answers to your questions.

If You Are Addicted to Something, Tell Your Doctor

Any substance that your body demands you take daily could be an addictive one. Some addictions complicate cancer treatment. You cannot be effectively treated for cancer until your doctor knows about any addiction you may have.

Patients who are addicted to illegal drugs or who take legal drugs in some illegal way and who disclose this to their oncologist don't go to jail for it. They get effective help, either at the hospital or with a nearby referral group like Alcoholics Anonymous or Narcotics Anonymous. Of course, if you've been robbing banks to support your habit, you may be sent to the slammer for that little indiscretion—just hope it doesn't come out until you have finished cancer treatment. Penal medicine is not a preferred course.

Exercise Regularly

"The benefits of regular physical activity for preventing chronic diseases such as heart disease, type II diabetes, and cancer, are well documented. Specifically, regular physical activity reduces the risk of colon and breast cancer and helps maintain a healthy body weight . . . [and] also decreases the risk for cancer of the pancreas, prostate, lung, and endometrium," according to the American Cancer Society's 2003 report *Cancer Prevention and Early Detection: Facts and Figures.*

The report notes that, overall, 41 percent of women and 36 percent of men in the U.S. population have no leisure-time physical activity. Couch potatoes are easy prey for cancer. They contract it more often and, once afflicted, have lowered defenses. If any of this is giving you guilt pangs, resolve to do something about it.

The chart "Moderate Physical Activity" (see box) was put together for the benefit of people with cancer who feel basically fit. If you as a patient are capable of exercising, consider making a few of these activities a regular part of your lifestyle.

Many cancer patients need further guidance as a result of any of several causes, which may include their illness and treatment side effects. See the designated person on your medical team. The point is not which type of physical exercise is best for you. The point is to find something physical to do, if at all possible—making certain your oncologist approves, of course. (You can go to Chapter 28 for more on this.)

Moderate Physical Activity Examples*

Washing and waxing a car for 45-60 minutes

Washing windows or floors for 45-60 minutes

Playing volleyball for 45 minutes

Playing touch football for 30-45 minutes

Gardening for 30-45 minutes

Wheeling self in wheelchair for 30-45minutes

Walking 1 3/4 miles in 35 minutes (20 minutes per mile)

Basketball (shooting baskets) for 30 minutes

Bicycling 5 miles in 30 minutes

Dancing fast (social) for 30 minutes

Pushing a stroller 1 1/2 miles in 30 minutes

Raking leaves for 30 minutes

Walking 2 miles in 30 minutes (15 minutes per mile)

Water aerobics for 30 minutes

Swimming laps for 20 minutes

Wheelchair basketball for 20 minutes

Basketball (playing a game) for 15-20 minutes

Bicycling 4 miles in 15 minutes

Jumping rope for 15 minutes

Running 1 1/2 miles in 15 minutes (10 minutes per mile)

Shoveling snow for 15 minutes

Stair walking for 15 minutes

Less Vigorous, More Time

↑
↓

More Vigorous, Less Time

*The amount of physical activity is influenced by its duration, intensity and frequency The same amount of activity can be obtained in longer sessions of moderately intense activities (such as brisk walking) as in shorter sessions of more strenuous activities (such as running). This chart adapted from Chronic Disease Notes and Reports, a publication of the Centers for Disease Control and Prevention, by the American Cancer Society

Get Health Checkups

For the same reason that you'd pay attention if you were in a cage with a hungry tiger, you must watch your disease. Your sense of physical well-being is an excellent indicator, but it is not completely reliable. You must see your doctors regularly. You must take the tests, even the ones that hurt physically or fiscally.

Don't bargain with your doctor over this. Don't compromise or cheat. Take the most conservative path and be just as grateful as you can be that the tiger is still pacing on the other side of the cage and that you've got a program in place to protect you from it.

Pay Attention to Your Diet

There is a mighty chorus of advisors who want you to follow diet guidelines of this kind or that. One or more of these diets will likely help you combat your disease. Other diets can be expensive—and take a lot of the enjoyment out of eating—without any particular benefit. Some foods and food supplements may cause you unnecessary physical pain, interfere with medicines, or set your recovery back in some other way. So diet is important. But it is something for you to work on with the help of your medical team. This often leads to the ministrations of a qualified oncology nutritionist.

Diet, nutrition, food supplements—paired with exercise—are the subjects of Chapter 28, which will help you put the comments of your medical team in greater perspective. If, as often happens, nutrition and exercise don't come up during the initial phases of your diagnosis and treatments, Chapter 28 will be particularly important.

New Things and Places

If your only experience with torture is flying coach on a major airline, cancer will broaden your horizon. The test-and-evaluation phase of diagnosis will very likely introduce you to equipment and procedures you don't like. There isn't much you can do about time spent fruitlessly in waiting rooms. Bring this book along and read another chapter. There are other parts of this and subsequent treatment phases where knowing a bit about what's coming will be very helpful.

Anesthetics. Do not expect to drive a car or to be much of a bon vivant after any procedure that requires a strong anesthetic. You may also be given medicines to take beforehand. You will be forewarned. Follow directions.

Any unfamiliar test or treatment procedure. Any time a test or procedure comes up that has not been explained to you, it is your obligation to ask what it is all about. Your team probably just forgot to brief you or thought you knew what it was. No matter. Be sure you get all the information you need to: (1) know what is involved; (2) know what benefit you will derive; (3) agree that it is worthwhile; (4) know if there are insurance approvals or other administrative details to take care of first; and (5) know about side effects.

Blood and similar tests. Some staff are better at drawing blood, taking a biopsy sample, or installing an intravenous line. Always compliment a person who does a fast, painless job for you. It is important PR. If this is a procedure you will have to repeat, ask for him or her next time. You may even be able to make an appointment.

Catheter. Ask the nurse what to expect ahead of time if you will need a catheter. Sometimes the clothes you wear to the experience need to have certain features. People find amazing places to insert these tubes in you. The experience may be more embarrassing than uncomfortable.

Feeding tube. One of the early preparations for treatment of a cancer in the head or neck may be the installation of a feeding tube (see Chapter 28, "Nutrition and Fitness," for more).

Chemotherapy. The chemotherapy experience will probably not be as bad as you have heard. Chemo today is not like it was even ten years ago (for details, see Chapters 27 and 33).

Imaging. Most of the equipment that looks inside you is easy to use, safe, and not painful. At worst it may be cold to the touch.

There are also body scanners with little tunnels in the middle. You lie down on a table, and they slide you inside. There you stay for up to an hour, serenaded by grunts and bangs from the equipment. Most people easily deal with it. Severe claustrophobics and some children can't. There are alternative ways for your medical team to get imaging data, if you require it.

Giving you a chemical cocktail to drink or an injection may improve the contrast between internal soft tissues or the features of an organ. This is a definite NBD (no big deal).

Ostomy. An intestinal or urinary tract diversion into a bag requires surgery. Get your medical team to coach you thoroughly ahead of time. You can also seek the advice of someone in the United Ostomy Association (see Reference Center listing at the back of this book).

Radiation. Radiation is usually fast and painless. Always ask the nurse in charge if there is anything you need to know, or if there is any precaution to take, before beginning an unfamiliar radiation treatment (see much more on this in Chapter 27).

Uncomfortable tests. If you suspect that a test will hurt, ask what can be done to minimize your discomfort. Sometimes a medication that must be taken before your visit will help. There may also be dietary guidelines.

Children may receive less insulation from pain than adults. It is harder to give them effective anesthesia.

How to Be a Better Patient

Nobody in his or her right mind wants to excel at being sick. But cancer is not like tooth decay. There are no assurances that you will be fixed, nor have you any idea how long this experience will persist or at what price. The quality of your eventual recovery can largely depend on your being a dutiful, communicative, conscientious patient. You need to be easy to read by those diagnosing you. You need to understand and follow orders. You need to be predictable. You need to be respected. Frankly, you also need to be liked.

The idea that a patient who is more likable will get better treatment may get a protest from your new doctor. But later, after your medical team knows (and likes) you, you may get a shy smile of agreement. Hey, people are people, and nobody looks forward to unnecessary challenges or encounters with churlish patients.

Make Yourself More Effectively Treatable

Staff at the best cancer-treatment centers will see all the patients possible, which means you will get as much attention as the treatment team feels is necessary, plus maybe a courtesy thirty seconds. Time is in short supply. No offense, but you can't take more of it than your case warrants. The rest belongs to other, equally needy patients.

While there's no time to socialize, you don't deserve to receive less than enough time for proper care either. So learn the techniques you think are necessary to get the most value from treatment meetings. For example, learn how to identify which parts of your physical condition are of greatest concern to your medical team. It isn't hard. Simply observe and ask questions about what's going on. When both you and your medical team are on the same page, so to speak, you will get better results.

Parts of this process should be important and interesting. For instance, learning how to interpret enough test data to follow the progress of a treatment will matter to you (see Chapter 6). Whether the news is good, bad, or indifferent, you get a better sense of how the game is progressing.

Another thing you'll be coached to do as part of learning the lingo (Chapter 6) is pick up a few words of doctor-speak. If medicine is a bit far afield from your previous life, words like "hematology" and "oncology" may seem intimidating. They get even more mysterious when you find out that they refer to medical sciences that no one completely understands. Perhaps knowing that you're not the only ignoramus in the room is the best reason for you to feel completely at home with a medical vocabulary that describes your condition and its treatments.

Your interest and attempt to get familiar with the language will also pry out more information than you would otherwise have gotten from your medical team, and it will evoke just a teensy bit more attention to your case. Like chicken soup, it can't hurt.

Make It Safer to Be a Patient

The process of training to become a medical professional, be it physician, nurse, or another member of your treatment team, is partly designed to eliminate people who should not be entrusted with the welfare of the sick. But even pros fumble the ball.

Before we continue with this discussion, which is meant to alarm you, a reminder: Cancer care in the United States is more effective than it is anywhere else in the world, and its procedures are very, very safe. Cancer care has never been better than it is presently. It continues to improve in both effectiveness and safety. As you should expect, more of those who can afford cancer treatment anywhere in the world choose the United States than any other country.

That said, let's get to the scary part. Medicine is imperfect. A 2004 study by Health Grades, Inc., a respected health-care consulting firm, estimates that about 195,000 people died in the United States the previous year due to "preventable hospital errors." We can safely infer that hundreds of thousands more were made sick, injured, or maimed. This is not a cancer statistic. It includes emergency-room medicine and many other high-risk therapies and protocols. But it does include cancer medicine. And it is not seriously questioned at the National Institutes of Health or by any association of medical professionals.

If you understand gambling odds, you know that every exposure to the same risk gives you about an equal shot at a random happenstance. The odds that you will receive unintended harm are about the same every time you undergo treatment. So the more often you visit a doctor, the more exposure you get. You have cancer. You'll get lots of exposure.

Okay. The first part of the point is made. Now let's back away from the subject a little and come at it from a different direction.

There are people who go to health appointments with their revenge ready and a trial lawyer on their cell-phone speed-dial setting. This added burden to health professionals' liability insurance partly explains how Tylenol administered to a hospitalized patient has gotten to ten dollars a pill. Don't be among these people. This mindset makes a less than optimal experience more likely. A tension enters the doctor-patient relationship that obfuscates. You have a critical illness. Do nothing to lessen the quality of your care.

Instead, take some simple steps to reduce the chance that one of the people caring for you will make a mistake. There are records and an appointment calendar you should make a habit of carrying with you. There are signposts and indicators for you to remind the doctors and nurses about (see Chapter 11). There may be times when your antennae just begin to twitch. You know what is supposed to happen, and a different result is evident. You need to be self-assured enough to tug on a sleeve or smile at a nurse and ask a question.

You are much more apt to be clobbered on the way to the appointment than to suffer because of a mistake in a clinic. But you must keep your wits about you or, when you're too sick to be attentive, you need a partner who knows what's going on to support your medical team's treatment process on your behalf.

Tools for Staying in Touch with Normality

The first thing cancer tries to do to you is take away pieces of your normal life. It takes your time and money. It tells you there are things you can't do anymore. It can hurt or disfigure you.

Just knowing that your disease has these objectives is going to help you fight it more effectively. Several chapters here will help you with specific related issues. But beyond all the things cancer will try to take, nothing is worse than the strain it puts on relationships. Those closest to you will be the first to suffer unless you make a concerted effort to keep this from happening. Even then, cancer will win some of the time. When you hurt, for example, people who love you will hurt too. There's nothing you can or should do. Cancer wins the round. Just learn more about pain management, or get your health back, or both. Don't hide the pain.

You can also expect to deal with disruptions, even chaos. Your disease will affect every aspect of your life, including your profession (see Chapter 12). But knowing that cancer will make these moves on you is the first long step toward the countermeasures you can have ready. Your preparation robs cancer of the element of surprise.

Homelife changes could occur as your cancer becomes more insistent and aggressive. You may need a place for a nurse to stay. Structural modifications may be necessary. Rooms may need to be reorganized or their functions changed. You may already be imagining a grab bar over the tub or a toilet-seat modification. You might need help climbing stairs or wider doors for wheelchair passage. Some people even open a home office for disease management (for more on care at home, see Chapter 43).

You may decide that a van or an SUV is more practical than a standard sedan. Commercial travel could provide more challenges. It may become more interesting too. And possibly cheaper some of the time (see "Transportation" in the Reference Center "Yellow Pages"). Movie, restaurant, church, and other congregate experiences may become more complicated.

Oxygen bottles and other bottles and bags you may need, as well as changing physical limitations, can also require some preparation. Your cancer causes some of these inconveniences. Your treatments will cause others. Recovery may literally become a royal pain in your backside. None of it is good, but it will be better if you understand what is happening and know how to make the best of the hand you've been dealt. Looked at in another practical way: You don't ever want to be surprised because of lack of preparation. At a minimum, it could be embarrassing. At worst, a silly mistake or something your ego tells you to do could maim or kill you.

Improve Your Comfort

You are not required to have cancer *and* a hair shirt. There are three messages here: First, don't suffer needlessly. (Chapter 40, "Dealing with Pain and Nausea," may become important.) You will also be unintentionally physically hurt by those near to you. You will prefer to endure some of it. A hug from a person you love very much, for instance, may hurt a lot. But not getting the hug could be worse. You also have a right, a duty, to let people know what pains you.

Second, don't let things that haven't happened ruin your day. "I'm an old man, with many troubles," Mark Twain once wrote, "most of which haven't happened to me yet." Many people around you, including some doctors, may want to tell you about how bad things could get later. You should probably—but not necessarily—pay attention. It depends on the credibility of the witness. In some cases, people scare you when all they really intended was to relate their own experience in a dramatic way. The folks who do this probably wouldn't if they stopped to think about what they were saying. In any case, don't let gloomy predictions of what might happen in the future ruin today.

Don't tomorrow today.

This advice isn't easy to follow. That old saying, "Sticks and stones may break my bones, but words will never hurt me," isn't true. There are predictions that can hurt you, scare you, make you crazy. If what people say to you becomes really bothersome, help is available. Sometimes books, tapes, and CDs featuring the curative powers of laughter take care of it. There are also specialists whose counsel can help in times like these. Your medical team probably has a name and phone number. The Reference Center has listings, too.

Make the things you have to do as simple and comfortable as possible. Equally, don't try to do something the way you used to do it when cancer or a treatment makes it hard. For example, if you're tired of walking, sit down and rest or ask for a wheelchair.

Reduce Unknowns

Cancer may not change everything, but it will try. Discovery, including a rigorous questioning process by which you shine a light into every corner of the experience, will be an important part of each step you take through this time. See everything that's coming. Many things may lie ahead, so do not focus your discovery beam narrowly.

Now, stop. Put a bookmark right here and turn to the Contents. Look at chapter after chapter that speaks to unknowns of one sort or another. Some of them will never affect you, but others will. There is a road ahead, and it has potholes. Knowing that problems lie out there and having some idea of which will come your way should make you better able to adjust your speed and to swerve when necessary.

All right. Now read on.

Improve the Quality of Your Recovery

With all the tools and pharmaceuticals, with all the new discoveries, with the exceptional talents of the medical teams—the likelihood is that you will get through this thing. The question is, How well? How much of your precancer self will you have left? Hair gone? Not a very big deal in the cosmic scope of things. It will probably grow back thicker, anyway. A breast lost? A lung? A leg? Different story. Maybe not as bad as you think. See Chapters 27, "Treatments," and Chapter 29, "Implants and Replacement Parts." The guidance is tried and true. The options may surprise you.

More broadly, you can vastly improve the quality of your recovery by learning from those who endured the processes before you. There are groups you can join. Your hospital or clinic has people on staff who want to help. Some of them are good at it. All of them mean to be. There are counselors, books, and Web sites to learn about too. See the Reference Center for leads.

5   Know the Illness

"Cancer" is the family name for hundreds of diseases.

Facts People Think They Know about Cancer

A patina of serious misunderstandings crusts cancer's image. Some of them are so offbeat, they seem funny. But we laugh for the same reason we laugh at a clown's pratfall. Later you might wonder why the clown thought his injury would be entertaining—and what laughing at it says about us.

It is possible that you are too recently diagnosed to have experienced some of the common things people say about your affliction. This seems to be a good time to list a few. There's no point in your getting blindsided.

Cancer is invincible. Wrong. About ten million Americans have survived cancer. The number grows all the time. You have every reason for optimism. (This statistic doesn't include the basal and squamous-cell skin cancers, which are rarely fatal.)

Life ends with diagnosis. Cancer deserves your attention. It is a serious condition. But don't let it ruin your life. Fear's unhealthy.

Be comforted by the quality of your medical team. Talk to cancer survivors. Let the support of friends and family lift you up.

Cancer is contagious. Nope. You can hug and kiss, share cutlery and toilet seats.

Cancer is hereditary. There is evidence that some kinds of cancer follow bloodlines. The chance that a cancer patient's children or grandchildren may get the same disease is greater in these cases, but there is no certainty.

Cancer is shameful. There are people who believe that cancer is a sign of God's displeasure. Shame on them.

Nothing a person can do will increase the chance for recovery. You are holding a book full of things you can do to improve both the quality of the life you will live during cancer treatment and the likelihood that you will recover.

Once cancer is discovered, you must turn your life over to others. This time, like none before it, demands that you take greater charge of your life. Listen to the experts. Work with your partner and care team. Listen to your heart. Don't, whatever you do, leave the firing line.

You are to blame. We have all engaged in risky behaviors. Some of us have gotten cancer. Most haven't. There's no proof of blame.

Someone else is to blame and you should sue them. Go get 'em. Just keep in mind that legal action of this kind is emotionally taxing and may require investment. It may take longer for the courts to settle than a normal lifetime. There are also class-action cases, finished and waiting for injured parties to apply for settlements (see Chapter 16).

The "Yes, I Had Breast Cancer Too" Mistake

Most of us aren't scientists. We don't want to be burdened by minutiae from some laboratory. Neither do we expect to be treated like nincompoops. When a detail matters, we want to know it.

Details matter when identifying cancer. You need to know where in the body the cancer originated, which is how it receives its general name. Cancer originating in the breast, for example, is called "breast cancer." So it's just fine for a former patient to say to someone in treatment, "I had breast cancer too." The problem comes when these two people assume that they are discussing the same disease, treatable in the same ways. More than thirty different cancers originate in the breast. Even the same cancer can act differently and need different remedies in different people.

For purposes of illustration, let's say two people think they are on the same page. Now let's say that the former patient benefited from less-radical sur-

The beginning of wisdom is to call things by their right names.

Chinese proverb

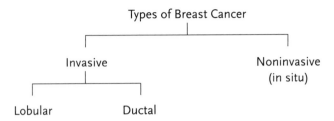

5.1 Types of breast cancer (includes more than thirty different physical forms)

gery than has been recommended for the current patient. Suddenly, doubt about a key treatment decision has been raised. In a case where the cancer is aggressive and the surgical team is ready to go, the resulting confusion could have serious consequences. It may stop something that needs to move forward and, maybe, damage confidence in the medical team.

You need to be sure that you know your exact type of cancer cell. Continuing with our hypothetical breast-cancer example, let us say that the new patient's specific tumor was one of the infiltrating ductal cancers, whereas the former patient's was noninvasive. Each case leads to its own further classifications and subclassifications as the supervising physician sorts through and identifies characteristics. There's much, much more. You get the idea.

Even though surgery is usually the prime treatment in breast cancer, the location and extent of the surgical procedure, types and locations of radiation, and types and protocols of chemotherapy are specifically based on detailed diagnosis.

The fine points missing in the comment, "Yes, I had breast cancer too," are unimportant at a social gathering. But a lot more has to be known before treatment decisions are made. Although the rate of survival is better than it was, about forty thousand women in the United States will lose the battle to a breast cancer this year.

Among the many excellent Web sites offering term definitions and treatment explanations, the National Cancer Institute provides one of the most successful: cancer.gov.

If you don't have access to the Internet from home, or you feel your access skills may be inadequate, go to your public library for help and Internet access.

Understanding Mechanics of the Disease

Cancer is a general term for cells in the body that grow in abnormal ways and multiply, instead of being detected by the immune system and destroyed, which is usual. The conventional wisdom is that this activity is caused by malfunctions in chromosomes, which are part of every cell. These abnormal cells become one of the malignancies of blood, bone, or tissue that are called cancer. Your tests and treatments are intended to get rid of the one of these that you have.

The term "conventional wisdom" was meant to signal a general reservation of the scientific community. While cancers are being stopped—or at least stymied—with regularity, there remains much that is not understood about them. Now that you have a particular reason for noticing, you'll see and hear about new medicines, new discoveries, and new theories all the time.

Patients burning with curiosity need something close to heavy-duty medical research into their disease. A much larger number of cancer patients would like to know as much as possible at a lay level. If you fall into either of these categories, ask your oncologist to recommend the best book, brochure, videotape, or DVD for you. You may augment the recommendation with a trip to the Reference Center at the back of this book for further resources. But let your starting point be your doc or the person on your doctor's medical team who's responsible for helping with educational matters. Come back to use this person as a sounding board every so often. You need a firm foundation so that you have a general guide for separating fact from fiction. Then venture into the Internet jungle if it appeals to you. Observe the mixed choruses from everywhere else in life that often provide more passion than illumination. Marvel at the gems you come across (also see Part V, "The Illness").

Understanding Diagnosis

Treatment of very early stage cancer is the most likely to be successful. This often means—but not always—that your medical team wants to move ahead without delay. This is a very deliberative process. Step one is to carefully identify and then target the object.

General Symptoms

In general, your oncologist begins by checking your symptoms against those that provide a signature for cancer. Pain, swelling, bleeding, a sore that won't heal, persistent cold or flu, trouble with a body function, or a change in the way an organ works are signs that point to specific kinds of cancers—along with many, many other conditions. The fact that you have one of these conditions is just a warning, not conclusive evidence of cancer.

Physical Exam

The next step is usually a complete physical examination. Areas of greatest interest include the nose and throat; lymph nodes in the neck, under the arms and in the pelvic region; women's breasts and pelvis; men's prostate gland; abdominal organs; rectum. Chest X-rays and scans via equipment with names like CAT, PET, and MRI are sometimes used.

Blood Tests

Blood tests are important clues to body chemistry. If the basic components of your blood, which are some of the most complex substances studied, test normal, you are probably in good shape. Blood also carries many things that may be tested for. You will need to ask your medical team for specifics to know anything further about why you are having blood tests.

Tests of Stool, Urine, Spit, Bile, and So On

Stool and urine samples can reveal all kinds of problems. These are the garbage cans your body fills with its refuse. The things you have too much of, the chemical indicators of battles your system won or lost, things like blood that shouldn't be there—all tell tales on you.

Other critical elements, such as spinal fluid, stomach fluid, and bone marrow, may also be required. These are never extracted unless the physician has a sound reason for it. Be very concerned if you learn that one or more of these tests has been ordered for you. Ask for an explanation. Expect some discomfort.

Imaging

It is always troubling to have someone drape you in lead, then dash from the room, telling you that everything is just fine and "Don't move!" The trusty X-ray is Stone Age technology compared to other ways now in use for imaging. Sometimes you drink stuff before the event, which makes this organ or that more photogenic. There are further levels of imaging in which you enter a tunnel on a table. Sound is sometimes shot into you in place of nuclear particles. Some of the sound-wave techniques produce movies.

Imaging is now an advanced medical specialty. It may have been a physician specializing in this science who first confirmed your cancer diagnosis.

Endoscopy

As exams go, this is one of the easiest to endure. It has also saved many lives. Things grow on the walls of the lower intestine. The examiner takes care of them painlessly. The worst of these examinations takes place the day before, when you drink a gallon of foul-tasting stuff that acts like Drano on steroids.

Bronchoscope, Cystoscope, and Other Intruders

Flexible fiber-optic probes have been developed to navigate just about any passage from your body into the outside world. The practice is generally easier to take than the idea of what the technicians propose to do to you. The resulting information is magical, due to the wonders of teeny-tiny lenses, other sensors, and microcomputing.

Biopsy

Examining a small piece taken from what doctors call the "region of interest" reveals the "characteristic patterns and cell types defined as cancer." This is often a surgical procedure. Sometimes the sample is removed by inserting a needle and sucking out a fragment. Scrapings get samples from the mouth and other cavities. Blood, bone marrow, and other working fluids of the body may also be subjects of biopsies.

Advanced Lab Work

Of the many sophisticated studies now carried out in the lab, the physical study of cells, cytology, is one of the most amazing and important to cancer diagnoses. This work is so sophisticated, it can now perform studies at the individual-cell level. Findings can provide a developmental history of the cancer since long before it was detectable. These studies may also forecast how quickly the cancer-cell population will grow and reveal new body locations it plans to attack.

There are a great many other types of diagnostic research in cancer labs. The supporting equipment is equally advanced. Watch the results of your tests come in and ask questions. The firepower your medical team uses against your cancer is awesome.

6   Learn the Lingo

You've stepped through the looking glass and here you are.

Welcome to Cancerland

What we need right here is the theme from *Sesame Street* and a couple of those plush characters to convince you that learning a foreign language will be easy and fun. So just pretend you're three years old again, sitting cross-legged two feet in front of the TV, singing along with an animated stethoscope and a pill bottle in a hula skirt.

Maybe this isn't the first time that you've been someplace that the people spoke a language you didn't understand. There is nothing quite as frustrating as losing out on what everyone is saying, especially when some of it is about you. Welcome to Cancerland. Where they don't speak your language. (Fade *Sesame Street* theme music.)

No Tourist Accommodations

One golden rule we all understand is "He who has the gold, rules." You are the patient. You control the gold. Besides, you're sick. You have a right to expect that the people who serve you will speak in language you understand.

Let's test that theory in Cancerland. You've already been to several medical professionals. You've experienced their effusive attempts to explain your condition to you. You know you are not the first one they practiced on. Did your gold help? Did your condition? If your experiences were average, the answer is that you saw great concern and effort in their eyes, but there were words in their language that they couldn't translate into yours. And that left you with a sense of bewilderment that you really didn't need on top of everything else.

Clearly, these people can't make it to your side of the language barrier. You're going to have to learn at least pidgin doctor-speak.

The Sleeping Dictionary

The Great War, World War I, was the first opportunity that Americans had to be reenergized by European culture and language after about 150 years of isolation. Family and friends were amazed to find that remarkable numbers of our soldiers understood French or some other new tongue when they returned home. How, one might ask, could such a transformation take place?

A prime motivation for the doughboy was the mademoiselle. The resulting language skill was sometimes obliquely explained as a benefit of having had a "sleeping dictionary." Back home, the locals presumed that to be a reference to some machine that, ah, drilled the GI while he slept. *Au contraire.*

You, too, have been involuntarily transported to a perilous place and there immersed in a foreign language. The need for you to catch on is equally rewarding. Fortunately, you will enjoy the same rapid learning curve if you just pay attention.

Tips for Fast Learning

For most people, careful listening is enough. Those so inclined can take a tape recorder or notebook along. Either way, when you hear a word or phrase that you don't understand, stop the process to ask what it means. Repeat back the word or phrase and what you believe you were just told about it. Get somebody on your medical team to confirm that you have properly learned the lesson.

Do not be disheartened if you forget. Relax. Continue the exercise. That lesson is still in the back of your head. It will leap out and surprise you later.

Practical Results of Your New Skills

All medicos, doctors especially, are inclined to be selective. They feel pressed for time and don't want to be trapped into situations where a long-winded explanation may be needed or a patient's eruption into anger or tears could take place. If the doctor believes you are up to speed or a quick study and are reasonably in control of your emotions, you are much more apt to get the regular detailed reports that keep the treatment picture colored in. As you become more able to manage your short list of new words and your body's role as a battlefield, your medical team hears a person emerging whom they are more comfortable providing with technical situation briefings.

You may be one of the great many patients who do not want the play-by-play analysis, just the big picture. Reducing the detail of information is easy: When you have heard enough, say so. But don't use this as a reason to avoid understanding. Learn the vocabulary. You still need it.

The result of your linguistic transformation is that your medical team treats you less like an inanimate object and more like a peer. No one intends to put this prerequisite on your relationship with your medical team. But it's there, particularly if English is a second language or if you are a shy person by nature, a youth, or a senior citizen.

Improved Care

This is heresy that your medical team may hotly deny, but here it is: When you use the proper wording and terms, treatment staff will presume that you and your partner know the difference between first class and steerage. You will receive more prompt, higher-quality care. It may not be dramatically different from the attention given to other patients. It may be just a smidgen better. But being pleasant and up to speed oils the machinery.

It's simple human nature. The nurse who believes that the woman in chair three knows the difference between a good procedure and a sloppy one—a patient who may later mention that she got a good "stick" from Jones—is going to be more careful to earn your approval.

You do not need to make a grand demonstration of your medical vocabulary to succeed at this. Simply show, through your courteous interest in the services being provided, that you know and appreciate the difference good people are making in your treatment.

Always say thanks for a job well done. Especially one that hurts. Your nurse knew it would cause you pain, which increased the pressure to do as well as possible. Minimizing the hurt to you by being highly skilled and professionally focused deserves your accolade. Even when bestowed through clenched teeth. Especially when you know how much worse the procedure could have been in the hands of someone who cared less or had fewer skills.

Lingo Not to Learn

"Can I pay you to spend extra time with me?"

An oncologist remembers:

We had occasion to admit one of our hospital's directors. In addition to being on our board, he was a very prominent, very wealthy member of the business community. He was also gravely ill.

During his initial examination, he motioned me close. "I know how busy you are, and I appreciate the care and concern you have for all your patients. So I wonder, can you make arrangements to give me a little extra time, that I, of course, would pay you for?"

I had to fight down my surprise and anger. The implication that I might not give every patient—including him—every bit necessary was shocking.

And then I pictured the scene in which this trustee, sitting with the rest of the board in plenary session, learned that members of the staff had created multiple levels of care for patients, based on their ability to pay or station in life. The moral and business questions that cascaded from that scene left me chilled.

Then I squeezed my patient's hand and smiled. "Don't worry about a thing," I told him. "I'll see that you get world-class care."

Finding Translators

When things happen that you don't understand, make a habit of getting an answer fast. Speed is important because you are in the process of learning something. The sooner you find help, the more completely you will learn the lesson and the better you are apt to remember it.

Medical Staff

Events move quickly in treatment centers. Your time in Radiation may have been so rushed that you had no time to ask the question that came up. You need someone or someplace to go for help. The most likely person to help you is the one you were with when the question occurred to you. Make eye contact or touch them to get their attention. Immediately ask your question. If for any reason you need more information than that person can give you, ask the next person you see. Try to get immediate satisfaction while all the details are fresh in your mind. Still not satisfied? Ask where you can look for the explanation you need. Be a persistent and intense questioner. Get your medical team in the habit of explaining things to you. In the same spirit, always listen carefully to what they say.

Peer Counselors

There are parts of your treatment experience that you may feel more comfortable discussing with other patients or informed third parties than with your medical team. The Reference Center lists organizations dedicated to helping you. Find an appropriate phone number and make a toll-free call. The people who answer the phone are often present or former cancer patients who are trained to help you. They have been exactly where you are, or they can find someone who has been. Some of them have medical training. Most have only medical experiences. With a bit of persistence, you will find a buddy who will happily fill you in on hosts of issues, including nomenclature.

Cancer Books

There are mountains of terrific books that attempt to provide explanations. If your cancer is in one of the fifteen to twenty most common classes of the disease, your primary oncologist or someone on staff probably pointed you toward a specific reference book a while back. They did so because, when a question comes up, it's apt to give you a suitable answer.

There are also general books that may be extremely good for reference. Go to your nearest library to see if *Everyone's Guide to Cancer Therapy*, by Malin Dollinger, Ernest H. Rosenbaum and Greg Cable, suits you. If it does, buy a copy and keep it handy. If you don't get along with *Everyone's Guide*, there were at least half a dozen other books of the same genre beside it on the library shelf. Pick one of them. Ask somebody on your medical team if it's right for you.

Understanding Your Tests

People have begun testing you in multiple ways. They take blood samples. They take biopsies. They do imaging. You can be certain that each test has a specific purpose. You will be a better, more confident patient when you know at least a few of the details.

To illustrate one of the several ways to go about this, let us imagine that a nurse has asked you for some blood. (We'll use the name of a common test as an example. If you never hear of it again, no matter.)

YOU: What are you going to do with my blood sample?
NURSE: CBC.
YOU: What is a CBC?
NURSE: We look at the amounts of various things in your blood to see how you're doing.
YOU: What do the CBC initials stand for?
NURSE: [To her, the initials are a triviality she hasn't thought of since school. It is still an excellent question.] "Gee, I don't know."

There is some calling around the room. "Anybody know what CBC stands for?" The staff in the room laughs. You caught 'em. "We only do a *million* of these tests a day." Finally, somebody comes up with it.

SOMEONE, *reading from a pamphlet*: "CBC is a comprehensive blood count test. The resulting analysis provides a fast, general look at the health of your blood, your immune system, and the performance of certain drugs you may take."
YOU: What are you testing my blood for?
NURSE: Your treatments frequently cause your white blood-cell count to fall below normal range. If it does, we give you shots to bring it back up.

The conversation goes on to reveal the numeric range that your white cell count should fall into and the name of the shot that they give you when your count is too low. You may also learn of other constituents of blood that are affected by your disease or its treatments and how the test scores them.

That information graduates you from being a blindfolded passenger in the backseat to a participant in a process. You have a sense of why and what. In a small but significant way, you have taken a piece of yourself back from your disease.

You are also helping people remember to help you. When you pay critical attention to your tests and their results, they will too. If you are a patient in a small clinic, "helping people remember" you will sound strange. But if you are receiving services at a large regional medical center, where hundreds, even thousands, of patient tests are managed every day, this can be an important issue.

You will know your interest in the testing process is producing the right result when your medical team brings printout test results to you for discussion. Accept this as the positive act of work sharing it is. If they offer you copies for your files, thank them and accept. You have just learned that a record of this particular test is a good thing to have, that you may benefit by collecting your own set, and that your medical team now thinks of you as a peer on an important new level.

Testing Your Powers of Observation

There once was a guy sleeping with his burro in the town square. If someone asked him what time it was, he would lift the burro's tail, stare intently, and give an accurate answer. An intrigued observer finally asked him how he could tell time by lifting the burro's tail. "Because, when I lift it, I can see the clock on the wall over there," the burro master replied.

In the same way, you may think you know by observation what your doctor or one of the nurses is doing and why. Ask anyway. You will be surprised by the number of times the obvious wasn't obvious at all, or you learned about some further part of a process, because you asked.

Collateral Benefits

By learning the lingo and the things that go along with it, such as what's important about tests that are frequently taken, you become a fully formed face in the crowd. The team remembers you, even though you are only one of the many who pass through a treatment center every day. They will do more to preserve your dignity, which heaven knows is easy to lose on a day when you get examined by half the staff. Your medical team also talks to you, not past you. You will find that people have more concern for your comfort, and for the amount of time they keep you waiting, too.

More Options

Funny thing about learning the lingo: Even though you think you only sound like you know what you're talking about, you will discover that you actually do know more. You will also make progressively better-informed decisions. This is a growth process that is going to save you money, time, aggravation, and health.

Personal Key-Word Strategies

You need to develop key-word strategies that will positively control the outcome of discussions you have about your cancer with family, friends and coworkers.

Here are a few predictable situations, with suggested courses of action.

Lingo and Personal Truth

Practice complete truthfulness about everything related to your cancer except when it may needlessly hurt someone you care for. When you do not want to be truthful, use silence as your first alternative. Either say nothing, literally, change the subject, or take charge: "Let's not talk about that right now."

"You Feel Better Now, Don't You?"

Do not accept invitations from friends and family to tell untruths, as when you are asked if you "feel better" when you don't, or if you are pleased with your progress when you're not. Questions of this sort are others' attempts to feel better about you at your expense. If you perform for them once, they will ask for more and more. You don't need this annoyance.

"Do You See God's Hand in This?"

Even if you believe it, do not agree with those who say that your disease or your recovery are the works of God or the devil. A great theologian who has none of the effects of cancer to tote around might be able to hold his or her own in an ensuing debate. You are not apt to, nor is there any value to trying.

"You Know Smoking's Done This to You, Don't You?"

Carefully consider before agreeing—or disagreeing—with those who want to identify the cause of your disease. Maybe you have smoked heavily over a long period of time. Maybe you have regularly consumed alcoholic beverages. Maybe you worked in construction or a coal mine. Maybe you are a few pounds overweight. Maybe cancer has struck others in your family, so it looks like you were more at risk than other people are.

Don't accept any of these possibilities as conclusive. You don't have scientific fact to prove your cancer's origin, even if the indicators are pretty certain. Once you open the door to this kind of speculation, it makes cancer a crime you committed. This increases the sport of discussing your illness. More people will happily join in. You may even find people punishing you in small ways for this thing, as in, "You've done this to yourself." Don't let people beat on you in this way or give them reason to cluck about you behind your back.

Testifying, Particularly to Children

Sometimes cancer provides an opportunity to help influence someone else's lifestyle choices. You get the chance to deliver an important message because cancer is thought to have given you special insight. "Don't smoke." "Power of prayer." That sort of thing.

Lay it out as you truly believe it. Say only what you believe. Stop short of using your illness as an example of consequences. The fact that you believe it wholeheartedly is the essential part of your testimony. Beating on yourself adds nothing.

In all too many cases, the so-called truth is something that someone is prompting you to say that you do not honestly know to be fact. Decline the invitation. It would be dishonest for you to affirm it. There is no need to compromise your standards at this critical point in your life. Besides, children, in particular, sense insincerity.

III Team Building

People Don't Beat Cancer;
Teams of People Do

7 Deciding Where to Have Treatment

Several thousand hospitals are available. One of them is perfect for you.

Back when they were common, butcher shops featured scales with the promise, "Fair weight. No springs." This chapter is devoted to a core issue that needs the fairest consideration possible without permitting the vagaries of springs—or the butcher's thumb.

You will be relieved to know that, momentous as the choice of a treatment center is, most people later believe they got it right. You will be able to validate this for yourself when you compare notes with fellow patients at the place you end up. But we're getting a little ahead of ourselves.

Making the Decision

The first step toward picking your primary treatment center is to decide who takes responsibility for the final decision. The answer is obviously not the same in every case. But the foremost nominee, the one who must be comfortable with the decision now and later, is the patient.

Accept all the help available. Listen to all sides if there is a debate. Sort out the merits. Use your heart, as well as your head. Give it time. Then pick a road. Try not to look back.

If you leave the choice to others, you are handing them a burden they may eternally regret if, or when, there's an unhappy conclusion. You, the patient, are the only one who can make the decision without concern for criticism later.

This may be difficult if you are distracted by your illness. It is worse if you have a parent or partner who normally makes the close calls within the family circle. Someone may have already made the decision for you, presuming—not even bothering to ask—that you are to be led. But in this case, maybe for the first time in your life, your parents' or your partner's set of issues is different from yours. Their love and concern override other factors influencing the decision. They do not have your balanced view.

Don't Complicate a No-Brainer

If your medical advisors agree that you have a treatable condition, and if they agree on what that treatment should be, and if they tell you that they can provide it, the likelihood is that you are in the right place with the right people helping you. If an independent second opinion confirms the finding, you have probably read as far in this chapter as you need to. Go sign on. Get fixed.

Checking Out Your Hospital before Checking In

Several important health-care standard-bearers want to help you make sure that the hospital you choose is the best available to you. Medicare leads the way, with a general evaluation process that includes all but some 60 of the nation's 4,200 general hospitals. The Leapfrog Group and Health Grades, Inc., also provide general information designed to compare hospital services fairly. Hospital Compare, the Medicare site, is at www.hospitalcompare .hhs.gov.

A Hierarchy of Complications

We turn now from ranking specific treatment centers to a general discussion of how you are apt to do in the hands of the oncology center you choose. We'll begin with a bit of background.

Information about the "success rate" of treating your type of cancer is influenced by the cancer's stage of development. Sometimes this changes the treatment options. In other cases, treatment options are complicated by worries about disfigurement or loss of body function.

As you read on, it may be helpful to make notes in the margin about how your cancer and its treatment relate to the points raised. It may be even more important to identify questions you realize you will need to ask.

Success Rate

There are tables that quote, on a percentage basis, the likelihood of the patient's survival from a general type of cancer. If the medical group that provided your first diagnosis did not give you this information, you may find it on charts at either the National Cancer Institute's Web site, www.cancer .gov, or at the Web site of the American Cancer Society, www.cancer.org.

This success rate is general, for a family of diseases. As an example, you may find only one number for "breast cancer," which is actually more than thirty widely different diseases. Some are more responsive to treatments than the success-rate percentage would indicate. Some are less. Some require different treatments than others. A success-rate percentage gives you an indicator, nothing more. But it's a start, an input into the decision-making process.

Stage of Development

The development of cancer is measured in four stages. Stage I describes a small tumor of cells at its original site. Stage IV describes a cancer whose cells can be found in many places throughout the body. Stages II and III describe the intermediate steps between. Stage I development is often a condition that the doctors feel confident in treating. Stage IV development is generally much more difficult. Remission rather than cure is often the goal.

But there are complications. Some Stage I cancers offer almost no hope. Treatments of some stage IV cancers in the leukemia and lymphoma families have high success rates. Age can also confuse the issue. Children under a certain age almost always survive types of cancer that take the lives of older people. Other cancers, when they occur in the elderly, progress so slowly that the patient outlives them without treatment.

Treatment Options

There are a variety of ways to treat cancers. Surgery is part of about 60 percent of all remediation, according to a 2005 survey of the National Cancer Institute. Chemotherapy, including all its variants such as immunotherapy, is a treatment that may require the support of a sophisticated medical institution—or may not, depending on many factors. Radiation therapies come in many forms and types, from electron beam to seed implant.

Nontraditional healing practices and non-proscribed compounds are also common. Those who keep track of these things report that many patients use substances, medallions, and megavita-this or -that along with mainstream medicine. The oncology team is usually okay with it. Exceptions are when something directly interferes with a treatment program, or when the patient is harmed.

Most of those who use nontraditional healing practices as primary cancer treatments live in third-world countries. Western medicine is very interested in what goes on there. It in no way discounts these practices and potions, but there is skepticism. A huge effort is under way to document results. Those living in the United States who rely on nontraditional medicine often started with more conventional treatments. The objectives they hoped for weren't achieved. They now face a pessimistic prognosis. The switch to a nontraditional healing program is the last-ditch effort, a "Hail Mary" pass with time running out.

Many common cancer problems have multiple treatment options—surgery, radiation, chemotherapy, seed implants, "do nothing and hope it stays passive." Each has its good and bad points. Some options are riskier than others but may offer greater reward if successful. For example, men who elect radical surgery for prostate cancer have selected a likely means of eradicating the cancer but risk incontinence and loss of the ability to perform sexually. There are at least five other roads open to most prostate-cancer patients. The outcome may be a bit more in doubt, but the risks are fewer too.

Simplifying a Complex Calculation

You have just skimmed through the broadest and most general look at the complexities that go into a patient's treatment-location decision. If the discussion leaves you feeling that your treatment needs can be met at a local hospital, there's a good chance that they can be.

If your situation is more puzzling, it is probably more perilous as well. There may still be a simple way to come to the right decision: Look your trusty family physician directly in the eye and ask, "What would you do if this were your spouse/child/parent?" If this is a friend, and if you get a straight answer to the question, it will more than likely be a reliable guide. It came from a talented professional who knows you, knows the cancer world, is used to its complexities, and has read enough clinical papers to have a pretty good idea where the A-Team for your condition hangs its hat.

If you don't get a recommendation, or if your medical advisor honestly doesn't know, there are other ways of finding good answers to the "where" question. We'll examine a couple.

Doing a Factors Assessment

The status of your disease can be generally figured out by evaluating the success rate, stage of development, and treatment options you know about. Make a list. If your cancer has a low percentage success rate and if it is at a level of development higher than stage I, your concerns have to be increased. If you find your treatment options baffling—or chilling—it is more likely that you need to find a team noted for research into the treatment of your specific illness.

Once this analysis is complete, consult with your family doctor or the specialist you have been referred to—a qualified person you are comfortable talking to. Discuss this calculation you've made. Did you do it right? Are there factors you forgot to include? Does your expert agree on the severity of the situation? If no, would this person say your condition was more in need of a leading specialist, or less? Does any of this bring other ideas or solutions to mind?

A Next Step That May Satisfy You

Back when telephones had dials instead of keypads, during the mass discharge of men coming home from World War II, it was possible to dial O and get the voice of a strange woman in your ear. A venturesome gent could introduce himself and an adventuresome telephone operator might agree to meet him for a cup of coffee after her shift. "Faint heart never met fair maiden," they used to say.

If you are feeling venturesome, go to the Reference Center. Look up one of the service groups concerned with your type of cancer. Call a peer counselor. Tell this person you've never met, and probably never will, about your disease. The discussion that follows will need your careful evaluation. It could be one of the most important of your life. Close the conversation by getting a referral. Call a second and maybe a third place. You'll be talking to people who, by sharing their own experiences with you, may show you how to get out of your quandary. They may provide whole new levels of sophistication in the way you view your situation too. Or you may be wholly unsatisfied by the experience.

The Scholarly Approach

We are preparing to discuss a process that your third-grade teacher introduced you to when the class made that first trip to the library. "Look at all these books, children. Why don't you pick one out, go sit at a table,

Paid Research Services

You can pay for help. The quality of results will vary. It is best to use a person or company with a verifiable track record. For candidates to start with, turn to the Reference Center "Yellow Pages" under "Research Services (fee charged)." You can also ask for a researcher at your local public library.

and read." Later: "Wasn't that fun?" Well, no. But you weren't going to tell Mrs. Schultz that.

There are cancer patients who, by academic inclination and intellectual curiosity, are motivated to put great energy into medical exploration. Most of them don't charge far down this path. The mountains of esoteric material and the complexities of the science become discouraging quickly. Then illness sucks away stamina. You're also apt to be hammered by the blues, which everybody gets.

This is where a partner or a friend can step in. Research is a noble endeavor that scratches that academic itch deep down and satisfies their need to do something about your predicament.

Searching for Centers of Excellence by Cancer Type

All the top-gun cancer centers in the United States excel in specific areas of treatment and research. Get on the Internet. Call up the search engine of your preference, type the name of your cancer on the "Search" line and hit "Go." The organization most often named, the employer of the greatest number of research scientists, based on published papers and news reports of achievement, is a good treatment center for you to consider. Also take a look at the second- and third-most-named institutions.

Capture the names of the doctors most often associated with your disease, however they come up in this Internet search. Set a short list of these aside for later.

Now go to the Reference Center. Do a longer, more exhaustive version of the telephone survey touched on a few paragraphs ago.

Look up every organization that might be qualified to help you. Talk to the peer reviewers. Do a quick survey of what these soldiers with trench-warfare experience think of the situation you're facing and the hospitals and the doctors you have on your list. The path to enlightenment should be evident.

Satisfaction isn't guaranteed. There is no reviewed and recommended selection process that works for patients in these difficult situations. If a better scheme becomes apparent during this exercise, use it, of course.

One final suggestion. If the treatment center or the physician of choice cannot accept the patient, get a referral and a specific reason for it before you give up the dialog with choice number one. Go back to the Internet search engine. Add the new referral as a basis for a new investigation. Then go through the winnowing and qualifying process again.

Leaving Home for Treatment

If your evaluation of places for treatment leads you to decide on one that requires travel, try not to be dissuaded by the extra cost and trouble. You arrived at this decision based on higher priorities—survival, and the quality of life to follow. These are priceless objectives. Besides, people and organizations stand ready to minimize the costs and inconveniences (see Part IV, "Supporting Resources"; Chapter 48, "Travel for Medical Purposes"; and the Reference Center).

Not Leaving Home for Treatment

There may be people who desperately want you to go someplace they think is really spiffy. But you don't want to. You see enthusiasm in their eyes. But you are more comfortable here, with the medical staff you have come to feel confident in.

Your cheering section is doing everything it can think of to encourage you to make just one little visit. You see only added exhaustion and discomfort to no particular purpose. And you do not have the energy to argue much about it.

If you have already made this decision, put this book down. Get your mom, dad, spouse, partner, kid, right now, and tell them. "I've decided. This is what I want to do." Further assure these dearly loved ones that there is no reason you cannot change your mind later. But no trip now.

Tell them. Don't ask. Tell them. Then tell them not to argue.

Clinical Trials and Other Misleading Selection Criteria

Poor reasons to choose a treatment center:

- Equipment of any kind, including something no other facility has
- Advertised claims that clinical trial slots are open for its patients
- Size of hospital or staff
- Religious affiliation or the lack of one
- Collocation with a teaching institution
- Gardens or beautiful buildings
- Swimming pools and horse trails
- Celebrity endorsements
- Weekend special rates

A great reason to choose a treatment center:

- Clinical success with the specific form of cancer you have

The voices that extol the virtues of this place or that based on any of the first set of features are doubtless sincere. But, bluntly put, you're not going for the golf or the weather. Clinical trials and advanced diagnostics are available to the team you choose, not the other way around.

Go for the people with the best track record. They obviously know all about how to get the right equipment and drugs.

8 Medical Teams

Who was that masked man?

The White Coats Are Coming!

There used to be a golf course beside the Royal Thai Army Base in Korat, Thailand, with fourteen tees for eighteen fairways. If soldiers did not learn instinctive ducking anywhere else, they learned it there. The earliest phases of cancer care are like Korat's brand of full-contact golf. The patient moves from experience to experience, never knowing when another personal assault will occur. Like the Thai soldier, you get more than a little jumpy. Who are these people? How did they come up with so many ways to get into your pocket, scare you, take your time, hurt you?

Of course, the role of cancer patient isn't chaotic at all, so far as the docs are concerned. This seemingly random endless passage from one office to the next is a perfected, proven process for careful evaluation, diagnosis, consultation, and second-opinion gathering. Sometimes the demands of insurance companies and others further increase the number of holes you play before you finish this course.

It's Like Learning to Dance

The patient is the only one on this dance floor who doesn't know the steps, has never heard the music. Nor could you learn all there is to know overnight, even if you weren't sick. Surrender yourself to your medical teams. Look down at each partner's feet. Follow as best you can. Listen and learn. Remember Ginger Rogers. She learned to dance as well as Fred Astaire, backwards, in high heels.

The evening's young. Here's a brief rundown on some of the partners you'll shag and sha-na-na with.

Oncologist

If you look up "oncologist," the source will identify the medical specialty as having to do with the treatment of tumors. Cancer may not be mentioned. It's only one class of cell clusters. The medical oncologist also examines benign growths and precancers, plus a host of other conditions relating to tumor medicine.

If it hasn't happened yet, an oncologist should eventually take charge of your case. This person will be the quarterback on your healing team, the person who calls the signals and initiates the key plays.

Phlebotomist

A nurse or a technician may use this title, which refers to a person with special training in the taking of blood samples and certain blood-related materials such as bone marrow. A phlebotomist performs a service that is necessary to the diagnosis and treatment of your disease.

If you want to have a little fun with your phlebotomist, bring up the past. Two hundred years ago, most phlebotomists were physicians. They believed that disease and fever could be relieved by opening a patient's vein, allowing blood to carry the malady out of the body. As we know today, the theory was flawed. The country's first president, George Washington, was bled to death by phlebotomists.

Surgeon

Surgery is considered the most certain road to successful recovery if the cancer is completely removed. Surgery is frequently necessary to help during the diagnostic phase of your case too. Samples called biopsies may have to be taken of some internal part of your body. In other cases, surgery is necessary to treat some problem in addition to the cancer. More than 60 percent of all cancer patients receive at least one surgical procedure at some point during treatment.

Radiologist

About half of all cancer patients receive radiation therapy. Its purpose is to kill cancer cells through a process called ionization that either fries the little buggers or neuters them so they can't reproduce.

"Radiation" is a general term for any of a great many ways that deliver X-rays or electrons to the area of the cancer. Another branch of the same healing art, nuclear medicine, uses radioactive isotopes. Sometimes seeds of radioactive materials are implanted near tumors to kill them. In other cases, radioactive cocktails and injected potions are used to attack cancers, including those in the blood.

Beam-radiation treatments are generally fast and painless except for some treatments in the stomach and intestines. Hair loss, if any, is limited to the skin area that the beam passes through to reach the cancer. Patients are sometimes slightly radioactive after treatment. It doesn't last long, and you don't glow in the dark (for a little more on this, see "Treatments," Chapter 27). Your best and most pertinent information will come from your radiologist during your pretreatment meeting.

A cure is sometimes the objective of radiation therapy. In other cases, radiation is used to help make chemotherapy or surgery more effective. Radiation therapy may also be a palliative treatment, meaning that the objective is to relieve symptoms such as pain, not to cure.

It is essential for you, as a patient, to know the objectives of a radiation therapy you receive. Patients commonly hear what they want to hear, rather than what the doctor is telling them. If the explanation you get is not clear to

Do surgeons swear while operating?

Yes, based on observations during a hundred consecutive operations at a British hospital.

Most profane: orthopedists

Least profane: ear, nose, and throat specialists

If you believe you are receiving a radiation treatment that could cure you, when the objective is something else, and if you are then told that the procedure was "successful," you are on the cusp of a dangerous misunderstanding.

you, stop the proceedings. Get clarification. Perhaps because of the impressive size of the equipment, it is easy to assume that there will be more lasting benefit than may be the case.

Nurse

Nurses manage the doctors, the Chemo Room, and many other areas of cancer care. It is an unofficial sort of administration, much the same as the way sergeants and warrant officers run the armed services. Nurses are your best early-warning system when pain or nausea may be coming. They can get you in when there are no time slots left. They can slip you a care package of extra bandages or booties or skin conditioner. When you face a major treatment question, they will have a good idea of what your options are, if you ask. Stay close to these key players on your medical teams. Remember their names. Get the direct phone number for the nurses' station, for emergencies. Nurses like little things you do for them, like giving them chocolates and flowers. Don't go overboard. Err on the side of less rather than more. Be certain not to cross the line between a token and a bribe. Always cherish, never tip, a nurse.

Anesthesiologist (Physician Pain Specialist)

Some cancer patients get along just fine without ever needing the expertise of a pain specialist. The oncologist manages the discomforts. The patient has no additional complicating physical conditions.

Other patients find that pain is a major adversary that a specialist must help them with. The oncologist has anesthesiologists on call. Ask for one if you need to.

It is not wise to ignore pain or to keep it to yourself when you hurt. Pain relief contributes to healing. Pain is also a signpost that points to something the doctor probably needs to know about.

Pain may conjure up images of drug dependency, which is of concern to both doctor and patient (see Chapter 40, "Dealing with Pain and Nausea"). The short version is that pain is bad. Relief is necessary. Don't let fear of addiction or cost or some other objection get in the way of your healing program.

Pathologist

A highly specialized physician, a pathologist examines samples taken from the human body. Cells and tissue today are tested in widely different and sophisticated ways to identify cancers and their origins in the body. A pathologist may also forecast the speed of cancer development and other factors that directly influence the oncologist's treatment choices.

Psychiatrist

The emotional impact of cancer can be extremely serious. Those closely related to the patient may also experience anger, fatigue, fear, uncertainty, melancholy, and a host of other feelings that a physician specializing in

Many well-meaning, smart people will claim or imply that some food or food supplement may cure you. Linus Pauling, eminent physical scientist and history's only recipient of two Nobel prizes, made this claim for vitamin C. There are recovered cancer patients who also claim it. The jury's still out so far as most of mainstream medicine is concerned, because good results cannot be duplicated in controlled laboratory or clinical trial settings.

The vast majority of those who elect to rely on nutrition for a cure do not survive the experience. Accept the term "help" as plausible. Be aware that "hurt" may also be a consequence. But "cure" is probably a misunderstanding of the facts on somebody's part (see Chapter 28, "Nutrition and Fitness," for more on this).

mental illnesses can treat. Related specialties include psychology, family counseling, and psychiatric nursing.

Nutritionist

An oncology nutritionist comes forward when diet can help in your fight against cancer. The nutritionist may work with you to overcome a diet deficiency or to prepare your body to withstand some part of your cancer-fighting experience yet to come.

Nutrition is a tool. It comes out of the toolbox only when it is needed, and that is not all the time. Cancers and the people they attack create an almost incalculable number of nutrition-oriented variables. Don't try to second-guess the nutritionist. Ask questions and be led.

Physical Therapist

A physical therapist helps the body recover from damage. In cancer circles, physical therapy (PT) is a normal part of restoration after surgery. For example, after a mastectomy, swimming helps remaining chest muscles readapt and reduces pain. PT may also be part of making adjustments to the new you, as when a patient must learn about walking on a new leg or developing new speech ability after losing the tongue or voice box.

If you are recovering from an extensive surgery, you are apt to meet your first physical therapist before you leave the hospital. Their ministrations may be somewhat painful. They may be frustrating. Muscles they know about that you didn't and things you will do that you didn't believe were possible will also impress you.

Physical therapy tends to be a slow, multipart process that goes on longer than you thought it might. If the place you began this work becomes inconvenient, or if your insurance carrier is sensitive to the cost and is encouraging a transition for economy, you may be able to make a change without any program setback. You may find nicer facilities, a great babe or hunk to work with. The field is competitive. You may even be offered free gym or pool access after you have completed the therapy.

Other Specialized Physicians

Cancer treatments can invite other diseases and conditions. It is common to require the help of other medical specialties during treatment. Just be certain, particularly in a medical emergency, to let the caregivers know you are a cancer patient. Also provide a complete list of current prescription drugs you take, plus the name and phone number of your oncologist.

Four Don'ts That Screw Up Good Patient Care

The patient, the partner, and the lead oncologist constantly battle four insidious cancer-treatment conditions. It is important that all three work together to see the problems coming as far ahead as possible—then to defeat them.

Apply a rule of reasonableness before acting. There are literally millions of people besides you currently in cancer treatment. Medical facilities and staff have not been able to keep up. So if you experience one of the "don'ts" and if you can tolerate it, let it go. Cooperate. Hope that your example will guide a staff member or another patient to make room for you when the tables are turned. The don'ts:

- Don't allow unreasonable delays between appointments. If your doctor has told you that you need to come back next week, but the person at the desk suggests two weeks, repeat the doctor's instructions. If the person with the appointment book persists, take the problem back to the doctor.
- Don't allow schedule slips. An emergency may cause an office to reschedule an appointment. A pattern of frequent changes in appointments is a symptom of something more seriously wrong with the care unit. An aggressive cancer marches right along. Test and treatment delays matter.
- Don't allow unexplained treatment shortcuts. They are unprofessional and may be dangerous.
- Don't allow disinterest. Force eye contact. Use smiles and personal questions to create conscious attention. Learn about the staff member's family or about something going on in the clinic that you can chat about each time you're in. Never, never just sit there. Especially if you are feeling quite ill.

Dealing with Don'ts

The patient's first countermeasure is a smile and some version of, "Are you sure there's no way we can't . . . " (stick to the original schedule; complete all the parts of the exercise; go with the doctor's order; expedite the prescription authorization)? If not, why is that? (Keep smiling. Keep smiling.)

You Need Prompt Referral Appointments

Your current doc is probably going to want you to see a colleague or specialist for something. The person will probably have a busy practice. If you try to make the appointment, you may not get the prompt attention that your current doc has in mind. For that reason, always ask your medical team to make referral appointments for you. In circumstances that require it, your oncologist or one of the key nurses on staff has the power to whip out a cell phone, ring the right person, and request a professional courtesy.

Your Cancer Team

In many cases, cancer is discovered at an early, treatable stage. The discovery process moves as smoothly as these things can be expected to. Extraordinarily wonderful medicine, which is the norm for cancer treatment today, moves into place through the process that has been described to this point. Your teams, perhaps after a terrible fight against your cancer, perhaps after losses, nevertheless carry the day.

This is the general profile of cancer medicine in urban settings throughout the United States today. Rural medicine is frequently the same, though if you are a rural person, you must be prepared to adjust if your oncologist believes that the minimum acceptable treatment option for you is located somewhere away from home.

The Turn in the Road That No One Wants to Come To

Sometimes cancer

- that is normally defeated refuses to surrender.
- that went into "remission" comes back.
- evolves into a nastier type or is joined by another one. (Now you have two cancers.)
- is not discovered until it has advanced to an "untreatable" stage.
- is one of those that rarely respond to treatment.
- baffles your oncologist, who tells you so.

A turn in the road is not the end of the road unless you fail to make the turn.

If one or more of these happen to you, surprise and shock are understandable reactions. If you were allowed a day or two to get used to the original diagnosis, this time take no more than ten minutes. Your cancer team needs major reinforcements. Presume that time is more critical at this juncture unless you are assured that it is not.

Do not think small. Do not waste time experimenting with minor treatment changes. Call for the cavalry, John Wayne, Gatling guns, the war wagon. Do not rest. Do not allow delays. Take no prisoners. Spare no expense.

A part of Chapter 7 suggests ways of locating and qualifying advanced medical teams. That section was about how to find the right one. What follows is about what you will find when you get there.

You Can Tell Who They Are by the Way They Get off the Bus

Every profession has its top 5 percent. Everyone who makes it to the penthouse of achievement recognizes everybody else who's there. With exceptions, they've learned how to put the rest of us at ease. If you are observant, the travel itinerary, the plaque on the wall, the small Cézanne in the alcove, the deference of a colleague—any of these gives them away, even though modesty demands that they try to hide their superstar status.

This is important to mention here because people of this caliber are found at the medical centers that have the greatest success treating the hardest cancer cases. One, maybe several, of these people could end up consulting on your case. How do you act when the very best in the world, the eminent doctor whose name is on the building, on the book, on the lips of everybody else, who invented the technique, was honored by Congress strides into your examination room and says, "Hi! I'm Doctor ——"?

You act normal. You act pleased. You relax. You get down to business. Toward the end of the meeting, it is absolutely fine to ask the doctor to autograph your copy of the doctor's book that you brought along. (It is bad form to ask for a free copy of the book.)

The reasons these people reach the top of their profession are many. Aside from the fact that there are no stupid stars, generalizations don't fit very well. They tend to be highly confident, and they tend to have individual style. One of them tape records every key patient conference and then gives the tape to the patient! Unheard of. Everything you need for a multimillion-dollar malpractice settlement. Others give patients their private e-mail address, their home phone or cell phone numbers. While a typical too-busy doc may have four layers of people you must go through before making direct contact, some of the great ones will call you. During a break in a conference. From Singapore.

Top-Drawer Hospitals

The very finest medical teams, at the very finest hospitals, do not save all their cancer patients. Some lose more than their share because of the high-risk nature of the patients they serve.

These places tend to be quite large, with further construction always under way. A slight hint of dust and disorganization will shimmer over the place at a tasteful distance. Parking will be inadequate.

The staff shows cohesion and purpose. Everybody in the city knows about the place. Everybody has a story to tell you about it.

The hospital has its own sewage system, parks, medevac facility, travel agency, discount deals with local hotels. Your health insurer will know all about this place—which may not be good news but usually is. You will sit beside patients from all over the world and one or two celebrities. If it is in your nature to make new friends, you will, and they will be highly interesting people. Young patients will have their own section or even their own floor. Some old person will be playing a grand piano beautifully in a nice reception area. Volunteers will offer you coffee or punch. Later, after you return home, you will discover that your bill is screwed up. It will be your only complaint.

Dance with the Ones Who Brung Ya

Amid all the terror and hurry, do not neglect the fine base of health professionals that you relied on before this cancer thing messed up your life. They brought you this far. They were the first advisors to help you find cancer specialists.

They care about you. You need to keep them informed. They include your:

Family GP
Gynecologist
Ophthalmologist
Other specialized MDs you see
Dentist
Pharmacist
Acupuncturist
Herbalist
Chiropractor
Psychiatrist, family counselor

Be sure you talk to all of them about your current situation soon. Your dentist and pharmacist will have immediate concerns to discuss with you, particularly if you are scheduled for chemotherapy anytime soon. Your dentist will want to complete any necessary hygienics or treatments beforehand. This eliminates a major point of attack by infections. Your pharmacist will be interested in reviewing your medications for compatibility. The others may also have important issues to help you resolve or reasons to consult with your oncology teams.

Physical mail will probably be too much trouble, but if the home team will give you e-mail addresses, there may be an easy way to send periodic status reports to everyone. It's in your best interest. They will appreciate it. Maybe your partner can do this or another friend who would like to help you.

Folk Medicine

If you are culturally oriented away from modern healing practices, perhaps accustomed to Native American health support or the guidance of a religious healer, discuss your cancer with this specialist by all means. Navajo medicine, for example, pulls off some healing tricks that baffle the folks from the big-deal medical schools. But be aware that you are involving your body in a clash between lifestyles. Many treatments and herbs may be effective, but your oncologist will remain skeptical until a scientifically sound study provides the necessary reassurance. "I'm going to hold such treatments to the same standard that I hold the drug companies to," is the typical oncologist's view.

9   The Partner

Required reading for partners and those considering partnership.

Partners during Cancer Care

You can go to the dentist by yourself. You may not look forward to the experience, but it's over before the Novocain wears off, and you get a new toothbrush.

A cancer patient should not go to any part of the examination, testing, or treatment process alone. The reasons abound. Here are a few:

- The patient is really sick and probably weaker than usual. Help on the trip to and from may be more than a luxury.
- A cancer patient can be made sicker by exertion beyond a reasonable level. Help should not be considered optional, even if the patient protests.
- A potentially fatal disease will be discussed. A little loving support matters.
- Two people need to listen to what the doctor says to be sure that all the information is retained and that none of it is distorted or misunderstood. In cases when there is really bad news, it is vital that a partner be there to continue careful listening after the patient's ears begin to ring and heart to pound.
- Examinations and treatments go better with pleasant company.
- Sometimes medications have to be administered that make it dangerous for the patient to travel alone. These treatments and their effects are not always predictable in advance. Having a partner there is smart insurance.
- Sometimes the partner can take care of business-office matters while the patient is in treatment. This lifts another burden from the patient.
- Afterward, a meal, a laugh, or a movie with a friend takes some of the curse off a rotten, maybe painful, day.
- Compassionate listening—ears open, mouth shut—always helps.

Helping and Not

"Oh, don't bother." As testing and treatment planning begin for a new cancer patient, someone usually suggests they go along to help. Patients often instinctively respond, "Oh, don't bother; I can take care of this myself. " They haven't figured out yet that this is not routine medicine. Ignore the patient's protest. Bore right in: "It's no problem. I want to do it. When shall I pick you up?" Months from now, when the patient looks back on this moment, the partner is likely to be thanked for "the hand-holding and TLC you gave me when I was lost and had no idea what I was getting into."

"Listen to me: I would rather go alone." There may be situations when the patient really doesn't want the partner along. After a partner has done as

forceful a sales job as is pleasantly possible, the patient's continued no means no. Let it go.

After being left at home a couple of times, the partner should ask the patient if someone else would be a better partner. Another strong possibility is that the patient would like different partners for different parts of the medical experience. Either way, a partner must respect an informed patient's wishes. Don't show offense, especially when your feelings really have been hurt. The patient needs support, not friction.

Good Partnering Practices

The patient-partner relationship has to be taken seriously and nurtured, or it will fray. Giving the process of going to medical events some formal structure may help. The partner may want to take the lead here. The patient, who has both mental and physical distractions, retains the option of contributing— or not.

- Treatments and exams have a way of becoming monotonous after a while. Patients, particularly if they are not feeling their best, may go through this stuff like zombies. When that happens, the intensity necessary to stay ahead of the cancer's assault is lost. Important changes can be missed. To avoid this, the partner and patient need to mentally prepare, as the medical staff does, for each event. Briefly discuss what is going to happen and what the result is expected to be. Write down any questions or ideas the partnership plans to discuss with the attending physician. Agree on errands that also need to be run and maybe on a reward at the end of the day for having gone through all this.
- During the event, the partner needs to remain focused on what the patient is going through. Don't bury your nose in a magazine or go outside to make phone calls. The partner's focused attentiveness helps the patient stay on point. This is not to suggest that a partner should keep a patient alert at all times during treatment. Patients can't always be alert. The point is that, by being an aware observer, the partner is setting the tone for the patient. This visually reminds the patient that, even in highly repetitive, boring therapies, something important is being accomplished. Mental and physical benefits result.
- When the event is over, patient and partner should go through a debriefing process. It may be only seconds long, but it formally caps the event in the professional way the patient's disease deserves.
- Patient and partner should not be together all the time. They need to pursue separate interests so that they can come back to the cancer fight refreshed.

I think the big lesson I learned about my wife's battle with cancer is that people handle this disease in many different ways. Liz wanted to know the complete good and bad about her future. She didn't want to have a spin on it to make her feel better. . . . I found this very hard as a partner and an optimistic person.

Jim Nentwig

Note: Liz Nentwig, mother of three, dearly beloved, was lost to liver cancer at age forty.

Attributes of a Partner

The patient, the patient's loved ones, friends, business associates, and medical teams will all grade the performance of the partner. Each patient has needs. If the partner serves them, the partner has great value. If not, the partner's a speed bump, to be navigated around whenever possible

A partner must also possess certain personal character attributes, and be prepared to acquire certain skills. If the standards are not met, family members or the medical team will hound the partner from office. If the skills fall short, the patient may be in trouble.

Absolute Trustworthiness

A promise the partner makes must be a promise kept. Doctors and nurses will either work with the partner on behalf of the patient, or not. A partner who loses the confidence of the medical team is reduced to the role of chauffeur.

The partner may need to take over some management of the patient's money. There can be no hint of impropriety (also see "Management of Patient Assets" further on in this chapter).

As the partner exercises the authority this trust invests, there will be great temptations to make decisions or interpretations in the patient's name without discussing them with the patient. This is the first step down a slippery slope that can end with patient and partner going separate ways if the patient believes the partner is being domineering or dismissive.

Full Commitment

If the patient becomes very sick, the partner may be suddenly handed the management of the patient's entire life for an extended period. This can happen despite any agreement that the patient and partner made beforehand. The partner's own job and personal plans get sucked into a black hole.

Incidental Burden Relief

The patient may look to the partner to take over all manner of jobs and responsibilities. In a marriage, that may include activities the partner has spent considerable effort avoiding. Managing the checkbook or mowing the grass, for instance.

The partner, married to the patient or not, could be handed the management of financial portfolios, court proceedings, bill collections (for more on this, see Part VII, "Relationships"). Be warned in advance not to count on one comprehensive discussion of such needs. New surprises come with each passing day.

Nursing Skills

Partners frequently need to learn how to take temperatures and blood pressure. They may also have to chart blood tests, collect samples of body wastes, measure and monitor pain medications, or give shots with a needle. They might need to take care of tubes and change bags coming from or going to some of the darnedest places. Assisting with adult diapers and sponge bathing may be necessary.

A partner cannot count on the nurse to take care of these things. Cancer sometimes creates very demanding situations. The partner may need to be at least available as a fully qualified backup to be certain the patient is well cared for.

As challenging or distasteful as these jobs may sound, a partner can do them. Possibly with pride in the skill developed. A nurse will demonstrate the techniques.

Decision Making

Changing conditions may dictate the organization of a new plan to care for the patient. This need may come at a point when the patient is not competent to help with decisions. The demand to act may be accompanied by the conflicting voices of family members and other influential interests. Demands may be accompanied by threats. The partner, and maybe an attorney, ends up doing the critical divination.

Three of the most common arrangements involve selecting and negotiating with a nursing home, organizing home care, and arranging for hospice services. Each is quite distinct (for insights, see Chapter 43, "Care at Home"). For conversations with authorities and caregivers who have traveled these long, dusty roads, see the Reference Center "Yellow Pages" under "Nursing at Home."

Sickness Administration

Someone has to keep track of the paperwork. Since budgeting and bill paying are vital parts of the process, the family's financial head may want this responsibility. If the finance manager is also the cancer patient, the partner may fall heir to the job. Maybe someone else is the natural person to be responsible. The partner needs to be certain that *someone* is. The job is an absolute necessity, best attended to a day at a time. Not keeping records current or not putting pieces of paper where they ought to go—right away—can lead to frustration later. The size and complexity of this job depend on many variables (see Chapter 11, "The Patient's Personal Organization," for a discussion).

Helping a Sick Friend Who's Having a Bad Day

Basics

When a patient is functioning at 20 percent, the support group has to find an extra 80 percent to keep wind beneath the wings. There is no better time to remember that working smarter beats working harder. Involve enough helpers so that no one takes on too heavy a burden. Make note of things that helped the patient through the situation, so that there is a lesson learned for next time.

Verbal and Nonverbal Messages

When a patient gets sicker, it becomes more important to pay attention to real wants and needs. It may seem harder to satisfy them. Or the discomfort the patient appears to show may instead be delirium. Pain medications may be needed. Sometimes mood-altering drugs are suggested. It is important to be sure that any substance administered is intended to help the patient. Caregivers must never use medication just to quiet a patient.

News from the Doctor

If the partner receives medical news about the patient that the patient deserves to hear directly, ask the doctor repeat it to the patient immediately. Explain that the patient may have questions, or that the facts could be distorted in the retelling. Carefully evaluate any extenuating circumstances. Discuss the possibility that other specialists or clergy may also be needed in the room. Wonder if there are family members who should to be present. Consider the possibility that a second opinion may be needed before any of this is taken as gospel.

Bandits at Six O'Clock

A partner may find that family members or others close to the patient use the cover of illness to mount an attack. They want attention. They want an argument settled. They want money. They think this is the time to receive the patient's property. ("You know I'm getting married, and that china has to stay on our side of the family. Supposing he dies and she remarries?") Just as a head's up, the ploys people use to accomplish these aims can be direct or brilliantly devious.

There are too many possible scenarios to detail solutions here. A partner who is a spouse has the clout to deal with much of this. A partner who is less well positioned needs support. The police will tell you that the most dangerous assignment they get is to break up a domestic dispute. Even with weapons and body armor, they don't want any part of these.

Bandits at Twelve O'Clock

Earlier, the need for the partner to remain consciously alert to the effects and implications of treatments was discussed. There are also at least six groups of toxic people to be aware of. Some of them inhabit medical centers. Others appear at church, at school, at work.

Naysayers and Critics

At any stage of the disease, whatever the prognosis, type of treatment, or location of the treatment center, self-appointed experts will show up with urgent recommendations for patient or partner. "A guy at work died in the parking lot after one of those treatments." "It's much better in Puerto San Pablo, where they don't have FDA restrictions." "You'll lose your hair unnecessarily." "We met this couple . . . " Whatever.

This is a permanent state of affairs. It will remain as long as cancer continues to be the unpredictable, highly serious condition it is. Naysayers and critics enjoy an open season.

A person with unlimited time and resources might feel obliged to investigate each of the major charges brought against the patient's treatment program. An alternative is to find a highly qualified sounding board to bounce this flack off of. The patient's oncologist is certainly going to want to hear about major criticisms and to respond. Other advisors may surface to help with this information processing. If not, there's the Reference Center. It is not a good idea simply to ignore the critics. One or more of them may have made an important, constructive point.

I'd Like to Help but My Nails Are Wet

This is a type. The guy trying to look busy while playing solitaire on his computer comes from the same mold. They're putting in their time. You're interrupting.

Be pleasantly persistent until you get the thing you need. When you do, double check. It's probably fouled up.

Don't go on a crusade. It's somebody else's mess. People don't come to this level of bored disinterest without the permission of incompetent supervision.

Speed-Bump Builders

When someone says, "You can't," pause and reflect. When someone says, "Slow down," be certain you know why. People sometimes impose artificial barriers for their own convenience. Even critical conditions can lose their urgency for people who have no personal investment in your welfare. Patients become faceless numbers.

Suppose you hear: "We limit the center to fifteen cases a day. You would be number sixteen. But I can schedule you for a week from Thursday." Go immediately back to the doc. Be certain a week from Thursday is acceptable. Always question the necessity of an obstacle when it might impact recovery.

The Walking Dead

There are people who turn their minds off when they clock in. They stay on autopilot during their shift, then come back to life at the exit. Others, fatigued or hungover, slip into a trance. They perform by rote.

There are also particular times of the workweek, such as Friday evening or just before the end of a long shift, when patients need to be protected from people who are asleep on their feet. Their eyes don't really register. They have no sense of humor. You're a number, not a name.

Sometimes touching a person's bare arm will wake him or her up. Sometimes a joke works. Or a question that requires thought. But do something to snap the person out of it or don't accept service.

Shortcut Specialists

You will run into people, mostly in medical support roles, who like shortcuts. They sometimes leave out parts of a service they are supposed to perform because, in their opinion, it doesn't matter. There are others who get paid by the piece. The more people they process, the more money they make. You are probably not going to recognize the work of a shortcut specialist, although people who are bent on rushing the patient through may stand out. But be aware that these folks are out there. If a test comes back with an inconclusive or clearly wrong result, the possibility of a mistake by a shortcut specialist is another reason to demand a review or a retest.

Poor Health-Service Organizations

There is no intent to portray most HMO, Welfare, or VA-sponsored health services as substandard or indifferent to patients. But some are.

There are institutions, notably among health-maintenance organizations, that believe their patients are captives. A few of the most infamous are associated with welfare or VA medicine. Many more are low-ball private insurers. Give careful thought to accepting services at these places. There is a chance that they may deny necessary testing, skills, or medicines for a nonmedical reason, such as cost.

The Partner as Public Spokesperson

The partner should defer all inquiries on health and related matters to the patient except when another spokesperson has been appointed. In general, the partner should be as silent as events will allow. But sometimes the patient is otherwise occupied, asks the partner to take a piece of this load, or is too ill to deal with it.

Here are some brief guidelines for the partner who becomes a public spokesperson:

- When in doubt, say so or say nothing.
- Never speculate, particularly to groups that have vested interests such as the family or people at the patient's workplace.
- Defer medical speculation to an authority.
- Try never to make a significant announcement—either bad news or good—unless the patient wants you to.

Information for Friends and the Inner Circle

A partner who is a blood relative to all concerned is expected to tell all the truth that is available. Discretion is still advised. In general, anything said to one party will have a way of making the rounds to everyone else.

Code Words

Most of the time, the correct answer to a health question from a casual acquaintance is to say that the patient is "fine," or "about the same," or "better now." All the questioner really wants to know is that the disaster is no worse, even when it is. For this crowd, "had a bad day" or "recovering from chemo this week" are graphic, intimate details. There will rarely be a need to be more specific.

Cancers differ from each other. Find a set of code words that describes the general course of events in this case. Expect that they will satisfy most of those who ask about the patient.

Questions from People with Health-Care Training

People in the biz talk shop. Friends and family familiar with cancer medicine will ask technical questions. Answer as best you can. It will provide extra assurance that the patient is in good hands: Even the partner has a grasp of what's going on.

If such discussions reveal intimate details of the patient's condition that the partnership has decided should not become general knowledge, explain this and ask for confidentiality.

Pointed, Personal Questions

It is generally believed that a woman with breast cancer is going to lose a breast and that a man with prostate cancer will become incontinent and lose the ability to perform sexually. There is also the general morbid suspicion that if a person gets cancer, the end is probably near. None of this is necessarily true, of course.

People ask partners about these things more often than they ask the patient. The partner needs to have answers worked out and cleared with the patient. It doesn't matter so much what the answers are, so long as they are always the same, and so long as they preserve a truthful spirit.

Oncologists and people on their teams have a lot of experience coming up with satisfactory answers to these questions for the specific type of cancer involved. Former patients on the hot lines listed in the Reference Center are also experienced and may be a little more in touch than the docs with the sensitivities of the world you live in.

Questions from Children and the Fragile Elderly

The children of a cancer patient and elderly friends or relatives past the point of prime mental acuity need carefully constructed answers to their concerns. It is not wise to misconstrue the truth. But the form of the message needs to consider the audience.

Management of Patient Assets

The personal and financial property of the patient may have to be put under the control of the partner. This is usual when the patient is the spouse. Elderly patients with few if any blood relatives may also require it.

If the patient is alert, work through a plan for management of assets. Suggested parts of the plan include:

Durable power of attorney
Advanced directive about treatment contingencies
Appointment of someone to manage the estate
Funded operations budget and instructions
Inventory of possessions
Plan for gifts in near term
Instructions for settlement of pending legal matters
Instructions for disposal of business assets
A will
Appointment of a supervising attorney, if appropriate
List of bank accounts, with contents
Plan for disposal of property
Trust funds
Funded plan for funeral

A plan to conserve the estate needs to be written down and formally agreed to by the patient. If the estate is significant, copies of the plan need to be put into the hands of those who share estate management and conservation duties.

If the patient is not alert, the family must do its best to agree collectively on a similar list of issues.

The partner who is not a member of the immediate family would be wise to stay out of the decision-making process and to demand a formal appointment to the caregiver role. No handshake arrangements. Everything on paper, with signatures and witnesses.

Burnout

A partner must prepare to make the role long lasting. Involve others, as makes sense under the circumstances. Make provision for regular breaks and for vacations from the job. Also make sure that everyone agrees on who pays each cost and when, down to gas, parking, postage, and tips. Financial matters must be managed and settled in a crisp, businesslike manner or the partner will be stressed—big time.

10 God

Carefully consider inviting this applicant to be on your team.

The God Button

You are trapped inside a body invaded by cancer. Think of it as a tall building that has been broken into. There's serious damage, possibly more than you know. You've got a lot of people helping you fix things up. You think all the damage is repairable. You certainly don't want your building to be condemned.

Picture yourself on a floor of this building that needs a lot of work. You want to get some of your people on it, but the workforce is scattered on several other floors. You aren't certain whom you need, or where they're working at the moment. You'll have to search. You find the elevator. There are several buttons you can push. One of them is labeled "God."

You wonder, Does this button work? If it does, will it take me to the help I need?

The Scientific Case for God

From the beginning of human awareness of the Creator, people have prayed for healing and believed that their prayers were answered. There has also been skepticism, buttressed by notable voices in physical and psychiatric medicine. In general, the naysayers have prevailed during the last 150-odd years. The notion that God can heal on request was beaten out of most medical students by their professors—until very recently, when computers, munching on huge databases of facts about cancer patients in the 1980s and 1990s, began isolating "recovery factors" having to do with "religiosity."

Case Histories

More than 1,200 scientific studies in the United States since 1975 have focused on the therapeutic effects of active worship, according to Dwight L. Carlson, MD, prominent psychiatrist and best-selling author. More than 800 of them documented a positive result. "Documented" is a word medical parlance reserves to describe something that has withstood rigorous questioning, using scientific methodology, and proved to be potent. Simply and directly stated, scientists have certified that an active relationship with your higher power is an effective cancer fighter.

If you have a faith, cancer may have shaken it. Others come to this page with long-held skepticism. Both views are welcome, healthy points from which to examine the evidence.

Here are digests of a few of the studies that Dr. Carlson was referring to, selected for the high quality of the investigative tools used.

Effects of Intercessory Prayer in Coronary Care

Randolph C. Byrd, with John Sherrill, found that heart patients who were actively prayed for had less congestive heart failure, required less diuretic and antibiotic therapy, had fewer episodes of pneumonia, and had fewer cardiac arrests, according to an article the *Southern Medical Journal,* July 1988.

The Healing Power of Spirituality

Kath Colon, an oncologist, observed that patients he treated who demonstrated spirituality, a sense of purpose, goals, and meaning in their lives had more satisfactory treatment experiences and higher recovery rates, he reported in *Minnesota Medicine,* December 1996.

Spiritual Recovery Movements and Contemporary Medical Care

Marc Galanter, in the fall 1997 issue of *Psychiatry,* reported that a religious or spiritual orientation is an effective buffer against psychiatric symptoms. This was notably true of patients with cancers that had spread and were thus unlikely to be cured. These metastatic cancer patients had an appreciatively longer mean survival time than similar patients with no religious belief.

The Healing Connection

Harold G. Koenig, with Gregg Lewis, discussed more than 850 research studies examining the relationship of mental health to religious belief and practice in *The Healing Connection,* released by Word Publishing, Nashville, 2000. They found "enormous, credible scientific evidence that shows a connection between faith and better mental health."

Religious Commitment and Health

Dale A. Matthews and his research team found a direct connection between religious commitment and better medical treatment outcomes in 80 percent of the cases they studied, as reported in *Archives of Family Medicine,* March/April 1998.

Effects of Intercessory Prayer upon Patients with Rheumatoid Arthritis

Patients who received in-person intercessory prayer showed significant overall improvement over a one-year period, according to a study by Dale A. Matthews published in the *Southern Medical Journal,* December 2000.

The Role of Religion in Recovery of Adult Burn Patients

An exhaustive search of current literature showed that people who are religious have a better outcome in both general and mental health therapies than those who do not, reports Sherrill K. A. Larson in the *Southern Medical Journal*, 1988.

Prayer in Medicine

Shimon Waldfogel reported in *Primary Care*, December 1997, that patients who prayed recovered from their illness more quickly and completely than did others.

U.S. News and World Report, July 2, 2001

The cover story, "Drugs, Scalpel . . . and Faith?" compiled by the magazine's editorial staff reported that two-thirds of the nation's medical schools now include course work on spirituality because of its proven healing benefits to patients.

Rethinking Things

When W. C. Fields was dying of cancer at an Encino, California, rest home, a visitor found him reading a Bible. "Bill, you're an atheist. What are you doing?"

For I the Lord thy God will hold thy right hand, saying unto thee, Fear not; I will help thee.

Isaiah 41:13, King James Version

"Looking for loopholes," the great comic replied.

Struggling by yourself with either the Christian or Jewish Bible, notoriously hard reads, isn't necessary. (The Koran is no easier place to begin a spiritual walk.) People are standing by at toll-free phone numbers listed in the Reference Center to help you build the faith you need. If you drop the slightest hint of interest, your medical team will produce a chaplain. Call a friend who attends a place of worship. Flip open the Yellow Pages of your local telephone book. All you have to do is ask.

Going Back to a Place of Worship

If you once attended a place of worship and would like to revisit it, grab somebody for company or just go. These days, when worship centers all have phone info lines and Web sites, you can easily learn everything online, from where to park and which services offer child care to proper dress and types of services. If you remember the name of someone you used to see at services, make a phone call. See if they still attend. Maybe you can meet them.

Going back to a place of worship may be difficult. Even so, scientific evidence encourages you to take this step.

Faking It

Some people have never understood this God business. They never worshiped growing up. They can't relate to any of what has been discussed here except that getting God to help would be a darn good idea.

They have no religious preference. No place to start a journey toward recruiting the Big Guy.

Trust the notion that God is actively trying to get in touch with you. Let your friends know what you're looking for. Expect that you're going to learn about some worthy choices and that you'll be comfortable with most if not all of them. Look forward to meeting good people and having good times.

Jump in. If you have never prayed, no matter. If you have never been to a worship service, follow along with someone who has. Be sincere and honest. Get those healing juices flowing. Pretend to comprehend—get in there and fake it—until understanding comes to you.

> Though he slay me, yet will I trust in him.
>
> *Job 13:15, King James Version*
>
> I am a lapsed atheist.
>
> *C. S. Lewis*

Prayer

Insofar as prayer is concerned, it is better just to report for duty than to give God instructions, as beginners sometimes do. Find a quiet place. Maybe shut your eyes to improve your concentration and start a conversation. Say hi. Tell God what your situation is and how you feel. Tell him what your biggest problems and greatest needs are. That's literally all there is to it.

Be open and completely honest. Don't offer God deals. "Dear God, if you will just get rid of this cancer for me, I promise to . . . " kinds of bargaining are rather silly offers to make to the architect of the universe. Just tell him what's on your heart.

Allow times of silence during prayer. Give God a chance to minister to you. Examine the thoughts that come to you about your life, your loved ones, and your illness.

> For someone of your faith to speak with, see the Reference Center "Yellow Pages" under "Prayer."

Fringe Benefits

Worship should be a special time, with music, laughter, insights into life, the warmth of friends, and healing. You may discover people worshiping with you who have great experience with your illness and will help you. These contacts may turn out to be fringe benefits not of this new dimension of your life, but directly from God.

Common Ground for Patient and Partner

Teams have to be able to share intimacy and agreement. Patient and partner, and others in the patient's personal organization, must be simpatico with one another, both on the field and off. You need to agree on the fundamen-

> Two are better than one; because they have a good reward for their labor; . . . a threefold cord [patient, partner and God] is not quickly broken.
>
> *Ecclesiastes 4:9–12, King James Version*

tals, be equally yoked oxen, as they say. That's you, your partner, and God, minimum.

Sometimes reality bites hard during the active phase of treatment. The greater the difficulties, the more important it is for the three of you to have some common place you can meet to work on issues and solutions.

The greatest difficulties are most apt to be between patient and partner. If they can find a place of philosophical and physical agreement, God will be there. School cafeteria, synagogue, church, temple, park bench, Denny's— you pick it. God will be fine with it.

Why Me?

If someone did a study, the most common question cancer patients ask God may be: "Why me?" It is a cosmic question. Why do bad things happen to good people? Or is this a punishment?

"Why me?" is a very, very important matter to tie down. You *must* find satisfying answers in the writings of your faith and through discussions with a leader at your place of worship. Don't bother looking anywhere else. Other answers from other places have never been satisfying except perhaps momentarily.

Your search may not be easy. The answers may not come as quickly as you would like. But the person who asks, Why me? of anyone but God doesn't want an answer; he or she wants an argument. The time and energy for contention are luxuries you cannot afford right now. You need to understand this issue for the sake of your physical healing—and then move on to the next thing necessary to beat this assault on your body. Don't get stalled here. Don't let emotion or debate get in the way of action. Cancer's not going to wait for you.

11 The Patient's Personal Organization

Small, simple preparations will make the treatment process easier and more effective for you.

Paper Blizzard Ahead

Cancer is complex and expensive. It lasts a long time. It is a U.S. growth industry. It is ideally suited for regulation and taxation. These are perfect conditions for the attraction and propagation of paperwork.

As with everything else concerned with battling cancer, the paperwork can be important. It is also frequently hard to read, contradictory, confusing, infuriating, and billing-error prone. There are two tricks to surviving the cancer paper blizzard. First, create the simplest possible filing system: Use the KISS principle (Keep it simple, silly). Second, give the jobs of filling out paperwork and following the instructions to someone else.

Basic Record Keeping

Appointment Calendar

The patient and partner are going to need an appointment calendar. Get something with big spaces for notes. A month-at-a-glance calendar is one useful format to consider. Keep only one calendar. Everyone who makes entries is forced to work in the same spaces, which helps avoid scheduling conflicting appointments.

Keep the appointment calendar in a central, open place, like the family bulletin board. Make a rule that no one can move it except the patient or the partner. Perhaps take it to meetings that may require the scheduling of more appointments, but try not to move it. Remember what can happen if it is exposed to spillable substances or rain.

The appointment calendar should double as a diary. Add a word or two about the results of visits and treatments. The patient, and at least the family tax preparer, will need this information later.

Name and Address List

Write down the name of each person providing any kind of service related to your situation, with full address, phone and fax numbers, and e-mail address. Add a sentence or two that describes the person's general role—medical or nonmedical. Include a little map if getting to a location is tricky. Keep this list complete and legible, so that even a stranger could use it.

The Filing System

Dig out three of four boxes. Each should be large enough for a brochure or a press-kit folder to lie flat in the bottom, and maybe eighteen inches deep. Toss general categories of paper records into them, as best suits your situation. Keep them out of the way of pets and small children. After you have been at this for a week or two, you may want to reorganize your system. This may happen several times as you come to understand your evolving needs. Just resist the urge to get fancy. KISS.

The Billing and Treatment-Record Box

Throw every scrap of paper, from blood-test results to receipts for cafeteria ice cream into one of the boxes you have set aside. In time, you may graduate to a more segmented filing system, but the box will do for now. Its open mouth invites you to toss everything in, whereas file folders require thought. Stay with the easy thing. Completeness will be far more important than neatness until you learn which pieces of paper need to be kept and which can go bye-bye.

Handouts Boxes

You will need a box for all the stuff that health-service teams hand you and possibly another one for all the instructions coming from insurance companies, HMOs, your employer, and government agencies.

Sneak Attack (Pearl Harbor) File

Soon enough, you will make the disappointing discovery that some of your health providers or your health insurer have imperfect accounting systems. A foul-up will come back to you, and you will have to show, from pieces of paper you fish out of your boxes, just how the cow ate the cabbage. Failure to stay on top of this game could be maddening and expensive.

Experience will let you know how and when to set up your Pearl Harbor file. You won't need it at first. Just keep your eyes open because, on some fine day when you least expect it, some government or insurance or hospital bureaucrat will try a blindside. Little do they suspect that you will be ready.

Health Contract Records

At all cost, you must now keep in force your health insurance, dental coverage, life insurance, and similar protections that you pay for. If one were to lapse, the presence of cancer would probably disqualify the patient for reinstatement.

Make a list of them, with amounts and payment dates. As you make each payment, log it. If you pay by check, that month's bank statement and your returned canceled check are important proofs. If you pay by credit card or automated account withdrawal, an equally powerful record is created. Cash payments work too, if you receive and safeguard receipts.

Your Reference Library

Many hospitals and some support groups provide major reference works to the cancer patients they deal with. You will buy others. These books, tapes, brochures, and so forth will become a small but important reference library. This book belongs in it.

You will need to spend quality time in your library. Make sure the info you need is ready when you are. Don't lend anything to anybody. If others need to read something in your treasure trove, let them do it in a nearby easy chair.

Electronic Gadgetry

Computers, PDAs, copiers, faxes, scanners, and all those other marvelous technical tools can prove helpful for personal organization. The force also has a dark side. Someone must spend hours entering and manipulating all the data. That someone had better not be too sick to get it done and to keep it all updated. There had also better be another someone who knows the highways and byways of the system to manage it when backup is necessary.

The seasoned citizen with a produce-box filing system and a nephew who likes to work with confused insurance-claims adjusters will eat nobody's dust. Moreover, the administrator working on that account knows better than to request a fax or an e-mail or a digital image. Neither the patient nor the nephew can be tasked with this or endure the cost.

Things That Require Planning

Budget Forecasting

Cancer not only costs money but also gets in the way of work, which impedes the earning of more. Get help from someone familiar with your disease and the costs of combatting it. There are people with this skill on staff at many major treatment centers. The health insurer has a specialist with good insights. The agencies listed in the Reference Center have financial advisors and peer counselors. Put a team on this as quickly as possible.

A Word about Budget-Forecasting Bad News

If you do a thorough, realistic job of budgeting, you will see nothing but a sea of red ink ahead. Take heart. You will find many avenues for financial help in "Supporting Resources," Part IV. You will also find people with ideas for you in the Reference Center. Follow the instructions on Hellmann's mayo: Keep cool but do not freeze.

Taxes

Both the IRS and your state's taxing authority have guidance on how you can obtain the most tax relief based on medical cost deductions. While that's very nice of them, an experienced, professional tax preparer can help you save even more.

Health-Insurance and HMO Navigation

If you have evidence that your health-insurance coverage may omit some major part of your cancer treatment, you will need expert guidance and planning. You can get good, often free, help from public assistance law firms (see Chapter 15, "Public-Assistance Law," and the Reference Center "Yellow Pages" under "Legal Counsel"). Services provided may be severely time restricted and may require a wait of days or weeks. Get a commitment from someone to see the project through before you place your hope in the legals and paralegals (see Part IV, "Supporting Resources").

Cancer Nonprofits

Some cancer charities provide invaluable help. You may receive free prescription drugs, medical services, prostheses, air and ground travel, sickroom equipment, supplies, hot meals, even walking-around money during trips. You will also meet people who can answer questions and provide guidance, friendship, and support groups. Take advantage of all you can. Start now. Advanced planning helps this process a lot (see Part IV, "Supporting Resources").

Disability and Similar Changes in Your Living Status

The government pays some people tax-free monthly stipends and provides complete, free medical care. You qualify by age, impoverished condition, unfortunate family status, a diagnosis of certain specific types of cancer, and so forth. The attorneys providing legal services, the bureaucrats in the VA and Medicare organizations, and the volunteer cancer-support groups may all be helpful. Call toll-free numbers in the Reference Center until you reach the source you need.

You can also call your federal or state elected representative's local office. There are people on their staffs paid to provide effective help for their constituents. The numbers for these folks are in the front of your home telephone book under "Government Services."

Travel for Treatment

If you believe you will need to stay overnight at a treatment center and are without funds, look under "Yellow Pages" in the Reference Center for help. Also check out the comments about groups in the alphabetical listing of the Reference Center "White Pages."

Free transportation and housing at the treatment center, and free meals, are available at some locations. The treatment centers typically know about these sweet deals and how to qualify for them. Call the clinic's general number and ask for travel services (also see Part IV, "Supporting Resources").

The Leukemia and Lymphoma Society and other groups that support patients with specific kinds of cancer may have travel-cost rebates you can apply for.

If the patient is a veteran, the military may offer free travel and other services. You are most apt to receive approval by asking through the office of your favorite elected representative. Do not be shy about mentioning combat service or medals. They aren't prerequisites, but sexy stuff always appeals.

Legal Issues

Trial lawyers specialize in representing those who may have cancer through the fault of someone or something with deep pockets (see Chapter 16, "Private Attorney Services").

Clinical Trials

An advanced treatment program that features free medicines may be offered to you. While "free" means the price is right, "effective" is the only adjective that matters. The offer is probably wonderful. But be certain to have your oncologist explain the entire clinical trial program to you. Be certain to ask about side effects and dissenting opinions if they aren't presented.

A clinical trial is an experiment, though several worthwhile objectives are often clustered beneath the general umbrella of "research" (for more on this, see Chapter 44, "Clinical Trials"). And, by the way, clinical trials are not always free.

Friends

You and your partner need to keep a master list of everyone who is doing anything on your behalf. As with your master calendar, create only one list, to insure completeness and to avoid duplications. One part of the list should be organized by key tasks, to be sure that someone is covering every base. Alphabetize the list by name so that you know whom to thank for each thing they do for you.

Think of lots of ways to thank your friends. Save a very special place for the partner who is seeing you through this.

Hearts, like doors,
Ope' with ease,
To very, very, little keys.
And did you know
That two of these,
Are "Thank you, sir,"
And, "If you please . . . "?

Variously attributed

Research

Soon after the discovery of a cancer, many patients and their families spend time in research to find out as much about it as they can. This is a healthy, normal, and generally all-around good thing. Three relevant points should be kept in mind:

- You will make eye-opening discoveries. It's important for you that you do. You can also amaze friends, but it is not likely that your discoveries will inform your medical team. Share with your doctors anyway. At minimum it will improve the communications link. This also gives your medical team a chance to see where your areas of interest lie and to guide your further research.
- It is a good idea to know the professional qualifications of all the people on your medical team. They are amazing people. Somebody on the administrative side of things probably has biographical data you can have. Some of your team members may have contributed to scientific papers or books. Just for the heck of it, "Google" your treatment center, too.

- The greatest benefit of this research will be to increase your knowledge and that of your partner to a point that improves informed decision making.

For more on organizational matters, see Chapter 46, "Project Management Suggestions for Partners."

12   The Patient's Workplace

Cancer can destroy the careers of the unsuspecting.

Do I Need to Read This?

A lot of people are perfectly secure in their jobs, and their jobs are perfectly secure with them. These workers understand their organization's need to learn that they are ill. They know that every assistance possible will be available to them.

You tell your boss. A process kicks in, with you in its arms. As they say in Australia, "No worries, mate." You're taken care of.

If this is your situation, your only reason for reading further in this chapter would be to learn about other people's problems and to commiserate with the less fortunate.

Some Work-Based Considerations

One of the unfair things about the way cancer effects those who are employed is that it forces everybody to think like an office worker. Even the laws that provide rights and benefits to the seriously ill are couched in terms that are most familiar to people who sit at desks, with access to copiers and computers. This chapter reflects the office-worker bias because it must.

If you are one of the millions of employed Americans with a different work environment, pick through this chapter to get what you can from it. The principles, tips, and job-saving tactics should largely apply to you too.

Cancer's Effect on Even Ironclad Job Security

Cancer affects life at work differently than it does life at home. Work is more structured than homelife, with a more autocratic head who can punish, reduce pay, even terminate you under the properly provocative circumstances. This would be reason enough for a chapter on how cancer affects a job, but there's more.

Coworkers and Team-Performance Jitters

Coworkers may respond differently to the news that a person has cancer than other friends and relatives of a cancer patient do. There is less loving worry, more steely-eyed speculation about what your disability may do to the group's overall performance. This is a specific concern to be aware of as you consider how news of your affliction will be received at work. The anxiety of those who count on you may show up in any of several forms.

A Suggestion

What follows are pages of thoughts offered as experiences and reminders of the human condition in the workplace. There is no particular order, no implied relationship between topics except where a link is pointed out. The hope is that you will find help as you need it to guide you through the process of repairing the damage your disease has done—and will continue to do—to your professional life.

President Harry Truman grew tired of the head of his Office of Economic Advisors telling him, "On the one hand . . . ; but on the other hand . . . ." His famous request to his staff was to find a "one-armed economist." In the same way, you are apt to tire of the ifs, ands, and buts for dealing with work issues raised by your disease. What you need is one-handed counsel. You're already tired, sick, upset, worried, looking for some relief from this problem that isn't your fault. You do not need Zen imponderables.

There is at least one possibly easy way out of this swamp: the EAP solution, which follows. If this solution is unavailable to you or gives only partial relief, you are left with the bunch of reminders, tips, and tactics in the rest of this chapter. If you have to go there, think of them as flowers in a field. Pick the ones that most apply to the situation you face. Get help from your partner, care group, or anybody else you can rope in.

With apologies, untidy coaching for an untidy, unpredictable situation is the best that *Living with Cancer* has to offer.

The EAP Solution

A small but growing number of employers have employee advocates called employee-assistance professionals, EAPs, on payroll or on contract. Their training and certification is typically in family-assistance counseling and clinical social work.

If an EAP is available through either your work or your health insurer, visit with this person as soon as possible. You can be completely candid. Your EAP is ethically bound to shelter everything about your situation from everyone else, even the fact that you are ill. Cost will be low or nil.

Your EAP is trained to answer the entire gambit of questions and needs your disease has caused. He or she will help you with your feelings of loss and anger. A plan for disclosure to workmates and to your boss can be worked out. Legal and financial issues, health insurance, family matters, your personal feelings—you can take everything that relates to where you are right now to an EAP.

The EAP is a counselor with connections. If you also need family-law services or a second medical opinion or someone to help you negotiate benefits or apply for disability or get day care for your grandmother, the EAP has a mandate to find you help.

Patience in the Workplace

Be prepared for reactions besides the sympathy you deserve. People don't hear news like yours every day and they don't have much experience responding to it. Be prepared to be tolerant of people who respond to you in ways you don't understand. Stay neutral in tone. Don't get angry. Don't apologize, either.

You do this to allow the social circuitry that your news blew out to reset itself. Usually the person with a poor first reaction will, on reflection, have a more compassionate, more generous second thought. You just need to leave the door open to it.

The same pertains to bosses. In spades.

Your Boss May Not Appear to "Get It"

Your boss may surprise you by not reacting much to your news. If your relationship has always been impersonal, businesslike, and arm's length, a lack of emotion should not surprise you. Maybe your boss isn't able to show you compassion. Another possibility is that your news has compounded a problem your boss has with management higher-ups. Or maybe the shock of your news destroyed normal sensibilities. There are so many other possibilities that we do no good trying to list them. The sole point is that you have to notify your boss. While you should have every expectation of sympathy and cooperation, you must not rely on receiving them.

Repeating the message: You deserve but have no right to sympathetic cooperation. Think of this bit of shocking news as a building block. More snippets follow, until we have enough material gathered to build something helpful for you.

Your Boss May Not Be Able to Cope

Your boss, who is legally and operationally obligated to deal with situations like this, may try to make you responsible for the "problem." It's a widespread foible of career middle managers. Another common reaction of management is a complete disconnect. "I'll have to get back to you on that" can be either procrastination or a fair reply from a concerned person on unfamiliar ground. You know your boss. If a shallow excuse for deflecting the topic fits within the boss's predictable range of bad behaviors, you may have a problem. Politely but pointedly ask for a time when this meeting can be completed.

Be careful not to insist on the completion of the business in a way that makes your boss feel trapped. You don't want to deal with a cornered animal. Most times, people of goodwill can find ways to work through mutual problems like this one.

There are no good solutions if you do not get the positive support of your boss. Despite laws and the requirements of common decency, you end up in a tiff with a person of some power that you are going to have to work with after all this is over.

Provisions of labor law, specifically the Americans with Disability Act and the Family Medical Leave Act, give you rights and protection. If you work in a company large enough to have a human-resources (or personnel) department, it has people who are familiar with ADA and FMLA. They should be your next stop if your direct boss cannot or will not give you the support and assistance you need.

If you don't have an HR person in your company, go to the owner or president or whomever you trust with your last best chance. After that, from a practical standpoint, see Chapters 15 and 16 for legal recourse and expect to be back in the job market soon.

What about the "Don't Tell the Boss" Option?

You have just read a discussion that included a series of confrontational options, and none of it sounds like something you would do. This business about telling your boss and then maybe having to make waves to get help is much too emotionally stressful. As a matter of fact, after thinking about it, you've decided you're not going to tell anybody at work anything.

Sorry. The problem, your illness, is not going to go away. Delay in dealing with the help you need from your workplace favors your disease over you. Eventually your sickness is going to be evident. Coworkers or your boss will ask about it. So you're stuck unless you quit and run, which is a really, really bad idea.

If you cannot bring yourself to tell management about your illness, have someone close to you do it. You still have to be present when the notification is given, or be prepared to accept any decisions made on your behalf at that meeting.

Business Priorities before Compassion

We have all heard the phrase "a business decision." The usual implication is that something was done that is unsavory but excusable because a need of the company/agency/department superceded fair play. Beware, cancer patient, of a "business decision" based on someone's fear of your future diminished performance capacity. You could lose your livelihood and, a couple of years later, the last affordable health-care umbrella you'll be able to get until age sixty-five.

Isn't this kind of railroading illegal? Yes, in its most blatant forms, it is. This is still a threat to be aware of, and it comes in many guises: A compassionate furlough to permit recovery and the qualifying of a person for a state-sponsored disability program could be two of its disguises. There are probably as many more as there are inventive managers.

Career on Hold

Cancer therapy is going to require your attention before you can continue your career. Cancer literature sometimes portrays this hiatus for sickness and recovery as minimal. You may read: "I just dropped in for treatments during my lunch hour." Maybe. But don't plan on it. Unless your doctor assures you otherwise, expect your treatments to take much more than an hour of your day. Further, hold open the possibility that some or all of your doctoring will be too debilitating for you to make any meaningful contribution at work later in the day, and maybe for longer—for emotional, as well as physical, reasons.

In the midst of this, don't give up managing your career. Think through a positive plan that permits you to continue work contributions with informed allowances for this new dimension to your life. Consult with people you respect. Or locate wise heads who have been down this road ahead of you. Crisis counselors and support groups can make valuable input (see Chapter 19).

Minimizing the Economic Penalty

If you rely on employer-provided health insurance, the quality of coverage is going to be extremely important to you. Health insurance and other perks will probably pick up a big chunk of the tab for your treatments. But the strings attached to cancer care by the insurer and your employer may become critical to your future health and welfare—or to the loss of them.

The point of discussing this here is to remind you that there are options in employee-provided health care (see Chapter 14, "Health Insurance," for instance). You will ultimately be responsible for making the right choices. This process begins by your making sure that your employer and your health-insurance provider offer you all possible options.

Once you are past the initial announcement and negotiation process at work, take this whole subject to the person who provides you with personnel services. So you can study your options, ask for a summary of your sick leave, health-insurance options, life insurance, vacation time, other paid time off, ADA and FMLA options, state disability, Medicaid, and your spouse's resources. Also find out if you can still buy more health or life insurance. Knowing what they know, what would a professional benefits manager do in your place? Explore even the remotest possibilities.

Dealing with a Corporate Yenta

There's a succulent Yiddish descriptor, "yenta," that originally referred to a middle-aged woman who makes passionate, persistent sport of tending to everyone else's business. A yenta can be amusing—until he or she picks your affairs to meddle in.

You may find that a yenta is managing your company's health-care programs. Though it is strictly against the conduct code of the HR professional, this yenta may want to divert you from the health-care path you've chosen onto some other one. Beyond irritation, you face the problem that sometimes the unpalatable is also proper and constructive.

Similarly, a coworker may corner you to insist that you see some certain doctor or take some specific cure. Worse are supervisors to whom you report. The worst of these may use coercion. This problem is not uncommon and is complex to fix. The best *Living with Cancer* can do is alert you. Look to those in your personal support team for advice. Chapter 19, "Support Groups," may also be helpful.

Sphinxes

There may be people, such as your boss and the experts in HR, who have good, informed advice to offer but who wait for you to invite them to speak. They fear that their position in the company—or maybe some other factor, like a religious difference—would compromise an unsolicited comment. Their silence may be just what you want. But if their experience, training, or background might be of value, you'll need to invite their contribution.

Your Friend the Euphemism

"Cancer" is a frightening word. Some of its implications are distasteful, if not downright vulgar. In place of these terms and the matters they relate to, you and those around you will find expressions that make everybody more comfortable with the discussion. These words and terms move us from starkness into the wonderful, soft-focused world of the "euphemism," a word or phrase that is less direct, less distasteful, less offensive, more politically correct.

Euphemisms are an important contrivance. They are particularly helpful in discussions with one's parents and children. But in at least two circumstances, candor is necessary: when you are describing symptoms to a doctor or nurse, and when you are discussing the future of your job with decision makers at work. Eventual recovery of both health and professional standing benefit from clinical accuracy in these settings. This does not require you to verbally blow somebody's head off with graphic details. Just insure that your listener has enough accurate detail about your condition to make the discussion of matters that relate to it useful and productive.

Work Notification

You need to tell the key people at work about the cancer, face-to-face. This should happen in a private place in an environment that permits calm, thoughtful exploration of implications. From at least the patient's point of view, the planning and cooperation that evolve from this step may literally save the patient's place in the professional hierarchy while contributing six- or even seven-figure cash support to cancer recovery.

Conflicts between cancer and work are predictable. When illness takes time from the job, you pay at work. When you try to give time back to the job, cancer interrupts.

The employer may benefit as much, but don't count on your news making this possibility evident to your boss. Plan for this meeting carefully. Also read "A First-Announcement Tactic to Consider" a little farther along.

Preparation

Do not keep cancer a secret. It is a serious complication to your life. Hidden, it is likely to become an embarrassing surprise at exactly the wrong moment. Known, it is something others can help you with.

You can get help planning for your first work notification by input from your partner and personal supporters in recovery. Your doctor, by the way, may not be of much help beyond providing a precise diagnosis of your illness.

What to Say

Make up a list of the most important issues to take to your announcement meeting. You may decide that the notification will be best handled as a sole issue. In other circumstances, notification is just the prelude to a list of topics to be faced and dealt with all at once. There is no rule. Everything depends on the personalities, values, work priorities, and friendships already in the room at the time of the discussion.

When Not to Make Your Announcement

The gravity of your situation and your personal dignity demand that you pick a moment when the state of things around you is generally quiet. Pick a time when your audience can stop and focus on you. Don't interrupt a meeting of the board. Don't stop your boss who's running to catch the train.

Matters to Include

At some point during this meeting and its immediate aftermath, specific issues need to be settled. The strategy is yours to decide upon. One way to be certain you accomplish this task is have your list of topics on the table in front of you during this conversation. This is an important meeting. It deserves an agenda. If it is a meeting between close, friendly associates, give your boss a copy of the list too. But your best result usually comes by keeping your notes to yourself. At the end of the meeting, provide a written summary of your needs, a correct spelling of your disease diagnosis, and your oncologist's name.

High-Test Emotions

These meetings often become highly emotional. People frequently hug and shed tears, which is absolutely appropriate. Freedom of expression is one of the reasons you must insist on making your disclosure in a private meeting.

These events often conclude with an agreement that worker and supervisor should go see someone in HR immediately. There may be more tears in the second meeting. Don't be embarrassed. You deserve tears.

Core Issue: Your Cancer and Your View of Its Implications

Briefly tell the story of how you learned that you have cancer. Describe how you feel now, what your treatment program will be, and the parts of the outcome you have been told by your oncology team to expect. You won't know all that is to come. Don't be led into speculation. Guessing what's over the horizon could be the beginning of an intended or unintended trap that takes away pay or benefits.

In constructing this narrative, be aware that this version of what has happened to you will need to be repeated to others at work. It will also pass from those you tell to others. So keep it positive, simple, easy for people to remember, and to the point.

First Points to Make during the Meeting

- You expect to survive.
- You do not have a contagious disease.
- You are not now nor will you become mentally impaired.

You make these points to establish your turf and to nip in the bud some surprisingly common misconceptions people have about cancer. After covering these issues, ask for questions. Keep your answers brief and to the exact point raised. Keep in mind the story of the kid who asked his mommy where he came from. After a graphic, thirty-minute torture session, the child complained, "Gee, Sharon said she came from Cleveland. I just wondered if I did too."

Next Logical Areas of Concern

Either make a point of saying that you expect to remain with the work team and to continue to make more of the same valuable contributions to its mission, or avoid the topic. This is a critical moment in your relationship with your employer.

Organizational Implications of Your Illness

You will need time off for treatment and recovery. A temporary plan for support of team activities during your illness and recovery time will probably be necessary. Your positive thoughts and suggestions on details may also be valuable at this point in the discussion. For example, you may want to suggest a best division of your duties between other team members and department temps. Or you may suggest a strategy for working from home during recovery, or the delay of certain tasks until you return full-time.

Contract Replacements

Another solution is to reassign your duties temporarily. Another employee, a consultant, a subcontractor, or a temp may be able to take over until you have recovered. This type of arrangement may be workable for periods of as long as a year or two. You may be able to serve as a consultant to this temporary job holder to improve the effectiveness of the arrangement.

If your illness is causing your employer to cast about for ideas and this one hasn't come up, you may want to suggest it. This is a direct and open solution to a serious problem. And it can be fair to everyone. Further, it leaves the imprint of your name on your workstation, which is important for several obvious reasons.

Some months or a year from now, when you are ready to return, problems may arise. Companies change. Key people and departments rise or fall in favor. The person who took over for you may have changed the job to something that you are no longer qualified to shoulder. This is not a prediction. It is a cautionary note. A person who takes over for you with the understanding that the arrangement is temporary is still a far better solution to the problem your illness has caused than are some of the alternative scenarios.

Forecasting Physical Changes

If you know that cancer or its treatment will leave you with a physical impairment, God bless you. You may have to change the mix of things you do at work. Carefully consider how this news may affect the course of your future. There may be someone to whom you will want to disclose these special concerns first. An EAP counselor or a specialist in HR whom you know personally and trust could be a good choice. Or there may be a coworker, a religious leader, or a person on your medical oncology team who can give you the best advice. Think creatively to be sure you get the best help.

Reassignment Realities and Recourses

You can and will be moved or removed from your job if organizational mission goals require it. There is a good deal of concern over job discrimination these days. What's legal? What's not? And people as sick as you are do not

---

The Impact of Obtaining Legal Counsel

The moment your employer believes you have obtained the representation of an attorney, you will probably lose direct employer-employee contact. Your attorney will be required to talk to the employer's attorney. You and your boss won't be allowed to negotiate directly or even to discuss open issues. The net effect is that you two may not talk at all.

Bureaucrats with investigational or enforcement responsibilities who get into the act will also cause this schism between you and your management.

That you have taken the step of obtaining representation is also generally taken as a signal that trust has been lost. It probably has been.

---

deserve this extra body blow. But you surely also realize that a secretary who can't type or a salesperson who can't sell or a president who can't lead has to be moved aside, one way or another.

In deference to reality, your best hope may be for fair consideration and compensation. Most large organizations have worked out the details.

You may want to discuss this with your shop steward or an attorney, because these programs are not always generous or even fair (see Chapters 15 and 16). There are also subtleties that may benefit from a good negotiator's tweak on your behalf. Such high-value items as the continued availability of perks, ownership of future stock options, and partial vesting in retirement and benefit programs should be nailed down. Or you may want a preferred place in line to reenter the company's workforce after a prolonged furlough.

If you use the services of the shop steward, a government regulator, the office of an elected representative, or any lawyer, try not to let it be evident to your organization. See if you can get coaching behind the scenes. Third parties are natural enemies of management. Regardless of how it all works out, your use of any of these people, if known, will not be taken as a friendly act.

Other Announcement Timing and Preparation

If you do not intend to remain on the job, the right time to make that public is most likely after the details of lifetime health-insurance coverage, disability, and any other benefits you may be able to take with you have been ironed out. Lifetime health-insurance protection is particularly important to a person whose (expensive) disease may disqualify any further affordable health coverage this side of Medicare.

Medicaid, which has different names in many states, is also available for some kinds of cancer patients, as is immediate state disability status (see Chapter 22).

To prepare further, dig out the employee handbook you probably received when you joined the company. Remind yourself of the policies concerning leave of absence, vacation, sick leave, paid and unpaid time off. You need to be something of a barracks lawyer to figure this stuff out and to evaluate all of the provisions. Someone in HR should be able to give you all the help you need.

You can also refer to the company's HR policy manual for further details. It is a right you have as an employee. Be warned that in some corporations, these manuals take up major shelf space.

A First-Announcement Tactic to Consider

Here's a tactic for getting the most of the best in support and benefits from your company. It will work only when your condition has been a secret up to the moment of the meeting with your boss. This tactic should be particularly good for those who have no sales skills and hate confrontation.

Ask for a short private meeting on a personal matter that you wish to explain in hopes of receiving advice that you (and say it in these very words) "just know will be very good." Do not explain further. Provide no hint as to the topic. Neither lead nor mislead. If badgered about the subject, just keep repeating, "It's personal," "Very personal." Be prepared in case the boss says, "Okay, let's meet right now."

In the private setting, explain exactly, candidly, what your affliction is and when and how you received this bad news. Outline the doctor's recommended treatment plans. Do not speculate as to outcomes beyond what your oncology team has told you. Complete this narrative in less than three minutes. Then smile and say: "I know that you are experienced in matters like this. So tell me, what can you and the company do for me?"

Give the person a look of eager expectation and shut up. Shut up. Zip it. Say nothing more. Even if the boss takes a minute or more to reply, hold out. Once your boss begins to speak, do not interrupt. If the boss tries to toss the ball back to you by asking a diverting question, reply briefly and repeat a version of the key question. With a smile, in a very respectful tone: "What I really need to know—if there is any way you can possibly tell me—is what can you and the company do for me?"

The information and the offers that come forth are likely to be the most generous promises your company can make to you. In fact, the offers may be precedent setting.

There is no downside to this tactic, although an embarrassed supervisor may later be forced to retract an extravagant promise made in the heat of the moment.

Determining Your Health Benefits

There are twelve million entities in the United States with paid employees. Every one of them seems to differ in the details of its health-coverage policies. You need to make certain that you will be receiving all possible benefits from your employer's plan. Once your initial disclosure has been taken care of, you will probably learn everything you need to know by visiting the person responsible for managing your company's health-care program.

But among this vast number of organizations, some still don't have employee protection of the sort you need. If you discover that your employer is among those without a health plan or has one with exclusions or very low ceilings on benefit payments, there is a good chance you will not receive the financial help you need. Should that be the case, you are going to need to spend extra time in "Supporting Resources," Part IV.

Possible Recourse for Uncovered Workers

You may discover that generous health benefits and related perks, including extended furloughs and out-of-pocket health costs, are paid to executives of your company but not to the rank and file. If you can bring such an instance to light through an attorney, it may be worth exploring.

The downside is that, by blowing the whistle, you'll probably lose your job (though that's technically illegal). But you could have tens of thousands of dollars in medical bills paid and a labor-grievance settlement worth something more. The likely alternative is to keep a job you are too sick to perform and to shoulder a catastrophic debt or enter bankruptcy.

If you are in a union, give the issue of lack of health insurance to your steward. An employer with several locations may not provide the same health-insurance package at all sites. You could get covered in the interests of parity because employees at another location have the health coverage you need.

There may be a negotiation coming up that can include your case as an example of a general need. You can be covered after the fact, even with a pre-existing condition, though don't count on it. Unions can also conduct special fund-raisers.

Never give up simply because the first look was discouraging. Cancer affects many, many people. It is likely there is somebody at your workplace or a friend of a friend who has walked this same path ahead of you and who will be only too willing to help.

Rumor Control

Expect rumor, as well as fact, to circulate about you and your disease. Accurate accounts are not something you should try to do much about, even if the tales invade your privacy. The best course is to allow your condition its fifteen minutes of fame, after which some other topic will start the rounds and you will find peace.

False gossip is another matter, particularly a canard that hurts your place in a professional hierarchy. You will want to do something. Your supervisor should want to help.

Faced with such a rumor, Mark Twain cabled the Associated Press from London: "The reports of my death are greatly exaggerated." Humor is a terrific rumor suppressant. Try it, if humor works for you. Expressing anger, for some reason, does far less to shut up your problem children. A calm retelling of the essential facts seems to be the best middle course.

It will help to find the people most apt to circulate rumors about you and recruit them to stop the spread of garbage. If they like you and understand what vicious falsehood can do to you, rumor gets suppressed.

Keeping the Work Fires Burning

If your job and your employer are important to you, don't let them forget you. Keep in telephone or e-mail touch with your friends and especially with your supervisor. If illness has drained your attention and strength, ask your partner to make an occasional phone call for you. Consider sending short notes, a postcard from the clinic, or even a photo of your newly bald head to keep the troops stirred up.

To continue to make this effective, you need to be reachable by people who are interested in situation updates. This accessibility will also bring advice-seeking calls from others who have just learned that they or a loved one has cancer. As you will learn in the discussion of support groups (Chapter 19), one person's sharing of firsthand experiences with another is most helpful—and therapeutic.

A Job-Evaluation Opportunity

At the point where illness is going to take away your work option for awhile, some introspection about your career may be helpful. Has it been worth the time and effort you have given it? Have you enjoyed your job? Your boss? Your coworkers? Are you excited by the possible places your job could lead? Are you as well paid as you deserve to be? Do you like the place you have to live to keep your job?

Sometimes a crisis allows us the perspective to look critically at ourselves. This may be such a moment for you. Has cancer endangered things you place a value on? How great a value? Is this a chance to make a positive course correction toward a better life?

If, on the other hand, you find that cancer is tearing you away from a place and a team of people you love, you consciously need to see what you can do to keep your spot reserved until you can get back into the old swing of things. There are no rules for doing this well or poorly. Your success largely depends on how badly your talents will be missed.

A Few Simple Steps That May Preserve Your Job

- Speak to your supervisor about your interest in keeping your job, even though you may be incapacitated for a while. Be warned, as Yogi Berra says, that a verbal assurance isn't worth the paper it's written on.
- Ask for a letter from your supervisor and another from the president or the head of HR (or whoever the right person is) that promises to hold open a place for you and spells out any conditions. Get at least two letters from well-placed mainstays, because you never know who may be gone before you get back. A letter from a former big shot cuts no ice.
- As already noted, your employer may be able to fill your slot temporarily. Another employee, a consultant, or another type of worker such as a temp may perform your duties until you have recovered.
- Look into taking disability status. The responsibilities of your work are lifted from you, and cancer may qualify you for Medicaid.
- Caution: Many employers consider the act of accepting disability status irreversible. If you are offered disability and learn that by accepting it you can never revert to your old job status, disability is actually termination— with partial pay and, maybe, benefits for some period of time.
- On reflection, disability status may appeal to you. If it does not, you may have alternatives. See if you can accept furlough status, a consultant's contract, or another arrangement that keeps your taproot in the company. You must understand each of these options thoroughly, however. Continuing pay and the amount of it that you will actually receive are two key issues. Disability pay is tax free. Consultant pay may carry extra tax burdens, plus a double hit for Social Security and other up-front withholds. Even though disability pay is 60 percent of your normal gross, the net in your pocket may be a little more than you are used to getting because taxes are no longer withheld. Then again, you

may have exercised a pay option that now reduces disability to less than 60 percent.

- The terms of continued pay and health-insurance coverage may be highly technical. Have someone you trust help you understand them completely.
- When you begin the time away from the job that treatment and recovery require, take work with you that the company will look forward to seeing completed and returned. (Never take anything of a proprietary nature from your employer without specific enthusiastic encouragement.) Be aware that you are probably not going to accomplish a lot during your recovery time. Think of this as a symbolic gesture to which you can add some value if you feel up to it but won't have to. And don't charge a lot for it. Your company is already being very generous. One generally accepted plan is to keep a log of productive time, to be compensated at a fair hourly rate for your pay grade. If you are salaried, many companies calculate gross hourly rate as equal to annual salary divided by the 1,700 to 2,080 hours in the company's work year.

Shared Sick or Comp Time

As this cancer thing goes on, your sick time, comp time, vacation time, and whatever other kinds of paid time away from the job your boss may be able to arrange for you may dwindle. Time off without pay, or some other play on that general theme, may be coming soon. You may be able to hold it off by borrowing or buying time from a coworker. The HR people have to lend a hand for this to happen. They may not have thought of this wrinkle, or it may go against the philosophy of a manager, but it can be worth a try. Many of the Fortune 500 and some governmental organizations accept it. You could trigger the creation of an important new policy.

Buying comp or vacation time may seem like an odd concept. Purchasing it from a high-priced executive may not be either appropriate or affordable. But a person who works in the mailroom may deserve and appreciate a financial consideration. If you can buy a day of pay worth $160 to you for $70, the investment is a no-brainer.

Some Paid Time Off That Isn't

Workers earn several types of paid time off. Once accrued, this time belongs to the employee, though with certain strings attached. Paid vacation time falls in this category. It's yours, though how and when you use it has rules. The employer may also provide paid time off for contingencies and special events. If it isn't used, it goes away. Some sick time or compensatory (comp) time may be in this category. Jury-duty time is an example. Maybe you get your birthday off too, if work demands allow it.

Earned paid time off is a commodity another employee could give, trade, or sell you, with the cooperation of the HR department. If this happens, it may be a taxable transaction.

Available time that the company holds open as an accommodation to the employee who needs it cannot be transferred from one employee to another or pulled out of a department's time budget. Employees and departments don't own or control it; the company does, and there are all kinds of treaty, tax, and regulatory complications that get in the way of using it in any way other than the one for which it is intended.

It is not unusual for people to believe that the use of unearned comp time is their right. It is also customary, when employees discover that such time isn't theirs, to damn the employer, which is grossly unfair. Now that we have rained on your parade, go ahead and see if you can negotiate some of this extra paid time off anyway. To paraphrase Nikita Khruschev, rules, like piecrust, are made to be broken.

An Answer to "What Can I Do?"

Coworkers and friends will often ask, "What can I do?" If there are things you feel comfortable asking for, name them. Be aware that your coworker has made a gesture of concern and courtesy, not an offer of indentured servitude.

Consider asking for prayer. Prayer is a unique and effective way to keep your team together. Your request for it is absolutely without penalty, even when you ask it of an agnostic. It does not compromise any religion. Prayer is universal. And, as we have seen in Chapter 10, prayer works on many positive levels.

Cancer and its treatments are team sports, with laughter as a bonus for inventive behavior. Let your coworkers know you appreciate rides to appointments. These are a great opportunity to stay in touch. You also have somebody you know close at hand when you need help. As you know, you are not always energetic and attentive after tests and treatments. This is an easy gift you let a friend give you.

If You Are the CEO/Owner/Officer

There are a few differences in strategy between employee and employer that may be helpful to note. The idea that the cancer patient should first get a partner or partners remains sound. For purposes of planning this announcement, one or more key business associates or board members should also be involved.

Plan the Announcement of Your Illness

You will want to give the same story simultaneously to all the audiences that matter to your business. They include employees, customers, industry, CPA, attorney, community, outside organizations in which you are active, creditors, ex-spouses and others who count on your stability and longevity, and shareholders. Tell them all the same thing. (They will compare notes later.) Include in the announcement a plan for interim management of the company. Name some hazy time frame (like "next spring") in which you will return to pick up the reins.

You say these things as morale boosters and as stabilizing points of organizational reference. Try your best draft of this statement ahead of time on a business associate or consultant whom you trust. Make every effort to find any flaws that could raise fears about the future of your company. To be most effective, your announcement has to be bulletproof when it hits the street.

Put an Interim Leader in Place

You may want to retain the final say as board chair or CEO, but you will need to name a chief operating officer, empower a management committee, or hire an outsider to run day-to-day affairs. This is a bitter pill, beyond the countenance of some owners.

Order the Drafting of a Highly Confidential Contingency Plan

Internal things can go wrong. You probably know which, from sad experience. Direct your stand-in to prepare a contingency plan for dealing with the most obvious ones. It's a great exercise, and it prepares people to think for themselves but along the lines you have in mind.

You also need to think about what may need to be done if your market sours. If you don't know what to do or if treatments are too great a distraction, toss the ball to your most trusted aid and rely on Providence. Your health comes first.

13 Friends

He who has a thousand friends has not a friend to spare.

—Ali ibn-Abi-Talib

Friendship has medically proven powers. Family, people you worship with, associates from work, support-group members, people you play sports with—everyone you know who cares about you adds to your recuperative power through their acts of love and concern. Don't withdraw from friends. Find extra ways to be around all the friends you can. Find more friends among fellow patients at treatment centers. Let them help. Be of help.

Perhaps you are not a social person. Perhaps the friends you've had—including your life partner—are gone. You can still acquire the valuable gift of friends. Practice smiling at everyone. Introduce yourself. Show an interest in others and be pleasant to those who speak to you. People will be drawn to you, warts and all, and you will make friends.

Sustaining and Life-Improving Friendships

Cancer patients with active friendships live longer, happier lives than those with fewer social ties. Physicians who have studied and verified this finding point out that friendship and caring are powerful medicine for even the sickest of people.

An extensive group of physicians, scientists, and notables—once led by the late Norman Cousins—believes that happiness, laughter, and the generally positive feelings that come with friendship have physical healing powers. Studies support them with scientific evidence.

In "Social Networks, Host Resistance, and Mortality," Lisa Berkman and Leonard S. Syme report on a survey of 6,928 adults of average health who lived in Alameda County, California, over a nine-year period. The survey showed that people who lacked social and community ties—friends—were about two-and-a-half times more likely to die than those with social ties of any type. (Their report appeared in the *American Journal of Epidemiology*, vol. 109, no. 2, 1979, pp. 186–204.)

Barrie Cassileth led a group of researchers who found that friendship improves the length and quality of a terminal patient's life (see "Psychosocial Correlatives of Survival in Advanced Malignant Disease," *New England Journal of Medicine*, vol. 312, no. 24, June 13, 1985, pp. 1551–1555).

The article "Psychosocial Coping Mechanisms and Survival Time in Metastatic Breast Cancer" tells of a study of thirty-five women with metastatic breast cancer. Those with friends lived the longest, according to a study team led by Leonard Derogatis (see *the Journal of the American Medical Association*, vol. 242, no. 14, October 5, 1979, pp. 1504–1508). In an unrelated study, Sandra M. Levy found that happily married women endured their disease more successfully than did other women (see "Emotions and the Progression of Cancer" *Advances*, vol. 1, no. 1, Winter 1984, pp. 10–15).

Stress undermines but friendship increases resistance to disease and illness, according to Leon Eisenberg's article "What Makes Persons 'Patients' and Patients 'Well'?" in the *American Journal of Medicine*, vol. 69, August 1980, pp. 277–286.

Furry, Finned, and Feathered Friends

Cancer patients, particularly lonely ones, benefit from pets. The medical community, which agrees that petship heals, makes every effort to accommodate patient companions from the animal world—within obvious and reasonable limits. The unconditional friendship of a pet is a healthy thing for a sick person.

Faith Fitzgerald, writing in the *Western Medical Journal*, found that patients in a coronary care unit who could watch fish in an aquarium or who enjoyed the companionship of an animal were six times more likely to be alive one year later (see "The Therapeutic Value of Pets," vol. 144, no. 1, January 1986, pp. 103–105).

All those unhappy, hurried, expensive, scary, and sometimes painful things you have to endure go better with friends. All those misunderstandings about treatments and billings are easier if the folks you're dealing with are friends.

You will also heal more quickly because you feel less stress. And friendships outlast cancer.

In a study by Erika Friedman of critically ill coronary patients, 28 percent of those who did not own pets were dead within a year. Only 3 percent of pet-owning patients died during that time (see "Animal Companions and One-Year Survival of Patients after Discharge from a Coronary Care Unit," *Public Health Reports,* vol. 95, no. 4, July–August 1980, pp. 307–312).

Friendships with Your Medical and Support Teams

You must make a conscious effort to humanize and be friendly with your doctors, nurses, technicians, pharmacist, therapist, and insurance-claims adjusters, and with the folks in accounts payable and people from the government agency that supports you. Use friendliness and consideration to improve the quality of your care and to destroy apathy. Work on eye contact and smiles. Go quickly to first names, as your medical team does. If a first name is awkward, such as when you are speaking to a doctor who demands formality or when the name is unpronounceable, come up with a good nickname.

In whatever way you can, be positive and personal. Take cookies. Ask questions. Notice photos. Learn about birthdays and anniversaries. Send cards.

Prayer, an Act of Kinship

It has been proven that prayer heals in marvelous, powerful ways (see Chapter 10). Regularly remind your friends that prayer is a way they can help you. You must also find ways you can pray for them, their families, and their lives in general. Make notes and discuss the details—regularly—with God.

With that in mind, let us suppose that one of your medical team looks stressed in a meeting with you. As you have learned to do, you ask how the person is feeling, and you learn that someone has been hurt, or that something similarly distressing is preoccupying this friend of yours. Ask how you can help. Wonder aloud if you can pray for those involved. Maybe even take the person's hand and pray briefly on the spot if this is comfortable for you both. There is no place on earth that you cannot pray. There is no time when your God is not available. The healing forces that an act of friendship of this sort releases will astonish you—and your friend.

Farewells between Friends

You may need someone on your healing team to leave it. After efforts to correct a situation, it becomes clear that separation is best for the team. The most direct thing is for the patient to simply state the fact, with thanks to the person. If the patient can't do this, then the partner needs to. It can be hard. It may do damage to a family or business relationship. It still must be done to prevent a greater injury to the patient.

Often, the person who does not fit in realizes it and relinquishes the role without a word having to be said. In other cases, a remedy short of separation is a first step that may instead become a permanent repair. With a friend, you need to discuss any serious mistake. In the most positive way possible, the friend needs to agree to a change and a course of new action. You close by saying, "Well, what should we do if this happens again?" By answering that question, the friend prescribes a specific future term of association. If "it" happens again, the friend releases himself or herself from the relationship. Patient and partner can afford to keep the parting amicable.

The point is that farewells sometimes pass the point where they are optional. When a farewell is needed, it must take place. To procrastinate adds stress to the patient's life. If the farewell is hard on somebody else, that is regrettable but less important.

IV Supporting Resources

*An Inventory and Evaluation
of Available Tools*

14 Health Insurance

Think you're covered?

Please Proceed with Caution

You can expect four- and even five-figure medical bills very soon. You obviously feel fortunate to have insurance that covers all this, but don't relax just yet. There are things to know and do.

First, You need to make certain that your medical teams, your health-plan administrator, and the insurance company that approves the bills and writes the checks are working together. The greater the teamwork, the fewer the medical insurance conflicts.

Second, you need to have someone, preferably an expert, thoroughly vet your coverage to identify loopholes and exceptions that may apply specifically to your cancer-treatment program.

This time you're relying on your health insurance to keep you from financial ruin. This time you're not worried about how many cheap massages the system will allow you, or how many pairs of glasses you can get. This time you'll be maxing your deductibles at the speed of light. This time the caps and co-pays and exclusions will matter far more. This time everything has to be right.

Basics for Those Covered at Work

You must advise your insurance company and your human-resources department that you have been diagnosed, right away. Companies of any size have a health-insurance specialist or maybe an employee-assistance professional, usually called an EAP, who is trained to help you go forward from here (also see the related discussion of this topic in Chapter 12, "The Patient's Workplace"). If you work for a smaller company or are self-employed, call the people who issued the policy.

For Medicare and Medicaid information, please turn to Chapter 22, "Public Assistance."

In either the in-house or small insured-group instance, an organizational meeting is needed. Take with you the name of the doctor you have been working with, the address of the practice, and the phone number. The clerk who administers your health insurance and the clerk in your doctor's office need to begin working together. Expect to be loaded down with instructions, forms, and brochures by the end of the meeting.

At least one employee of your health-insurance company, often called a nurse-advocate, is tasked with making sure you know how to get the most protection from your health-insurance plan. The nurse-advocate tracks—and smoothes the way for—everyone with abnormal numbers of insurance claims or claims of unusual sorts. You'll have both.

In addition to help with insurance claims, the nurse-advocate and probably the EAP can answer practical treatment questions. They can:

- Direct you to the medical groups that have the most experience with your kind of cancer.
- Describe from a witness's eye-level what your treatment regimen is apt to be.
- Tell you about teams of specialists.
- Show you how to structure things so that insurance pays for them, instead of you.
- Let you know where you can buy the things that you will have to pay for, cheapest.

Beginning Steps for Those Covered through Nonwork Plans

If your health insurance is through some channel other than employment, someone identified in your policy is probably waiting to help you. If not, see your insurance agent.

Learn all you can about the features of your health-insurance plan. You also need to know how your plan's administrators are set up to work with you most efficiently. Don't be in a hurry for this meeting to end. Give your expert plenty of time to thoroughly brief you. At the end of the conversation, give the person one last chance to cover everything by wondering, "What should I have asked you about that hasn't come up?"

The Style of Your Health Insurance: Impact on Treatment

Your insurance plan has a style: HMO, PPO, POS, whatever. It came with books, brochures, forms, an identification card, maybe a video. Even though an employer may have selected it, and even though someone else may be paying part of the cost, you are the owner of this product, for purposes of your treatment program. You are responsible for your part in its agreements and procedures.

You and your insurance plan must agree on a specific treatment program by a specific medical team. The agreement has to include every detail that your insurance company may be expected to participate in financially. This will include matters related to your treatments that need to be cleared in advance to qualify for reimbursement. Your general reporting responsibilities are also important.

If you have a critical area of disagreement with your health-insurance provider, solve it as quickly as possible. Don't allow the insurance company or anyone else affected by this problem to dismiss it before it is solved to your satisfaction. Unless you nail it, it will come back at the absolutely worst time and nail you. If you find that outside help is necessary in this matter, consult with one of the cancer groups or support groups discussed later in this chapter or listed in the Reference Center.

Guides and Aids

A high-quality health-insurance provider will have a nurse-advocate available to lift large parts of the insurance burden from your shoulders. Stripped-down plans make do with toll-free numbers answered by a less informed rotating staff. The ability of people you reach to make beneficial decisions will also vary broadly from insurer to insurer. Obviously, the first level of service would be better for you than the second, but you can work with either. Just make certain that you are dealing with a decision maker. "No" is an answer that any management trainee can give you. "No" does not require the slightest familiarity with facts or case latitudes. Try hard not to deal below the level of people who have the power to say "yes."

Another possibility is that someone on your doctor's staff may take over large parts of the insurance-company liaison. Or you could get an EAP on the staff of the hospital or on the payroll of a public agency who helps at low or no cost.

All this searching and negotiating should not be demanded of a person with far more serious preoccupations. But there it is. Moreover, if this ordering and organizing and reporting and negotiating are not all properly accomplished, you're going to have extra trouble getting your bills paid.

The Next Thing to Do If You Have Health Insurance

Your health-insurance ID card has a toll-free phone number on it. Call and ask to speak to the nurse-advocate, advises Glenn Ridgway, area senior VP at Gallagher Benefit Services of Kansas City. Tell the nurse exactly what has happened. "This is a professional, trained to help you get the most from the resources that your health plan makes available to you," he advises. The nurse-advocate (also sometimes called a case nurse) will start a special file on your case to make the claims process as smooth as possible. As mentioned earlier, this person may also have powerful ideas or suggestions. But, unlike others you deal with at the beginning of your cancer odyssey, your nurse-advocate will also be there later should things get more complicated. For example, let us suppose that a special treatment or clinical trial may become highly advisable a year from now. But the treatment would require travel and residence away from home for some period of time. Your nurse-advocate should be able to tell you how to qualify your treatment for insurance coverage and to warn of any snares. (There are also charities to help with travel and lodging.)

Vetting Your Health-Insurance Policy

If you were covered for all health costs and contingencies, your policy could be printed on the back of your health-insurance ID—and would be. Instead, the "whereases" and "wherefores" run for chapters. Your complete health-care coverage agreement—which you have probably never seen—may take up a complete bookshelf (and you have the right to read it). So now the question is, Where and what are the surprises? Large employee health plans employ experts who look at situations like yours and flag problem areas.

Why didn't "they" cover . . . ?

Insurance companies exclude things that generally pass unnoticed or unappreciated by customers. Huge savings in payouts result. Companies forgo insurance options when they believe their cost is unnecessary or too high. Options are also an easy place to cut. It's hard to get worked up over the loss of a coverage that nobody expects to need.

The formal insurance-company appeals process is like being pecked to death by a duck. For more on this experience, see Chapter 26, "Nine Easy Ways to Shoot Yourself in the Foot," Way #5: "The insurance company won't allow . . ."

Ask your health-plan administrator at work to put this person on your case immediately.

If your health insurance is purchased directly, task your insurance agent with finding an expert you can trust. Large health-insurance brokerages have consultants available to serve their corporate group accounts. Maybe you can discuss your coverage with one of them. There are also public servants in state health-insurance commission offices that can help, if they will.

Possible Coverage Exclusions

More and more expensive and critical details of cancer treatments are being assigned caps well below true cost or excluded from coverage completely. Your policy may not pay for:

- transplants, including bone marrow or stem cells
- a search for donors, and type-matching costs
- pacemakers
- pretransplant heart pumps and similar life-support systems
- after first breast surgery, a mastectomy on a second breast
- prosthetic devices or fitting costs
- training in the use of a prosthetic device such as an arm or leg
- cancer "episode" treatment limits. In clearer language: If the cancer ever comes back, there is no coverage.
- drugs for any use not listed on the FDA-approved label. Off-label uses in cancer are frequent.
- drugs for hemophilia and for infectious or opportunistic diseases, such as hepatitis. In this way, you could lose all coverage for medications related to heart disease, a common unrelated condition in older patients.
- limits on numbers of visits for therapy or psychiatric care.
- treatments that are, in the insurance carrier's opinion, "experimental." This could eliminate coverage for clinical trials, certain surgical operations, drugs, therapies, and prosthetics.

General Notes on Negotiations with Your Insurance Company

If the review of your health-insurance coverage reveals one or more areas of financial concern, your first and best remedy is to resolve the matter directly between the affected parts of your health-care circle. Business is brief and to the point. For example, if your insurance company excludes coverage for something you need, your oncologist may be able to change your policy restriction with a phone call to the company. The option of making the disputed treatment part of a clinical trial or of finding some other umbrella that a research grant supports may also be open to your doc.

Your employer (or your broker) may be able to encourage a favorable reading or an exception by your insurance company. They have experience reasoning with health insurers and bring the clout of a larger piece of business to the bargaining table. Failing that, you may need to get a cancer-advocacy

Table 14.1 Insurance-Gap Resources

The Bone Marrow Foundation www.bonemarrow.org	212/838-3029 800/365-1336	Helps transplant patients pay costs
The National Marrow Donor Program www.marrow.org	888/999-6743	The Office of Patient Advocacy provides advice, support, and information
National Transplant Assistance Fund www.transplantfund.org	610/527-5056 800/642-8399	Helps donors with expenses
Patient Advocate Foundation www.patientadvocate.org	800/532-5274	Helps resolve insurance disputes between all parties
South-Eastern Organ Procurement Foundation www.seopf.org	804/323-9890 800/543-6399	Offers life, medical, and disability insurance to donors

group to intercede with your insurance company. Or help may come from your state insurance commissioner's office. Failing all those possibilities, consider going to an insurance-gap resource.

Insurance-Gap Resources

Big-money disputes between insurance companies, treatment providers, industry regulators, patients, creditors, and others have become a larger, more complex issue, as sophistication and innovations in treatment increase. In 2002, Nancy Davenport-Ennis, president of the Patient Advocate Foundation, estimated that about 80 percent of her company's twenty-five thousand current cases involved patient-policy limitations.

Low Insurance-Cap Situations

Legions of Americans have purchased "limited benefit" health insurance. It is cheap, perhaps less than $10 per week per person. The basic deductible is low, and the patient's co-pays for some medical needs are low. The trouble is that the maximum protection allowed per year may be as little as $1,000. You may need over $100,000—and you should have at least $1 million available, to be on the safe side.

In some ways, a low annual cap plan is worse than no insurance at all because it complicates the process of applying for the help you really need. If you have fallen into this trap, get the most out of your mistake by filing all the claims allowable.

Meanwhile, let your agent try to get you more insurance, making certain it includes cancer care. You can expect this effort to fail. You will be turned down as soon as your illness is mentioned. Carefully document at least three rejections. Then see "Your State Health-Care Pool" a little further along.

The "Preexisting Condition"

No insurance company happily covers a person for a disease he or she already has. This is usually indicated by a paragraph in the health-insurance policy that prohibits claims for "preexisting conditions."

How was it, then, that the Sands Hotel in Las Vegas could continue to purchase postdated fire insurance for five years after its disastrous fire? The answer is that loopholes and large amounts of cash can work wonders. The same twosome, involving large numbers of employees in big insurance-premium pools, has worked for others in your situation. Typically, those who receive this special treatment are senior executives or have some other high business value to those who have gone to bat for them. You may be in that category. If you are not, but you know someone who was and received this special treatment, an advocate will have an argument to make on your behalf.

A Possible Coverage Option

Consider changing jobs. Large companies and government agencies at all levels sometimes provide group health-insurance plans that new employees can join without exclusions for preexisting conditions. In other cases, there is a waiting period of from three to twenty-four months, with one year being the normal maximum wait for a cancer exclusion to go away. Despite the delay, a piece of your financial problem is solved, maybe a very big piece.

If you consider this route, be careful to explain your health condition fully to the new employer before accepting the job offer. Then work out the details of how and under what conditions you receive health insurance. Everybody's got to work together on this or the strategy can't succeed.

Job-Interruption Caution

If, for any reason, your group health-insurance coverage is interrupted for more than sixty-two days, you will probably lose all right to claim or reclaim any health insurance you may have had. This can most easily happen if you quit or lose your job, or if you forget to pay the bill. You will also lose the right to claim COBRA interim health-insurance coverage. You lose, too, any credit for time accrued toward expiration of a cancer exclusion.

Your State Health-Care Pool

Legal provisions may be on the books for a patient with your specific kind, or stage, of cancer. These could reduce your waiting time or cut the cost of your coverage. Be sure to ask.

Most states have health-care pools that will insure people with cancer, Glenn Ridgway advises. The applicant qualifies by showing two or three rejections from other insurers. This insurance will be more expensive, perhaps a lot more expensive, than a competitive premium would be. It will still be far less than the costs of treatment you are hoping to find shelter from.

There may be an exclusion for a preexisting condition here too. In the states where this provision is part of the deal, you are expected to join and pay and wait, knowing that the exclusion will be lifted after a previously agreed period of time.

To apply for the health-care pool, contact your state insurance commissioner's local office. See the front section of your local phone book under "Government Services." Someone there will know how to advise you.

Long-Term-Care Insurance

If your condition demands an extended stay somewhere, even if it is far less pretentious than a hospital, the base cost is still apt to start somewhere above $150 a day. If any part of this need is covered by your health insurance, it will be strictly short term. After that, home care may be your most attractive alternative (see Chapter 43, "Care at Home," for lots of options and cost-saving ideas).

For more on a need to stay in a place that provides some level of medical care, talk to your oncologist. There is undoubtedly a long-term-care facility associated with a nearby hospital that you can enter. If what you are offered doesn't suit you, here are two pretty good resources: *Planning for Long-Term Care,* published by the National Council on Aging, $19.50 (call 800/373-4906 for more information or to order); call the Eldercare Locator Hotline, 800/677-1116, M–F, 9 A.M.–8 P.M., East Coast time, or visit www.eldercare .gov. One or both of these sources may have the information or contacts you need, whether you meet the age qualification or not.

Long-Term Care for the Terminally Ill

Those diagnosed as being in the last six months of life qualify for fully paid hospice care through the federal Department of Health and Human Services. Local private-party contractors usually manage hospice services. Patients and their families are generally served with compassion and skill. The oncologist will know how to obtain this coverage (see Chapter 43, "Care at Home," for more details).

An Expert's Insurance Strategy

"When Rose and I retire," Ridgway says, "I will purchase a $5,000-deductible health-insurance plan with a one or two million dollar cap for each of us." While the first $5,000 would hurt, he says, it's the hundreds of thousands of dollars later, for something like cancer or a bad traffic accident, that cost you the house and the nest egg. "It'll be about $75 each, a month [in 2003 dollars]," Ridgway predicts. In addition, he plans to keep a couple of thousand dollars in a bank account so that the couple can pay cash for minor medical costs and dental and eye care as necessary. Should a major medical expense exceed $5,000, the policy pays a flat 80 percent to its cap, which could still leave a stiff balance for the Ridgways. "It's all we need until Medicare kicks in at age 65."

By contrast, a typical health-insurance policy with a $750 deductible, pharmacy co-pay, and a reasonable major-medical cost umbrella costs $450 or more per month for a healthy fifty- to sixty-year-old. If there are major illness claims, such as for heart disease or cancer, the monthly cost of an individual policy can exceed $1,000.

15 Public-Assistance Law

Yes, there is an expert you can phone.

Partners and friends of patients—

Looking for a way to be of great help to the patient? Working with an attorney on a dispute could be it.

The big-money, enormously complex insurance and social services, and other disruptions that one person's sickness brings to the lives of others can be confounding. Just finding the right treatments or qualifying for them can be a major problem. Fortunately, several highly specialized groups have organized in recent years to help you cope with these issues.

Tens of thousands of people bring Gordian knots to public-assistance law groups every year. Often, a simple explanation—or a phone call on the patient's behalf—takes care of a problem that appeared unsolvable. In other cases, illness has reminded the patient that personal decisions need to be made and set out in legally binding form.

Carefully consider the extent of any problem of the sorts listed here. If you have some doubt that you will quickly and easily resolve the matter, discuss it with a public-assistance law group. These services are subsidized. The needs of the humble and the mighty receive equal thoroughness.

Issues of Law That Affect Cancer Patients

Workplace Topics

1. Cancer has caused you to be discriminated against.
2. You need an expert who will work on your behalf to explain more about the Family Medical Leave Act, Americans with Disabilities Act, Health Insurance Portability and Accountability Act, or some other provision of the law.
3. Your employer wants to help with your issues but doesn't know how.

Health Insurance

1. You are having difficulty receiving benefits from existing insurance.
2. You need help getting coverage.

Navigating Managed Care

According to a Kaiser Family Survey, one in two Americans reported a problem with their health-insurance plan in 1999–2000.

1. You need someone to explain your situation to you and help you understand alternatives and their implications.
2. Your insurance company is stalling your treatment program. You need someone to motivate action.
3. You and your insurance company differ on an important treatment issue. Your doc's recommendation didn't settle it. You need an effective advocate for your position.

4. Your insurance company wants to withhold services, perhaps by calling the treatment "experimental" or "off label," or by use of an unreasonable exclusionary treatment clause. This has become a debate over semantics between you and administrators. The issue of effective healing isn't being considered. Both sides need the help of an outside expert to arbitrate, right away.

Credit Negotiations

1. You need someone to help you negotiate credit problems, particularly those arising from disputed medical bills or errors that have shown up in your credit records. Or you need someone to effectively reverse the damage that the collection arm of a medical service provider has done to your credit history.
2. You have another financial matter caused by your illness that needs the help of someone who knows the law.

Trusts and Estate Matters

1. Estate- and tax-planning matters need to be explained to you.
2. You need a will, or you have another estate-related matter to resolve.

Custody and Guardianship

1. You need to have a guardianship created.
2. A custody matter must be worked out.

Government Benefits

1. You need help meeting the qualifications of a government program.
2. Your government benefits should be increased or kept from lapsing.

Advance Directive or Durable Power Instruments

1. An appropriate legal instrument needs to be created for you.
2. You need to be represented in a dispute.

Finding Legal Help

Several legal organizations specialize in providing help at little or no cost to the patient. Some of them are listed in the Reference Center "Yellow Pages" under "Legal and Procedural Counsel."

Resolution

The successful conclusion of any of these issues normally comes in the form of an agreement: You do something, the other party does something, and both sides are more-or-less satisfied. Agreement usually comes during negotiations, after tempers have cooled and before the case goes to court.

Perhaps the understanding will have a financial aspect, as when an insurance company agrees to pay for some treatment that you need or when a hospital amends a bill. But a win is not like hitting the jackpot. These case resolutions do not aim to provide the patient with large cash payments for things like punitive damages.

Some Perspective

Cancer creates life-and-death issues and big-time money disputes. Trouble gets attracted the way a picnic draws ants. Anger and misunderstanding are common parts of the mix. People start looking for lawyer gunslingers.

Legal matters require exponentially greater amounts of time than you can imagine. Some settlements take so long that they matter only to descendents. Be sure the stand you take and the decisions you make lead toward resolution, not away from it.

- Try never to say never. Leave room for reconsideration and reconciliation.
- Be aware that some fights, once started, have to be finished, despite escalating time, labor, cost, or other unintended consequences.
- Don't start a fight with someone who buys printing ink by the barrel.
- Understand that an attorney, who is providing subsidized services, may quit the fight short of the place you had in mind. He or she is serving interests in addition to yours.
- If you want to start a fight that is bigger than the one your subsidized attorney has in mind, be prepared to fund it.

National Program Advocacy

Some advocate groups in Washington, D.C., work with legislatures and federal agencies to improve understanding of cancer-care issues. Sometime after you have gotten control of your own health situation, you may wish to know more about who is doing what, for whom, and why. The major players representing your point of view and needs are listed in the Reference Center. Almost all of them gratefully accept help and donations.

16 Private-Attorney Services

Maybe you want to sue somebody because you're sick. Maybe you think of your illness as a golden opportunity. Maybe you're right. Maybe.

Did Someone Give Me Cancer?

It is generally agreed that cancer is not contagious. But there are known carcinogens, substances that can cause a person to get cancer. Anyone or any organization responsible for allowing someone else to be exposed to a carcinogen is answerable for it.

Should I Consider Legal Action?

You should discuss any question of exposure to carcinogens with at least two independent law firms. The consultations should be free. Make certain of it before visiting them.

Some law firms that specialize in cases like yours hold regular seminars open to the general public. You can enjoy the anonymity of being part of a small crowd. Listen to the experiences and questions of others in the room. Ask questions if you like, or open a personal conversation with a law-firm representative if you are comfortable doing it.

Isn't Suing Free?

You do not pay anything up front to sue, to finance the work necessary to arrive at a settlement, or to take a case through trial. A law firm will receive 33 percent or more of the eventual judgment as its fee.

You pay emotionally. You pay through time you might have preferred to spend in other ways. You pay significant out-of-pocket expenses. But you don't notice these because your lawyer incurs them and then takes the money out of your settlement check. You can also be countersued, which may or may not become a significant financial burden.

What Amount of Money Might I Get?

Successful class-action and individual lawsuits that relate to cancer have tended in the last few years to bring between $150,000 and $300,000 per plaintiff (that's you). All expenses come off the top of this settlement amount, as was just discussed. Also knock off 33 percent for your lawyer—to as high as 40 percent if the matter goes to trial. If you're fortunate, you get the balance. There is no income-tax liability on a court judgment. The math might look something like the numbers in the box "How Is Settlement Money Divided?"

What Are the Chances of Compensatory and Punitive Damages?

The financial settlement that follows a civil trial is calculated by totaling compensatory and punitive damages. Compensatory money is paid for your actual costs. Sometimes extra is paid to a plaintiff for "pain and suffering." The punitive part of an award is punishment, similar to a fine, that the defendant pays for wrongdoing. (Sometimes extra money is paid without admission of guilt. Draw your own conclusions.)

If this result produces a jumbo award, say something in seven or eight figures, the court may reduce the amount of the punitive part of the settlement if the judge thinks it is excessive. The defending company may negotiate a

How Settlement Money Is Divided

The total award to you	$200,000
Less all the costs	35,000[1]
	165,000
Less the attorney's fee	
(40 percent of the full award)	80,000[2]
You get	$85,000

Notes: Please do not take the numbers used in the example as other than hypothetical. Only you and your attorney can estimate the length of time a legal action may require, its fees, or the costs relevant to your situation.

[1] Costs could include travel and lodging for you, your family, attorneys or investigators; law-firm expenses, depositions, fees for expert witnesses, court fees, trial exhibits, fees to other attorneys, consultants; some of your doctor bills, medications, tests; other of your living costs—and much more, over a period of months to years.

[2] In this example, we have presumed that the adjudication lasted through preliminary hearings and a short trial, so the attorney's fee went up from the 33 percent for an out-of-court settlement to 40 percent.

dollar reduction with you too. Either way, you could end up with only a fraction of what the jury awarded you.

If the plaintiff dies before the matter is settled, any amount for pain and suffering is tossed out. An estate can receive the remaining settlement.

How Do I Find a Lawyer (or Change Lawyers)?

A personal referral is probably the most comfortable way to begin the search for legal representation. If you don't know anyone to ask, phone one of the bar associations listed under "Attorneys Guide" in the Yellow Pages, or go to the American Trial Lawyers Association Web site on the Internet. Bar associations follow strict ethical guidelines. The person who helps you will provide a short list of the most appropriate attorneys. You are expected to interview one or more of them and make a choice. Attorneys are comfortable with this selection process. Your initial calls on law firms should be interesting and pleasant. (If you are immobile for some reason, they'll come to you.)

An agreement you sign with a law firm can be changed if it must be. If you are forced to find another attorney in the midst of a lawsuit, you should not have great difficulty. Pick a new lawyer. Ask your replacement to dismiss the other firm. Expect a smooth transition.

What If More Than One Law Firm Gets Involved?

The settlement of a civil action produces only one attorney's fee. If more than one law firm has helped, you can be certain that the division of the fee has been privately discussed and agreed to among the attorneys. You should not be required to make any additional payment because you used multiple law

16.1 A newspaper ad typical of those run by attorneys who specialize in litigation on behalf of cancer patients

firms, nor should you have to pay for private investigators, testing labs, trial consultants, medical experts, or any other help with your legal action. Your law firm pays these costs. Later it takes the money out of your settlement check.

Are Doctors Liable for Mistakes They Make While Treating Cancer?

A physician is liable for any sort of error on the job. Understand a subtlety here: A mistake is not the same as misconduct. An honest mistake is apt to fall outside the range of things one can collect for in the way of high damages. Misconduct is worthy of financial recompense—maybe criminal action too. Mistakes by all members of the medical establishment take place—administrators, doctors, nurses, therapists, and lab techs. Some of these errors and omissions produce unfortunate consequences for patients. The really bone-headed stunts—like cutting off the wrong leg—certainly have severe economic consequences. But most mistakes and "acts of God" won't get you much more than an apology.

The oncology community adheres to high standards, even for the medical profession, which is itself strict. Impropriety is rare. Without evidence of deliberate malfeasance or gross incompetence, the chance of a successful lawsuit against some part of the oncology community is low.

What about Substances That Cause Cancer?

Many chemical compounds in the United States today can cause cancer. They can be found in our food, in the air we breathe, in water, and in our surroundings. Some are natural. Some have been put there. The details beyond those broad generalities are often hotly contested. For example, cigarettes are known to deliver carcinogens to all parts of the body, from the smoker's lips to anus. But is the more dilute gas exhaled by smokers and released by burning tobacco—so-called second-hand smoke—also a cause of cancer? Some say yes. Some say no. Conclusive scientific studies can be found to "prove" whatever position appeals to you. For this and the host of other questions about carcinogens that you may need answered, call a lawyer.

Is It Hard to Sue Large Organizations?

Any of the nation's few thousand largest business entities will be tough to sue. That includes utilities and nonprofits, as well as those in the for-profit world. It also applies to very wealthy individuals. Unless you can join a class-action lawsuit or the organization has shown a willingness to discuss your issue and has sympathy for your position, you will need big guns and plenty of patience to get your adversary out into the open.

The same is true of federal and state government units. The bureaucrats will lock you out or bury you in paperwork unless your legal representative has political clout or another way past the gatekeepers, or you can find a class-action bandwagon to jump on.

Cities and municipal districts such as water districts are sometimes easier to collect from. Just the hint of a lawsuit may send someone to see you with an open checkbook in hand. Obviously, this is not an invitation to go find a pigeon. First, you will need an attorney who has the confidence in your case to prosecute it on your behalf. Second, please carefully weigh the merits of spending time in litigation versus other things you might be doing at this point in your precious life.

Could I Qualify for Existing Settlement Funds?

Class-action settlements have already been reached for some of the most famous and obvious carcinogens, such as asbestos. An existing settlement fund may be open, just waiting for your attorney to request participation. If your attorney can qualify you—and if you find the financial settlement offer acceptable—you may be able to get a check in short order without negotiation or trial.

Why Bother with an Attorney?

The formal steps of a lawsuit may not seem necessary. A direct negotiation may look faster and more lucrative. Get an attorney anyway. Insist on adjudication. Your settlement should be a better one, including future protections and contingencies you might not have thought of. Your net compensation should also be greater, even after the attorney's cut and expenses.

Is There a Deadline for Court Action?

Attorneys find it comforting to note that, by law, a complaint must go to trial in superior court within five years of the date it is filed. Five years is also the measure of survival time after remission that often defines the word "cured" for a cancer patient. It is ironic that one entity considers this prompt action, while it may be a lifetime for the other.

17 Family Money

Things you need to know about your family's money.

A family is supposed to provide security and succor to its members. In a time of attack by serious illness, tradition says that family members should band together to provide love and care. So far, so good. But from the general principle to the specifics of an actual case, the going rapidly loses certainty. Those facing the situation must deal with the details of how much care—particularly of the financial sort—what kind, and for how long. Neither the law of the land nor religious custom offers detailed guidance except for law relating to the well-being of dependents, plus a bit about spouses. In general, family members who choose not to help have convenient exits.

Money to Those Who Are Not Legal Dependents

Giving financial support to someone who is not a legal dependent or a spouse is optional in the eyes of the law. When money is provided, the law generally classifies it as a gift. The giver gets no tax break. If the amount exceeds state or federal annual estate-distribution limits ($10,000 to $20,000), the recipient may be liable for income taxes. The income may affect certain pensions and the patient's qualification as a needy person for such programs as welfare or Medicaid. Unless collateral is specified in a formal loan agreement, there are few ways, if any, to enforce repayment.

Dependent Care

Though the details of the law vary from state to state, parents must take care of their dependent children. Must. Care is not optional. Financial and other types of assistance are available through an assortment of public and private institutions, many of which are listed in the Reference Center.

An important reminder: Get agreement from the organization that provides financial support before committing to the treatment. The greater the cost, the more important this little tip becomes.

What if you give up custody of the child? The strategy of giving up the custody of children so that a public or private institution becomes responsible for providing the necessary care should be the absolutely last resort. The consequences to both parent and child are severe. Irreparable harm to the love and trust in the relationship may be done. Moreover, when the parent has tangible assets, the state will garnishee what it can of the parent's resources on the child's behalf now or in the future. Later, when the parent wants the child back, there may be formidable opposition.

What if the needy child is in the custody of a former spouse? If you have money and your estranged family needs it to pay for medical bills, a court is probably going to demand that you write the check.

What if your sick child has millions and you're broke? There are many circumstances in which the kid's money isn't in play. In all cases, you remain financially responsible for the medical bills of your minor child.

What if you're sick and broke, but your underage child has millions? You are financially liable for your medical bills. Your child cannot be forced to pay a penny. So, for example, if the child has a trust fund, it cannot be tapped for your medical needs. Adult children have no legal responsibility to help with their parents' financial needs either.

The Needs of a Spouse

The legal and moral expectations of marriage in our society are that spouses share and share alike, for better or worse. Of course, there may be mitigating circumstances. Where there is a disagreement, an amount equal to the value of the couple's community property can probably be spent by either one, plus whatever liquid assets and credit the spender has control of. Under most circumstances, neither husband nor wife would spend such an amount unilaterally. Should treatment options become points of contention, there are advisors who have experience mediating solutions (see the legal assistance and disease-specific listings of the Reference Center). Help may also be available through your place of worship.

Common-Law Marriage

There is a saying among attorneys that hard cases make bad law. What they mean is that complex and ambiguous situations, endlessly argued, lead to messy, unhappy verdicts. Bluntly put, common-law marriage is a poor basis upon which to demand financial support. If the stakes are modest, the couple may be able to sort things out. If the cancer-treatment bills grow large and if there are assets on one side of the union that have become important—wealth that is not jointly controlled—the game and the viewpoints of its players may change. The amount of honey in the hive determines the number of bears that come callin' and the size of the swarm they stir up.

Common-law unions of same-sex partners usually face even more complex and uncertain issues than the common-law pairing of one man and one woman. If the legal basis of your union and the stewardship of its resources are issues of more than passing interest to you, and if you and your common-law partner are willing to take the matter to an attorney who practices family law, that's the suggested path to take.

Family Squabbles over Money

Disagreements and hurt feelings over money are common family problems. Mediation is a desirable strategy. Litigation is a poor thing to threaten and a worse thing to permit. In litigation, lawyers may be the only winners.

18 Charities

Giving and receiving through public charity is a highly refined U.S. art form.

Asking for Help

Most forms of cancer have dedicated nonprofits that support the specific type of disease: breast, brain, lung, leukemia, melanoma, and so forth. In addition, every treatment center has pockets of cash for its needy patients. Dwarfing both are broad-based regional and national cancer charities. The Jimmy Fund is a regional cancer charity of note. The national American Cancer Society is reputed to have the largest annual budget of any charity in the world. Each nonprofit—or charity, if you prefer—has a specific mission and benefits shaped exactly to suit those it serves.

Everyone with cancer is invited to seek support. The financial aspects of treatment become stunningly complicated. Take it on faith that as wealthy as you may be, and despite the superb quality of your medical insurance or HMO, there's at least one charity that will probably be an asset to you at some time during your bout with this thing. Look for more than money. The technical help and maybe the connections you receive can serve you in ways you never imagined. Go through the list of possibilities in the Reference Center. Call the ones you think might assist, even if calling makes you feel a bit awkward. There's no specific instruction for how to get help. Each group has a form or a Web site or a worker to help you. Make contact, get instructions, and do.

Let me count the ways . . .

You have no idea how many sorts of resources out there in the ether await your inspection. If you find the Reference Center or the aboutmycancer .com Web site impressive, you ain't seen nothin' yet. Go to the Internet Guide for Nonprofit Public Service Organizations.

U.S. Grassroots Giving

Americans are by far the most charitable people on the face of the earth. Contributions from all U.S. sources totaled $241 billion in 2002, a disappointing year because of 9/11 and a sluggish economy, according to "Giving USA," an annual report published by the American Association of Fundraising Counsel's Trust for Philanthropy. Individuals donated three-quarters of the total, $183.7 billion. The remainder came from corporations and foundations.

Organized charity has been traditional in the United States since we kicked out King George III. In 1840, Alexis de Tocqueville waxed eloquent on the subject and the "secondary associations" that bind citizens together outside government administration. He theorized that private charity is necessary to keep us from relying too heavily on our government, thus avoiding a descent into dictatorship or a return to sovereignty.

Qualifying for Help

For you to receive anything more than advice, your health condition must be verifiable through a treatment center that the charity recognizes. Make no presumption that diagnosis or treatment to this point will be respected. Different charities accept different centers and the opinions of different medical specialties. Your specific need must also be *within the scope* of the group you ask for help.

"Acceptable" as It Applies to a Charity

Charities are made up of people who have decided to use collected resources to achieve some objective. The charity's mission is probably fairly specific, such as fighting a type of the disease or helping with some particular treatment. It may support a hospital or a group of them. The focus may be on a certain kind of patient: children, hemophiliacs, amputees, the sightless. There are also community groups of service providers, such as Angel Flight, 4,500 owners of private aircraft who provide free transportation to treatment sites for cancer patients and their families.

To be successful in applying for help, you must ask for something that the charity is prepared to give. Equally, don't ask for anything besides what the organization offers, even if invited to do so. You'll confuse and delay things.

Two Fundamentals of Charity's Role

The first thing to be said about these nonprofits is that honesty, dedication, frugality, and the gratitude of cancer patients drive them. In a multibillion-dollar environment where the moving and shaking is always big time, sincerity displaces politics more often than a cynic might suppose.

The second fundamental is that charities are often one-trick ponies. Each has a specialty it is known for. It is a mistake to expect any one charity to offer something for everyone. That's what the big treatment centers and government agencies try to do—with mixed results.

Overall

There are hundreds of charitable nonprofits that have to do with improving some aspect of cancer:

Seek a cure
Educate or train
Maintain a professional society
Maintain a treatment facility
Provide a certain pharmaceutical
Help rehabilitate
Eradicate some harmful practice (like smoking) or carcinogen (like asbestos)
Help children who are patients
Help children in the families of patients
Help homosexual cancer patients
Help patients of a specific creed, color, ethnicity, or sex
Settle disputes

Develop better prosthetics

Lower a treatment cost

Match donors and recipients

Keep track of clinical trials

Pay for travel and housing away from home during treatment

Help with home care (food, volunteers, nurses, doctors, supplies)

Help those in the last six months of life

Increase public awareness and activism

Provide an Internet chat forum or data exchange

Fund research

Lobby Congress and state legislators

Take care of orphaned pets

For proof, turn to the Reference Center, which lists some of the more prominent national organizations of each type with the exception of orphaned pets (call the Society for the Prevention of Cruelty to Animals, SPCA). The massive array of charitable support is impressive and heartening, to most cancer patients.

A Three-Drawer Credenza

The cancer industry is a three-drawer affair. The top drawer is the most evident, with hospitals, medical teams, insurance, pharmaceuticals—all the stereotypical parts that people imagine. Like a piano with six million keys, it is impressive to contemplate and impossible to embrace. (You will eventually figure out which one or two octaves are best for you and ignore the rest.)

The second drawer has all the federal government arms and legs in it. Your tax dollars are working at a high and efficient rate here. Welfare and insurance programs suck up most of the juice. Regulatory, research, and information functions are not far behind. The Federal Drug Administration is the most vilified. The National Institutes of Health's National Cancer Institute is the most impressive and heartening.

The third drawer holds all the nonprofit organizations. Many have charitable intents. This drawer contains the breeding places for some of cancer-fighting's best new ideas, as well as the ancestral grounds where old elephants go to die. There is some government money in play. Most of the support for these organizations comes from their advocates. Ideas and organizations rise and fall as tides of enthusiasm take them. Organizations achieve national status primarily on the basis of merit. The Reference Center lists only national organizations with time in grade. (Other organizations of at least equal worth may have been omitted in error.)

This Is Not the Freaking Government

Many of us enjoy comprehensive help when we qualify for a federal program. By contrast, charitable activities, while compassionate, have austere limits. Most nonprofits are careful to tell you at the outset exactly what you'll get. If not, ask—and don't complain because it came plain instead of fancy. One of Winston Churchill's favorite stories strives to make this point: A boy falls from a boat but is saved by one of the sailors. The next day, a woman shows up. "Are you the fellow who rescued my son?" she asked. "Aye, that I am," replied the sailor. "Well, then, where's his hat?"

Charities Locate on Two-Way Streets

Almost certainly, one or more of the charities in the Reference Center will be of help to you. Later, when the crisis of disease has subsided and you are in a position to look back benevolently, please return what you can. Money is the mother's milk of any charity. Your volunteer labor and your public endorsement of the cause are also essential.

19 Support Groups

Some new friends want to meet you.

One of the terrible things about finding out that you or a loved one has cancer is the sense that there is no place to get a grip on the situation. There is no handle you can grab either to make a difference or even to hang on. A support group may provide the Velcro you need. There are support groups to help both patients and those active in the care of patients.

A support group is a place you can dump when a good dump is needed. It's your personal focus group where there is no such thing as a bad idea. It's a place where friends know exactly what you went through when nobody else in the world understands. It's a place to test a strategy. It's a place you may learn the answer to your problem. A place where you can say "cancer" right out loud, and nobody freaks out.

Catharsis

Psychiatrists and psychologists who have studied the issues generally agree that cancer patients who participate in face-to-face support groups (1) lead happier lives, (2) experience less stress and depression, (3) make better treatment decisions, and (4) suffer less physical discomfort. Support-group participants "learn how to live comfortably with unresolved problems," summarizes Karl Fleming, *Newsweek* magazine and CBS journalist. The remainder of the medical community and the vast majority of participating cancer patients agree.

How to Find a Support Group

The easy way to begin the search for a support group is to ask your medical team for direction. If that fails to do the trick, go to the Reference Center

"Yellow Pages" for leads under "Support Groups." Other patients in your cancer-treatment center may have suggestions. So may advisors you speak to at toll-free phone numbers in the "Yellow Pages" under your form of cancer. So may a leader at your place of worship.

Similarities That Matter

Look for a support group that has your kind of folks in it.

Don't take this as an absolute, but it is often helpful when others in the group are at about your stage of life with the same sorts of values and life experiences.

Similarities of disease help. Find a group that includes others with the same type of cancer you have.

Limiting a group to patients or to those close to the patient, has become policy for the Wellness Community and others that successfully sponsor support groups.

Some sponsors consider professional moderators important. Others limit seats to participants.

Some meetings have ground rules. Others are freewheeling. The choice of style doesn't seem to have much bearing on the success of the group.

The Three-Meeting Test

You'll probably know right away that a new support group is going to be valuable. But experiences vary. If the first visit leaves you unsure, try at least two more meetings before deciding not to continue. Keep the possibility in mind that you may have entered this trial with unrealistic expectations. Give yourself a chance before you abandon that support group.

Also keep in mind the possibility that you brought anger or fear into that first meeting. It will take a couple more meetings to mellow out. This will be particularly true if you didn't get along with someone in the meeting. Go back. Walk an extra mile with that person. Relationships strain easily in cramped quarters such as lifeboats. These sorts of friction are normal early parts of bonding.

Changing Support Groups

If you decide that you must change support groups, there is some risk that another one managed by the same organization will be no more fulfilling than the one you're leaving. Support groups generally take on the characteristics of their sponsors. If the patron of your first support group was, say, your hospital, there is a chance that none of the other support groups that the hospital offers will work out for you either. Instead, look for another sponsor's program. Try a Wellness Community offering. Churches and hosts of other organizations put energy and imagination into support groups. One of them may be right for you.

Virtual Support Groups

There are radio shows that feature talk between cancer patients. There are Internet chat rooms, too. These alternatives lose the dimension of face-to-face sharing and confidentiality. Some topics and questions are embarrassing in these more public venues. But they work for some people (see the Reference Center for alternative venues).

One-on-One Phone Counseling

The Reference Center lists telephone counselors in abundance. The people who answer your call are often survivors of the same sort of cancer with experiences and resources to share. This alternative moves a bit farther away from the core power of a support group. But telephone time is decidedly better than nothing. If you have no one else to talk to, get one or more of these guys and gals to help you over the rough spots for the moment. But you will also benefit from a real support group. Maybe your phone buddies can help you find a group nearby.

The Concerns of a Public Person

You may feel shy or constrained about going to a support group because you are well known in the community. The problem may prove far less than you imagine.

I stopped sitting at home saying "Why me?" or being depressed thinking I was the only one. I began to crawl to The Wellness Community like someone in search of an oasis in the desert. My car couldn't get me there fast enough. I couldn't walk fast enough from the parking lot. I couldn't get inside fast enough to be nourished by other cancer patients, and to know that I was not alone. I could hire people to be around me, I could pay groups of people to go through this with me, but I could never get what I got there, not ever.

Gilda Radner, It's Always Something *(Harper, 2000)*

Support-Group Dynamics

The characteristics of these support groups are generally the same, be it a Wellness Community–managed affair or one run by your hospital, your church, or your oncology team.

Optional Introduction

There may be an orientation meeting to set the tone for your experience. The idea is to relieve any anxiety you may feel and to explain a simple set of rules. Go. Sit. Smile. Meet the other participants. Don't feel awkward. You'll do fine.

Small

Ten to fifteen participants is common. Some of the groups are smaller or a little larger. The idea is to include sufficient people to have a good experience base for sharing, but few enough so that everyone has the chance to speak.

Intimate

An effective support group gets into the nitty-gritty right away and stays there. So same-sex groups are appropriate for patients with intimate (breast, prostate) problems. But a support group of people with less private disease implications (lung, head, stomach, blood) is apt to be mixed. That's a good thing. The sharing of men and women together is often more insightful than the thoughts of either sex alone.

Comfortable

The setting will be comfortable and private. Angst and hostility stay outside the door (though the room will probably be decently insulated). People make friends with one another. The confidential parts of what is discussed in the meeting stay in the meeting. Laughter is frequent.

Regular Schedule

The group will meet on a regular schedule. One meeting a week is quite typical. People tend to join, stay for a while, and then drift on after their needs have been met. Attendance, if taken, is for purely administrative purposes. Punctuality is a virtue.

Cost

In many cases, there are no costs for participating. Other meetings pass a hat to pay for coffee, cookies, office supplies, and room rental. This tradition of little to no cost has made it hard for family counselors and others to form and manage groups that they charge to lead.

There is no glaring reason that a for-profit support group would be any less successful than the other sort. Some group organizers argue that fees exclude those of very limited means. But the health insurance of many patients includes provision for paid counseling. There can also be special financial arrangements, such as paid scholarships. Pay or don't pay, as you choose.

Rules

Talk is what it's all about. Both the moderated support groups and those run by the participants have a few general rules to control and channel this verbal energy. Order needs to be maintained and fights avoided. People who need to

After joining a support group . . .	%
Feel less alone	88
Happier	87
Improved quality of life	83
Gained hope	82
More will to live	75
Improved family ties	72

Wellness Community survey

share must be encouraged. Limiting each person's comments makes it possible for more people to talk. Being quiet until one knows the rules is a wise and appreciated thing to do.

Further Activities

Many support groups solicit guest speakers. Other activities may include making book reports, joining in community activities, and helping in an oncology center. These gentle, love-based kinds of things add to the value of belonging to a support group.

Aid and Comfort

A support group is a place to go for shelter and comfort should things go badly. Its members may also help you with your family and friends.

Support groups give their members special tools for good times, too. The anniversaries of recovery milestones, for example, are often celebrated with a chorus of "Happy Birthday to You." In Milan, Italy, there is a retirement home for opera singers. As you sing, imagine a room full of crusty, showboat octogenarians. Belt it out as they would.

20 Fraternal Orders and Community-Service Groups

Some stand ready to help. Others are so focused on doing what they do that you can't get anyone's attention.

Ask for Help

Keep a lookout for fraternal-order and community-service projects that might benefit you in your fight against cancer. If you come across a program, telephone the people behind it and ask for the help you need. This direct, informal, immediate, verbal approach is a great tactic. Your directness and informality lower resistance. Yes or "I can try" is a much easier reply than no.

Good Luck

The problem with this suggestion is that it will probably prove wholly impractical and just a tad frustrating, first, because contacting these groups is not always as easy as one would assume. Second, you may be surprised to find that the group you appeal to is not prepared to respond. Service groups tend to create their own little worlds, which you may disrupt with your appeal. Nevertheless, expect a polite reception and a respectful hearing.

Your local Chamber of Commerce and church leaders will know how to contact some or most of the active service groups near you. Your community librarian may be able to expand the prospect list, probably with out-of-date contact names and phone numbers. You can drive to the city limits where there is usually a sign advertising the presence of local service groups, with locations and the times they get together. (The phone book may not help as much.)

Let's say you go through this location exercise. The possibility that you will come across a service group that is prepared to help you at this very moment is—remote, to be, uh, charitable. Perhaps the best result you could realistically hope for is to come across a community leader at one of these clubs who has cancer experience and can give you some pointers.

Tea and Sympathy

None of your local fraternal, community, and religiously based groups has a mission focused directly on cancer. "Well, I am certain a local Lions Club would be very considerate and compassionate," says a program-development spokesperson at Lions International headquarters. "It's up to the individual club to determine if it can help . . . " Her voice fades, and her desire to sound helpful without encouraging you to take your needs to a Lions Club is palpable. Each club has a giving program that features contributions to sight and hearing programs. In other words, the plate's full. Ditto Rotary, Elks, and the rest. They have all adopted other health causes.

General Technique to Improve Success

Tell people what you want the money for. Ask for an exact amount.

Let us say, for example, that you want help with travel to take part in a clinical trial. Itemize and price the airline ticket, hotel room for you and your companion, meals, ground transportation, and other costs. Add 15 percent contingency. Put the detailed budget on a piece of paper with your name, address, and phone number. Include a very brief statement of why you need the help— fifteen to twenty words. Your request will take on greater substance, making it more likely that you'll get help.

Neighbor-to-Neighbor Assistance

Having thoroughly discouraged you from seeking help through a local fraternal or service group, let's allow in a little sunlight. Local groups learn about the critical health needs of their friends and neighbors, and they help, all the time. "Lions make contributions to local foundations, and they support hospitals," explains the spokesperson. It isn't that people don't care. They do. Deeply. Other community groups may also be helpful, including businesses and schools.

A Perspective to Bring to the Hunt

In thinking about local contacts that you might make, knowing some of the basic characteristics of these groups will help you.

They tend to create, manage, and repeat programs. "Repeat" is the key. Expect a community service group that has supported cancer patients in the past to be more receptive to helping you than one that hasn't. There are no guarantees. This is just a good starting place.

If you or a close member of your family has an affiliation with your potential benefactor, your needs will probably receive first and more favorable consideration. (This is never an official policy. The Lions, among others, hotly deny it altogether.)

If you have been active in civic affairs leadership, you will be more likely to be served. Children get extra consideration too. (Again, these are not anyone's official policies.)

Before you open a discussion with the group, learn as much about any cancer case that it has supported previously as you can. The more closely your circumstance is like that in the previous case, the more likely you will receive help.

Be alert: Sometimes "help" is a multistep process. You may be told, "We don't have any money, but . . . " Pay close attention to what follows.

Know what your needs are and ask for specific help. It is always best to show a hard target. But stay loose. The group you have contacted may have far more experience at providing support than you have at receiving it. State your case and then listen, carefully and creatively.

Help from Local Corporations and Schools

There are large retailers and other businesses that want to give back to the communities they serve. Supermarkets, department stores, shopping malls, major employers, and fast-food chains can be very generous. Sometimes local news media help. Schools may hold fund-raisers. Then, as any of these groups provide you with help, others may bring further assistance out of the wings.

There is some chance that none of these organizations and institutions will benefit you directly. You certainly shouldn't count on them. Large corporations, in particular, do not feel comfortable providing people with direct help. They usually create charitable foundations to manage their giving programs. Ronald McDonald Houses and the Burger King Cancer Caring Center are nationally known examples. The many others may include a nearby help organization managed and financed entirely by your friends and neighbors. Local hospitals often create and support these enterprises, too.

The Eleemosynary Institution

Crossword-puzzle fans need never go clueless again for a twelve-letter word meaning "charitable." Knowledge of "eleemosynary" is also helpful when attempting to decipher annual report and Web-site jargon. Use of the word is a signpost pointing toward the programs and services that might serve you.

20.1 Hobo sign, chalked on a gate or tree during the Depression to signal other homeless that a residence was good for something to eat or a dry place to sleep

The use of the "e" word and of "foundation" also signal larger size and scope, possibly with the direct involvement of senior people in the organization.

Places to Look for Help

Looking for foundation and public service support requires you—if you'll excuse the baseball jargon—to get into the batter's box with a bat and swing at the ball. You cannot steal first base. But if you make the first valiant effort, help is more apt to come from any of those around you, including the pitcher. Here, then, are places to look for hits.

Religious-Based Community Groups

Catholic Charities is a biggie. So are the Mormon service groups. Your local B'Nai Brith is apt to be bountiful in terms of contacts and casseroles. Most large Protestant churches offer help in their communities. Plenty of religious organizations also run hospitals. Some offer low-cost, even free, care. But you should not make affordability the foremost basis of a decision to accept the help of a hospital. You have a disease that will kill you if it can. Unless that's okay with you, get the best possible medical team for your condition, and then address the economics of the situation.

Community-Service Organizations

Masonic organizations claim to spend $1.4 million a day on charitable causes worldwide. Rotary, Lions, Kiwanis, Shriners—each has a U.S. membership numbering in the hundreds of thousands. Each spends tens of millions on charitable causes. Any of them may choose to provide service or monetary support, although—as we know—each has a signature disease or other medical cause that it supports globally.

What we're saying is that (1) they've got the money, but (2) someone has to talk them into diverting some of it away from the place they had planned to spend it, and that (3) these cash diversions take place all the time, but (4) you are by no means assured of success, should you try for the brass ring.

To illustrate the most common way these diversions take place, several U.S. clubs of Rotary International (signature cause: polio vaccination in the third world) provide money and medical professionals to a cervical cancer clinic in Ciudad Juarez, Mexico, because the local club requested it. You could become the next Free Women's Health Clinic of Ciudad Juarez Frontera, but you'll probably need inside help and equivalent special circumstances.

Protective Orders

Group health insurance has many fathers, including Foresters, Order of Eagles, Knights of Pythias, Sons of Italy, Polish National Alliance, and Odd Fellows. Lodges explicitly for Jews, African Americans, and Hispanics, and Ladies of the Maccabees for women, were all dynamic and prosperous between 1900 and 1930. The New Deal, World War II, and political trends of the past sixty years have all contributed to their descent to present levels. But they're still there. You can join some of them, even though you are a cancer patient. Please make certain that you understand exactly what health benefits your membership in a protective order guarantees you.

Political Connections

Call your Congress member or senator—either state or federal. Explain your medical needs. See what sort of creative help surfaces. These folks can get the attention of the people at the Welfare Department, the Department of Social Services, and the VA in ways that you can't. You may receive more help, more quickly, than might otherwise have been the case. These congressional offices can also help you with the Hill-Burton hospitals and other H-B health-care providers in your area. (Don't know about Hill-Burton? Call 800/638-0742.)

Cities and large counties also have programs. A city council or county board of supervisors member may be able to provide you an entrée to a program you have never heard of or you thought was unavailable. One example: Some sister-city programs include health-program exchanges. Your city's hospital may have a special relationship with a major cancer clinic at a sister-city location.

Youth/Community

The YMCA and YWCA have health programs in many communities. Others may also, such as the Boy Scouts, Girl Scouts, and Boys and Girls Clubs. These programs provide counseling, direction to free or low-cost medical services, home care and home-delivered meals, rehabilitation, physical therapy programs, and similar benefits. Direct financial help is not likely, but in the process of applying for these other things, access to local philanthropy may open up.

Limitations

Each group with a giving program has a predetermined benefit list. It may be a cash amount or a free stay somewhere, help with telephone or utilities bills, or a pharmaceutical subsidization program. There may also be a policy that if you receive one thing, you lose eligibility for some other thing. The people who set up these rules don't consider the cruelty of the decisions these policies require. Benefactors are merely being practical and "fair."

In the same spirit, you need to decide which parts of whatever is available you will accept, and on what terms. Just as an aside, when you politely reject a bad offer, the giving organization may give its terms a much more critical reappraisal than a grumbling acceptance would engender. You lose nothing much and maybe force a change that helps the next person in your position.

21 Gifts and Givers

If you are five, there is a Santa Claus. If you are twelve, there isn't. By the time you're forty, you've seen enough acts of selfless kindness to believe all over again.

People threatened by cancer need things. Other people find themselves in a position to be helpful, and they are. There are no exceptions to this. You as a cancer patient will receive gifts during this illness.

This chapter is an attempt to help you understand when and how to deal with being a recipient. Beyond that, there are gifts you would like to receive. It would be good to know how to improve your chances. You will have to take it from there.

Day of the year when the most collect calls are made: Fathers Day

If They Only Knew

What you do about gifts and givers needs careful consideration. It's safe to presume that some of your potential benefactors will respond positively to the news that you need something. Your employer could be one of them. People at your church or club may band together to meet a need they learn of. Other possible givers may not be approachable because of family politics or some past twist on life's road. So the question of how much direction you can give to potential givers is individual and usually demands discretion.

In general, if in doubt, say nothing. There is a fine line between being needy and soliciting. If you're in desperate need, it may not matter. But understand that pressing the point is apt to weaken your friendship and your peer relationship with the person you appeal to.

Gifts from the Heart, a Fickle Place

The first thing to know about unsolicited good works is that you can't count on them. About the best you can do is be sure that your needs are visible and—equally—that you are doing everything possible to solve the problem yourself. A giver can come alongside, lend a shoulder to the problem, and leave without a fuss or further entanglement.

Need + Focused effort = Inviting situation

Gifts from Employers

If you work, you may have benefits that go beyond health insurance. There may be a welfare fund, for example, set aside to help those like yourself with special financial needs.

There may also be assets, products, or services of the organization that management can make available to you. This isn't part of any program, and it may require confidentiality. If management's detractors learned that extra costs were being slipped into overhead, there could be complications. You can still ask—gently—for help. You have a very justifiable need.

Do not be dissuaded because the sort of help you need may not be available to everybody in your organization. Perhaps you're benefiting from a prerogative of your position or your boss's. Perhaps you have been a particularly productive employee, or the company is having a better than average year. If you get right down to it, your employer may bend its customary practices a bit to help you. In any case, don't get too legal. Go for the benefit. Thank the giver, if silence isn't a precondition.

Here are gifts that organizations have given to cancer patients or their spouses, sometimes on condition of confidentiality:

    Paid leave of absence
    Salary bonus, by coincidence equal to a treatment cost
    Low- or no-interest loan
    Company car and driver to get to treatments
    Travel or meals on a company credit card
    Corporate aircraft transportation
    Additional vacation time
    Promotion to qualify for next-tier benefits
    Consultation with corporate health professionals
    Use of company premises for fund-raising activities
    Special exemption for disability retirement
    Return to normal employment status and accrued benefits some time
        after illness forced resignation

These sorts of humane extensions of normal practices are not limited to the private sector. Civil service organizations mix personnel practices with political serendipity quite commonly.

The Greater Corporate Circle

The gods living at the rarified level where organizations and even governments interact may respond to a paean from a peon. It can't hurt to let the upper reaches of your management and your community know about you. Here are benefits that really do come to cancer patients from time to time:

    Admission to clinical programs that have been closed
    Invitation to join a treatment program you had not applied for
    Debts paid
    Treatment costs waived
    Drugs made available
    Insurance-company coverage of the thing you need
    A job suitable for you or your spouse
    Sponsorship of you or your family by a service club

Help that comes to those in need from on high is not the result of an appeal or demand from you. About all you can do is place a brief, clear description of your case in the hands of someone influential. Could be an official. Could be a reporter.

The Drug Companies

The men and women in drug manufacture are well informed and compassionate. Every cancer drug on the market is provided at reduced or no charge to some of the most needy. The customers who buy these drugs for their patients—that is, the hospitals and physician groups—participate in these programs. Millions and millions of dollars' worth of the latest and best is given away to those in need every year.

Some critics disparage this generosity by pointing out that drug makers need good works to keep special-interest groups and legislators happy. It's an industry that deals in billions of dollars and enjoys excellent profit margins. Bottom line: So what? The more important point for you is that the people of the pharmaceutical industry understand your predicament and want to help if they can.

Quiet, Private Gifts in Times of Need

Probably every hospital in the country manages at least a few private financial support programs for needy patients. These are often trust funds in someone's name. Some are charities. Some are less formal and perhaps anonymous. As a rule, your medical team knows about these funds. In a few cases, volunteers like the woman who offered you coffee in the waiting room quietly manage them.

It is appropriate to ask your doc or your medical team's administrative staff for ways to apply for financial support, explaining why you need it. That's about all you can or should do. These funds, and the help of pharmaceutical manufacturers, are in place for needs like yours. Just—please—don't count on too much. Gifts come in all sizes.

The Most Important Gifts

Those who give you love, companionship, time, and energy are your real champions. The blood that's donated in your name and the sweatshirt earned at the fund-raiser are gifts of love, which is beyond price. So is the Internet research someone does for you. So are the phone calls a friend makes on your behalf. So is prayer.

Make Your Drugs Affordable

If the cost of meds is killing you, any of several great programs may come to the rescue. There's even help with excessive co-pays. Check out the Reference Center "Yellow Pages" under "Financial Assistance."

22 Public Assistance

> I want money quickly as I can get it. I have been in bed with the
> same doctor for two weeks, and he doesn't do any good. If things
> don't improve, I will have to get another doctor to help him.
>
> —*From a letter to the Welfare Department*

Please, Please, Please Connect Me to a Real Person

If you have recently tried to get service by phone from a public-assistance
agency, you have probably experienced frustration if not failure. People don't
answer the phone; computers do. Then you get to press more buttons that
take you to more prerecorded messages. If you persist, you end up on
hold listening to accordion music periodically interrupted by suggestions
that you hang up and go to some Internet Web site for further predigested
frustration.

Sometimes you can get to a real person by punching random buttons at
the "if you know the extension of the person you are trying to reach, you may
dial it now" cue. But if someone answers, you have to be instantly persuasive.
Public servants who are trapped into serving the public in this way tend to
be grouchy.

A Better Place to Start: The American Cancer Society

The ACS has people standing by to help you, 24-7. Call 800/227-2345, or go
to www.cancer.org. Tell the counselor what your circumstances are. Answer
some basic qualifying questions. Expect to learn what you need to know.

To receive help with your illness from a government office, it is best to
need kidney dialysis, have one of certain specified cancers in an advanced
stage, have a physical handicap, or be otherwise disabled, a veteran, a Social
Security recipient—or flat broke. Your ACS counselor should be able to lead
you through all that. If you qualify for a program, the counselor will let you
know what to do and how to do it.

It is also possible that your counselor knows about one of the growing
number of state-sponsored programs to help the uninsured. Maine, for
example, had a pilot program called Dirigo under development at the time
of this writing. New York, Michigan, Rhode Island, Texas, and California are
formulating programs, as are other states. Terms like "bare bones" describe
these efforts, which wax and wane with political vicissitudes and available
budgets.

Friends and relatives can also work with an ACS counselor to arrange
help for the patient. The ACS follows up with a free, individually assembled
booklet of advice and resources, which can be very valuable.

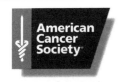

The information you requested is enclosed.

AMERICAN CANCER SOCIETY
1599 CLIFTON ROAD N.E.
ATLANTA, GA   30329

Your name
and address
will appear here

The American Cancer Society is the nationwide
community-based voluntary health organization
dedicated to eliminating cancer as a major health
problem by preventing cancer, saving lives and
diminishing suffering from cancer, through
research, education, advocacy and service.

Information, Inspiration, Ruminations, Recommendations -- find them in
ACS books at www.cancer.org/bookstore or call us at 800 ACS 2345

For additional assistance please contact your American Cancer Society
1•800•ACS•2345 or www.cancer.org

22.1 A free packet of help with government agencies and many other services is available from the American Cancer Society

Centers for Medicare and Medicaid Services

You are most apt to find the dollars that you're looking for through this arm of the Department of Health and Human Services. In the Reference Center, you can find the phone numbers and Web sites of the programs it manages that may specifically serve your needs. What follows are descriptions taken mostly verbatim from the agencies themselves.

Medicare

Medicare is an insurance program. Medical bills are paid from trust funds paid into by those covered. It serves people over sixty-five, whatever their income, and younger disabled people and dialysis patients. Patients pay part of costs through deductibles for hospital and other costs (with notable exceptions that you must watch out for). Small monthly premiums are required for nonhospital coverage. Medicare is a federal program. It is basically the same everywhere in the United States.

Medicaid

Medicaid is an assistance program. Medical bills are paid from federal, state, and local tax funds. It serves low-income people of every age. Patients usually pay no part of costs for covered medical expenses. A small co-payment is sometimes required. Medicaid varies from state to state, as do the names it operates under.

State Children's Health Insurance Program (SCHIP)

Free or low-cost health insurance is available for those under age nineteen. This can be a major find for the parents of a child with cancer. Your ACS counselor has probably told you everything you needed to know about this opportunity. If not, call 877/543-7669. If the number has changed, call the local office of one of your federal elected representatives for help.

Hill-Burton

Hill-Burton is a little-known program that provides free comprehensive medical care for the indigent. Hospitals and clinics all over the country are under contract to receive Hill-Burton patients and care for them. If you want to take a shot at this one, call 800/638-0742.

Social Security

If you can get your interviewer to agree that you are "disabled," you can get on Medicare in two years, no matter how much younger than sixty-five you will then be. This is a big benefit if health-insurance coverage is an issue, though the two-year wait is unconscionable. Your doctor knows how to present your case. So does the American Cancer Society.

Social Security Disability Income

A small amount is taken out of the paychecks of most Americans for Social Security Disability insurance. If you are too sick to work or if you meet other conditions, some of them rather arcane, you may qualify for disability benefits. This is not a big deal. The checks are small and don't begin arriving until the seventh month after you complete qualifications. The most important value, qualifying for Medicare in two years, has already been discussed.

Supplemental Security Income

Those who have not been in the labor force much and are without income can apply to Social Security for SSI. The amount you will get varies from state to state. Nowhere did it exceed $500 a month in 2004.

Veterans Administration Coverage

VA hospital medicine is theoretically available to any veteran with an honorable discharge. Cancer care of all sorts is offered. Your ACS counselor is a good first stop for information. The home office of one of your elected representatives is also likely to help with information. If you qualify for something that is available, your elected representative's staff can help get you into the program. A really poor third alternative is to contact the VA yourself. Like the welfare people, nobody comes to the phone willingly or ready to be of service.

The medical care facilities run by the Department of Veteran Affairs have been underfunded for decades. The result is not pretty. Presuming the veteran could get a bed, those with other options will likely prefer them.

Penal Care

Steve Lopez, a *Los Angeles Times* columnist, suggested that his parents "knock off a few banks" to get better health care. No insinuation, but there may also be parents so sick of the antics of their adult children that they might consider a failed bank heist just to get away from them. Others may look at the concept of penal care and see in it the ultimate retirement community. Given the size and quality of the condos in some retirement homes, the cells in selected penal institutions are competitive, a lot cheaper, and gated, the epitome of every high-toned joint.

All kidding aside, penal care is awful. Don't even think about going there.

Expatriate Health Care

Citizens of many other countries who live in the United States and Americans on fixed incomes who agree to emigrate have the option of

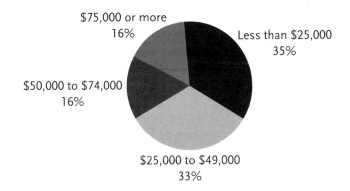

22.2 Household-income levels and percentages of Americans with no health insurance, 2002 (U.S. Census Bureau; NIHCM Foundation)

seeking essentially free health care outside the United States. It is only fair to add that cancer patients who live in these countries and can afford U.S. treatment centers prefer them. The Vancouver-based Fraser Institute ranked Canadian health care, perhaps the most visible expatriate option, on a par with that of Turkey, Hungary, and Poland.

Some Notes on Medicare

Medicare provides more than forty million Americans with a generally good preferred-provider plan, taking care of most treatment expenses through the doctors and hospitals you choose. Some help with drugs is also given, and this will improve significantly over the next few years. There is no cap on medical expenses under Medicare, which is a huge relief for cancer patients.

Medicare has deductibles, which may be covered by a Medigap supplemental health-insurance carrier. Should you as a cancer patient decide to look into a secondary insurer, more and more insurance companies are entering the competition for your dollars with more and more features and attractive payment schedules. Just beware the "preexisting condition" clause in some plans.

There are periodic campaigns, encouraged by Medicare, to move its covered patients into new HMO and private PPO insurance plans. These new options come with additional benefits that may include better pharmaceutical coverage and inducements such as trips and health-club memberships. If one of these options appears attractive, evaluate it carefully, keeping in mind the special requirements of a cancer patient.

Always begin your first meeting with a new care provider by making sure that it accepts your Medicare coverage. Medicare has periodic arguments with health providers over costs of treatment. Laudable as that is—a well-deserved response to the industry's occasional gross billing excesses—the schedules of what Medicare will pay sometimes dip below actual cost, according to health-care managers. As the patient in the middle, you could find that the team you choose will not perform the work you need because of a fight over money.

Some Notes on Medicaid

This is health care for the truly downtrodden. Even the ever-diplomatic American Cancer Society advises: "Not all health care providers accept Medicaid. This may limit your choices and, possibly, your quality of care."

The quality and availability of Medicaid will mirror the attitude of the state government toward the very poor. The luckiest Medicaid recipients live in one of the liberal eastern parts of the country or on the West Coast, during a time when the tax coffers runneth over.

23 Armed Services

The American military family does not leave casualties on the cancer battlefield.

If you are on active duty—U.S. Navy, Marines, Coast Guard, Army, Air Force—or the dependent of someone on active duty, if you are retired or the dependent or surviving spouse of a retired person, you qualify for cancer care by the numbers. The most important of these numbers is one. You're number one, so far as the system is concerned. You're going to receive the most comprehensive and thorough treatment your doctors can devise. No option is withheld. No cost is spared. No kidding.

The Process for Those on Active Duty

After cancer is discovered, the patient is referred to a regional military center with an oncology department. There, you will be seen by physicians who specialize in your type of cancer. Then a second opinion is automatically rendered through a medical team meeting called a tumor board. This is a sophisticated evaluation involving every medical specialty that can contribute to your evaluation and treatment. It's a process that was honed at the nation's finest civilian hospitals and is superior to cancer evaluations at typical clinics. Cost is not a consideration, and every case is family.

You will undergo a process called "staging." This is an assessment of how far your disease has spread within your body and may include further examinations, lab testing, and imaging. A treatment plan is created that may include surgery, radiation, chemotherapy—as necessary, to defeat your disease and to repair the damage it may do to you. Treatment continues through recovery, including prosthetic devices, cosmetic surgery, physical therapy. Should cancer leave you unable to continue on your military career path, you might be medically retired with disability benefits and medical coverage for the rest of your life, or be allowed to continue your military service in a new career field.

Timing

Civilian cancer medicine is often complicated by crowded appointment dockets. Though *nobody* lets a pernicious case of cancer go unattended, military care reduces time pressures at the appointment desk and again in the treatment rooms. "We make a point of keeping time open for extras and the unforeseen," explains Preston S. Gable, MD, Cdr., USN, and head of the Hematology/Oncology Division, Naval Medical Center, San Diego. Difficult diagnoses and medical emergencies still bring many pressures. But they are centered on wellness issues, never on time or cost.

The Limited-Duty Process

The initial diagnosis process leads to an estimation by the oncology staff of what's going to happen. In cases that are expected to result in a return to normal life, active-duty personnel are placed on "limited duty." The rules for sick leave become as liberal as necessary to accommodate treatment and recovery, including travel to multiple places for treatment when called for. The patient may remain in this status for up to two years.

In cases that are less predictable, the patient may be placed on a temporary disability-retirement list. The patient is effectively separated from the service, though scheduled contacts for treatment and evaluation continue. Active-duty pay stops and retirement pay begins, supplemented by disability checks from the Veterans Administration and a Social Security stipend. Though the gross amount may be less, income is no longer subject to taxes, making it possible for the net effect to be about the same as base pay on active duty.

Temporary disability retirement may last up to five years, but no longer. If fully recovered within this time, the patient can choose to return to active duty or continue disability retirement. If cancer persists, the disability retirement becomes permanent.

The Process for Retired and Dependents

After diagnosis, Tricare health insurance provides both guidance and the financial umbrella for treatment. You will be led through an evaluation process, followed by a treatment plan, by a Tricare case nurse. (For more on this, see "The Case Nurse" later in this chapter. It may also be helpful to read about ways that you can most effectively manage your health insurance in Chapter 14.)

You are covered by an exceptionally generous plan that will pay for any sort of treatment you may need without artificially imposed limits or the cap that many plans have. Depending on your particular form of cancer and related circumstances, you may decide to let the insurance system guide you through the experience. You also have treatment options. If you haven't already done so, thumb through "Orientation" and "Team Building," Parts II and III, taking special note of suggestions in Chapter 7, "Deciding Where to Have Treatment." You may also benefit from a discussion with a survivor of your form of cancer. You can locate one by looking in the Reference Center "Yellow Pages" under your cancer's general name.

Tricare (Formerly CHAMPUS)

This cost-sharing medical insurance program is intended to provide all necessary care to dependents and the retired. Its benefits go far beyond anything that the average civilian can afford or that the typical employer would offer. While you may feel the bite of the cost sharing, it maxes out at $3,000 per year or less, depending on your status and ability to pay. Considering that cancer treatment can easily climb above $100,000 per year—individual shots may cost more than a swank dinner in Tokyo—your savings are dramatic.

Tricare patients must resolve treatment-payment issues beforehand. It is unfortunate that Congress tied Tricare spending allowances to those of Medicare. Medicare goes through periods when some of its payment schedules are unacceptable to parts of the civilian medical establishment. The result is that before you go into a new treatment situation, you must identify yourself as a Tricare patient, making certain that the terms of your insurance are acceptable to the care provider. If this causes a problem, there is a resolution process. Talk to your case nurse.

The Case Nurse

Though the treatment processes are different for active-duty people and their dependents, there is a common Help button called a case nurse. When the patient is too sick to focus, when treatment matters become perplexing, when the intricacies of the paperwork have gotten to be too much and you need help with the rules of the road, ask your case nurse.

If the patient is in uniform, the case nurse will be on staff at the primary cancer-treatment facility. Expect to be contacted by this person, probably an experienced RN, shortly after your admission to the hospital. If you are not, ask your doctor for help getting a name and phone number.

If you are receiving help through Tricare, the case nurse will be at the prime contact phone number that appears on your Tricare policy paperwork. Case nurses pride themselves on knowing how to cut through the intricacies of even the most complex situation to get things done for you.

Cancer's Effects on Military Careers

Unlike the private sector, there is no performance prejudice connected with a past cancer in the military. "If a service member has a curable cancer, we make every effort to keep them on active duty," Dr. Gable says. Hearing aids, prosthetic devices? Absolutely. Retraining into a new military career? If that's what the patient wants, certainly. Career opportunities and promotions continue on a par with contemporaries.

"On the other hand," Gable continues, "we don't offer service members with incurable disease the option to continue on active service. They will be referred to the physical evaluation board. They can't opt out of this, although they may appeal the findings."

Qualifying Loved Ones

Sometimes, an elderly relative becomes a dependent and then becomes eligible for cancer care. In other cases, a person of foreign extraction, perhaps with children in tow, marries into the system. Should you need help to make certain that such a person or a child with medical needs will be served, speak candidly with a physician in the medical unit that provides your care.

24 Raising Cash

In the luck of the chase, comes the deer to my singing.

—*Navajo hunting song*

There is only one reason for reading this section. You need money. Added to the pressures of everything else going on in your life right now, finding cash probably seems a maddening exercise. Raising it may turn out to be difficult or impossible. Or it may not. Follow along for a page or two. Perhaps you'll see something that shows you how to move past this problem.

Raising money is hard work and takes time. Some patients have the stamina for it. Many do not. This chapter may be much better suited to the energies and ambition of someone who wants to help, rather than the patient. Even though the message is written with the patient in mind, the assumption is that others will be directly involved in this process. If you are that someone, welcome. Let us, as a Navajo might say, begin to sing for the deer.

Bite-Sizing It

The first thing you must do is break into small, discrete parts both your need and every way it might be paid for. Your goal is to identify and organize each so that it is a simple problem with a straightforward solution. Each needs to be clear and clean, completely thought through. Here is a sample of the type of problem you may encounter and a demonstration of this problem-solving process.

Making a Cost of Illness Manageable

This is how to break down a typical problem and tackle the cost.

Let us say—as an example—that you need $10,000 for travel and one month's living expenses to take advantage of a promising clinical trial in another state. Insurance or the hospital or the corporate sponsor of the clinical trial is paying all the other expenses related to this treatment. You are left to pay a pittance by comparison. But it is still a crippling, seemingly impossible slug of cash to come up with. Here's how you might manage it.

First, carefully and candidly identify every cost, eliminating frills:

Air travel	Two round trips	$ 700
Lodging	Modest motel @ $80/night for two	2,400
Car rental	Subcompact @ weekly rate, and gas	850
Food budget	Two people, one on a special diet	2,400

Miscellaneous	Personal needs, phone calls, tips, etc.	750
Cancer related	Medication	600
At home	Continuing costs: rent, utilities, phone, debt, etc.	2,300

Second, see if you can reduce or eliminate any line item. For "Air travel," for example, look in newspapers and on the Internet for lowest fares and travel specials. (Check buses and trains, though neither may result in any real cost saving.) The Reference Center lists supporters that offer free transportation, along with free housing and free or reduced-cost meals. In addition, treatment centers often have an in-house travel agency and an advisor to help visiting patients cope with these expenses. Ask for the hospital's concierge. See what happens.

Call the corporation behind the clinical trial you have been admitted to. Explain your need. Maybe there's a budget for patient travel expenses or a contingency fund. Call the charities that support your kind of cancer and other foundations discussed in Chapter 18. Some of those folks have travel-expense money for patients.

Ask your boss to cover your airplane tickets as corporate travel. It is easy for some companies to bury such a charge, which is a terrific saving for you. Not employed? Maybe the boss of a relative will consider picking this expense up. Or you could benefit from the corporate discount or frequent-flyer program.

Prepare to Be Effective

People must learn that you need help before they can provide it. You're going to have to tell them. Moreover, you are going to need to present your need in an attractive way. "I think anyone can become an effective communicator," says Roy Chitwood, world-renowned sales trainer and president of Max Sacks International. The main thing is to look at your situation through the eyes of the person before you.

Start by examining yourself. Are you someone this person would like to help? If you are not sure, Chitwood suggests, make certain that you are being sincere and respectful. Beyond that, is your request simple, straightforward, genuine, and realistic?

Chitwood has made it a mission to help people become well received by audiences. Here is his checklist of easy things you can do. These are general guidelines, Chitwood reminds us. You will not find an opportunity to practice them all in every situation. But forgetting to use each precept when you have the opportunity will diminish your effectiveness.

Smile. The preoccupations of cancer and its costs make it easy to start with a frown and a complaint, which will sour your audience. People may even think you are grouching at them.

Treat your audience like invited guests who have just arrived at your front door. Give your visitors the smile they deserve.

Be interested in them. People are more interested in those who are more interested in them, Chitwood advises. The more bread you cast on these waters, the more attention is apt to come back to you. Much more.

Speak in terms of your listeners' interests. When in Rome, do as the Romans do, and all that. Every way you differ from your audience is an additional impediment to agreement.

Use the person's name. People respond to hearing their name spoken.

Be complimentary when you can do so sincerely. Tell people when you see things or hear things about them that you like. If you are a quiet person, or if worry or pain is distracting you, this can be hard to remember to do. A conscious effort may be necessary.

Be a good listener. Listen attentively to people. Respond to the things they say. Ask questions, nod in agreement, laugh. Participate in the subject in other proper, positive ways. Good listeners also naturally remember more, which can be valuable to you.

Make the other person feel important. Pay positive attention to people. Be courteous. Acknowledge achievement. Don't demean or insult. Remember that all those things you learned about socializing when you were in kindergarten are still true.

Good Places to Look for Help

Moving on down the list of costs in the sample, let's take each item in turn.

For car rentals, call the car-rental companies. See if any of them have reduced-cost or free offers for patients with your disease, or for patients of the clinic you will be admitted to. You need to reach someone in or near top management. The counter people and their supervisors in a car-rental company can only rent you vehicles.

To deal with food and lodging costs, try the charity divisions of Denny's, McDonald's, and other national restaurant chains. These foundations, including the Ronald McDonald House and the Burger King Cancer Caring Center, may be good for free or discounted meals and free or low-cost places for a patient and a companion (or even a family) to stay.

A special tip in the search for help with meals and lodging: If the leads in the Reference Center do not produce a solution, go to your phone company's business office or to your local library. Get the phone book for the city you will be visiting. Turn to the business section and the Yellow Pages for leads and keep calling. Ask for help from the city's Salvation Army office, large local churches, the Red Cross, the major hotel chains, the airline you will use, the fraternal organizations (see Chapter 20). Important: If your respondent says no, ask for a referral before you let the person off the line. Say something like, "Well, you know my situation. Who would you call next?" Involve the person. Maybe you'll get a great lead or a cash donation.

The "Miscellaneous" and "Cancer-related" line items are amounts in a range that a local church or school or your employer could cover. Present your plan for treatment, supported by its written budget. This is a more powerful argument in your favor than you may realize. It shows that you have followed a thoughtful process from which a precise amount of money has been calculated. It is a packaged product. The decision maker can see a beginning and an end to the gift.

If your respondent says no, ask for a referral before you let the person off the line. Say something like, "Well, you know my situation. Who would *you* call next?"

If you explain your situation to your phone company and to your utilities (gas, power, and water), they are apt to offer you reduced rates.

If you have satellite or cable TV, cancel it for the duration of your travel. Explain why. Expect cooperation.

If you rent from a large corporation, you may be given some relief. Your city, county, or state may have a rent-relief program.

If you pay a mortgage to a large corporation, explain your situation and invite solutions. Many of these institutions have programs, as well as compassion. (Be careful that the option offered you is compassionate. Some mortgage-deferral programs have expensive and nasty repercussions.)

The Debt Alternative

When a person faces a major expense, covering it can easily lead to debt. In fact, you could probably put a $10,000 treatment expense on a credit card. This is an easy and convenient solution—one that credit-card companies and some health providers will encourage—but it may not be smart. As a rule, use debt as a very last alternative.

Negotiation Pointers

In many, many situations, it is not a good idea to let others know that you are hurting for money. Let's start with banks. As you know, financial institutions make low-cost loan and credit-card offers only to those who don't need the money. The moment you show want, the cost of the loan skyrockets, the interest rate triples, and the time to process the paperwork goes from one week to six. The same is true of everybody else. So long as they think you've got money in your pocket, they want to be buddies. The moment they think you're broke, they're gone.

> Nobody knows how badly you need the money but you . . . unless you tell 'em.

Good selling is largely attitude. If you offer people an attractive product at a fair price on a first-come, first-served basis, you're providing a good opportunity. If you hold a fire sale, a yard sale, an "Oh my God I don't know what I'm gonna do sale," the buyer thinks that paying you a dime on the dollar is doing you a favor. A used-furniture store cannot expect to get anything close to original retail for an item. The same piece in the hands of an interior decorator can bring twice the price. A person worth $6.25 per hour as a gardener can expect $50 an hour as a landscape designer. Bring your attitude and your money-raising strategy to a market where the customers expect to pay fairly for value received.

Inventory of Possibilities

Territorial differences, timing, the economy, and many other factors influence the value of things and the speed with which they sell. Here are brief comments and suggestions concerning some of the most popular items one might peddle or use as loan collateral.

Home Mortgage

You can investigate instruments known as first, second, third, and reverse mortgages. They are complex, so best examined with the help of a person in the business whom you trust. This money costs several thousand dollars to obtain. The total is usually buried in the loan document, but that makes it no less real. Rate changes also matter. Even small ones can add up to a lot before the loan is paid off.

Credit-Card Charges

The interest on credit-card charges has varied from 3 to 28 percent per annum in recent years. Credit cards issued to those with less than spotless credit usually charge a higher interest rate. Try to be sure that your credit-card debt has a fixed, rather than a variable, interest rate. Credit-card companies also offer easy ways to draw out cash and to add debt by transferring balances from other accounts. Few of these offers are bargains, but take a look anyway.

If you must borrow, and you have a credit history with your S&L or bank, investigate a loan through it, instead.

Stocks, Bonds, and Other Brokered Assets

The value one obtains, and the amount lost through commissions and fees, often depend on how much of a hurry you are in. Also consider borrowing against value instead of selling, which may be an option.

Life-Insurance Policy

There are companies that will pay a cancer patient between one-quarter and one-half of the face value of a life-insurance policy in good standing, in cash, immediately. To get the dough, you present medical evidence of your condition and make the company the beneficiary. If your life-insurance company doesn't offer this option, search for "viatical brokers" on the Internet. Don't take the first deal you are offered from any source. Get bids from at least two.

Your Stuff

Options include e-Bay, auction houses, tradio on rural radio stations, and other venues where personal items may be sold. Before choosing one of them, be sure of the commission structure and other fees. Old standbys include newspaper classifieds, company newsletters and bulletin boards, your church, supermarket bulletins, flyers, and yard sales. Be aware of the costs of advertising in newspapers, which may be excessive. Packaging and presentation dramatically affect your items' values.

Large-Item Donations

Cars, boats, and similar larger-ticket items can be donated to charity for major tax deductions. This practice is so profitable for the charities that in some parts of the country, the donor can also get up to half the appraised value of the item back in cash.

Projects Sponsored by Community Organizations

The Lions, Tigers, Elks, Eagles—and all those other fraternal animals—sponsor good works. Any of them may consider a venture that pays for something on your behalf. Others you may not have considered, such as your local supermarket or fast-food outlet, may be helpful.

Tax, Licenses, and Fees

Yard sales and other venues may require a license or permit. Expect it, if you hold more than one or two events at your home per year. A fee may also have to be paid to somebody for cleanup, security, or liability insurance, or for some other, often gratuitous, reason. There are things called long-term and short-term capital gains that your tax person should explain before you incur liability for either. Certain state and local sales taxes may also have to be paid on transactions. There are also penalties you can be tagged with later for ignoring taxability and related matters.

V The Illness

Help a Patient Can Use, and Things a Patient Should Know, to Make the Best of This

25 The Personal Side of Being Very Sick

This time in your life—and this illness—are new experiences.

You knew immediately that cancer was going to be a new experience. Its ultimate threat alone makes it different, of course. The kind of disease it is and the way it came out of nowhere are new and shocking. The unknowns about it are disturbing. The massive movements of people and resources that followed your diagnosis, the sophistication of all the apparatus, the money (Oh, my Lord, the money!)—all make it clear that this time and this illness are different.

You've been sick before. You've been in pain before. Always before, you and the doctor shared the confidence that you would recover. That is not the case today. People die of what you have. You can go to the Web site of the American Cancer Society or the National Cancer Institute, look up your brand of cancer, and learn what percentage of people who had your cancer died of it last year. There are no guarantees, but your chances for survival should be better than those statistics—because you are holding more information on survival in your hands right now than was available to those patients.

A Tougher Fight

We have all learned to disregard the parts of being sick that are inconvenient. You forget to take the medicine. You postpone the doctor visit if you need to. Sure, you want to get well, but neither you nor the doctor is all that concerned about any of it.

That was then. Cancer changed it. You now take care of your health. You take your medicines, and you meet with your healing team wherever and whenever your battle plan calls for it. You don't mess with this thing. It kills people. You give it no extra chances.

You Are Not a Victim

You have seen the term "cancer victim" in the press and in literature. It is pejorative. Use every means at your disposal to keep it from being applied to you. Victims are people who have lost control. Victims generate sympathy at the expense of respect. Victims lose their equality. When one person calls another a victim, the "victim" loses stature. Victims wait while others decide things for them. Victims get castoffs. Victims are poor, as in "poor Alice."

You are a cancer *patient*. A patient is a peer who is owed the best possible treatment. Being a cancer patient stands a $170 billion industry at attention to see what it can do for you. Being a victim sends you to a waiting area at

> Patients get better medical care than victims do.

County General. Don't allow anyone to steal your first-class ticket by calling you a victim.

Your Cancer-Treatment Options

A cancerous condition almost always has options. When considering them, be aware that there are truths, and that there are consequences in most cancer therapies. By selecting the treatment with the highest success rate, the patient may also have to endure the greatest loss. Disfigurement, even in this era of advanced prosthetics and plastic surgery, can be a deeply disturbing choice. Loss of body function—organ failure, sexual dysfunction, incontinence, or the loss of mobility, dexterity, speech, hearing, sight—is a terrible price to pay for recovery.

And so patients look at alternatives to such losses. Usually, the odds for recovery via these alternatives are lower. Sometimes, the odds for recovery are nil. But maybe the quality of the remaining life is greater. You literally pay your money and make your choices.

Frustration

People get sick of being sick—impatient because of not being able to do the things they used to do. Eager to get back to the old life. Pressured to earn money. Depression sometimes comes along to make matters worse. Then some clown begins forcing you to do things in therapy that are boring, that hurt, and that cost too much. Don't lose your positive outlook or your patience. There's precious little glamour to the recovery process. Fight on anyway.

It will help to set some personal goals and to reward yourself for attaining them. Maybe a ride around the block in the wheelchair appeals to you, or a movie, ice cream, decadent chocolate, a massage, a chance to fly the kite you made, a visit to a grandchild. Make up a list of your own rewards. Whatever you do, don't just stew about tough times. Also, find some humor in the situation somewhere.

Waiting and Delays

People should be on time. You should be. So should your medical team. Let us also acknowledge that in this imperfect world, the complexities of the game will cause delays and rescheduling by all parties from time to time.

You're going to miss appointments or be late. So will your doc. So long as there is mutual trust that every effort is being made to honor promptness, this occasional waiting and accommodation will be acceptable.

Work hard to be prompt or early. Your doc will appreciate it and reciprocate. Bring your good humor and this book along for the times when a fly falls into the ointment.

A positive attitude may not solve all your problems, but it will annoy enough people to make it worth the effort.

I have great sympathy for the patients I keep waiting. My administrative team and I are constantly working to avoid appointment delays. But my greatest concern is for the person in front of me during examination and treatment. If others aren't seen at the time of their appointments because I have taken more time than was planned with a prior patient, the only consolation I can offer is that each of them will also receive all of my attention, for as long as necessary, during our time together.

It makes no sense to me to stop in the middle of a procedure just because the time allocated for the person has run out. With apologies, I'm sometimes late. Without apology, I really am doing my best.

(Name withheld by request)

Prima Donnas

Oncology is a branch of medicine that congregates the best of the best and weeds out the rest. Those who are that good have no need to be prima donnas, to be showy, pretentious, phony. You will probably never meet a prima donna during your battle with cancer. If you should, run, don't walk, to any available alternative. A person so enthralled with him- or herself is not paying enough attention to your medical condition. Your recovery is at risk. Get out of Dodge.

Not the Time to Diet

People sometimes decide that, as long as they are sidetracked by cancer, a diet to shed a few pounds would be good. Don't go there. Cancers tend to strip off the weight whether you like it or not. You shouldn't be crazy about weight loss. Recuperative abilities can fade with the pounds, which is dangerous.

Weight gain can also occur. By all means, discuss weight change with your medical team. Controlling measures may exist. Then be prepared to accept the body that circumstances have willed for you.

A New Self

There are some general features of your disease that you should know about. All of these are possibilities, not probabilities. The amounts and intensities of each will differ. Don't expect them all at once.

1. You're going to lose some strength and stamina. You may experience shakiness. Cancer, your treatments, and changes in your lifestyle because you are a patient will all conspire. The information in Chapter 28, "Nutrition and Fitness," may be helpful, but you're not going to be your old self again for a while.

2. Nausea, a feeling like seasickness, and flulike symptoms are common. Both your cancer and its treatments can bring these on. Your oncologist has meds for these. Marinol is sometimes prescribed and is usually effective to combat these illnesses. It performs what is called a palliative role, meaning that it doesn't cure anything. It just takes away the feeling of sickness. Though the active ingredient, THC, is derived from marijuana, you won't get high, and there is no addictive side effect.

3. You are going to think about death, and it's going to scare you. The optimism of your doctor won't matter. If you don't have a spiritual advisor to speak with, your partner or a cancer survivor you relate to may be helpful. For goodness' sake, talk it out with someone.

4. Depression will most likely come along at some point. If there is a funny movie you love to watch, a dog to play Frisbee with, or some other way to snap yourself out of the blues, do it. Feeling happy and positive contributes to healing. If you can't get out of that bad place, consider spending time with a psychiatrist or psychologist with an oncology specialty. Serious, prolonged depression is an opportunistic affliction that you don't have to tolerate.

5. Other emotions may come along. Be particularly careful of anger and weeping. They are symptoms of depression. People who make you angry or sad may be getting the brunt of something undeserved.

6. You may find that your mental abilities are less acute. Lots of medications can be at fault. Some chemotherapy compounds have this side effect, too. They call it "chemo brain." Whatever the cause, mental sharpness will come back after your body has gotten over the chemical warfare.

7. You may not sleep as well as you used to. Your body is a battleground for major conflicts. Carefully question sleeping pills and alcoholic beverages as ways to get more sleep. There could be a pharmaceutical conflict. A sleep-aid dependency can also occur. It may be best to simply increase your stack of bedside-reading material and make good use of the extra time. It is always good to talk through this kind of thing with your oncologist. You may also get help from survivors of your cancer whom you meet in care groups or through one of the resources listed in the Reference Center.

8. Chemicals in your body cause constipation and diarrhea. Both can become painful, even dangerous, if ignored. Both may lead to irritating side effects. Should you experience either of them, talk to your doc right away.

9. Body odors may become a recurring problem. Aside from pesky 'pits, you can get stinky feet and spectacularly awful breath. You may be the last to know. Coach your close friends and partner to forget their manners and tell you. It may be as simple as changing soap, toothpaste, mouthwash, or deodorant. It may not. Your doc, perhaps led by suggestions from your pharmacist, may need to change medicines or add something.

10. Some cancer patients go through personality changes, or appear to. When a guy shaves his head or grows a beard, his appearance radically

alters. When a woman's hair turns from long, luxurious brown to white peach fuzz, and she drops from a size 12 to a size 6, she gives a whole new visual meaning to herself. Some observers may read more into the new appearance than is actually there. You, the cancer patient, have to be aware that you could shock your parents or scare small children. You may need a thoughtful way to compensate. A smile, a wig, a game, a joke.

Lifestyle Decisions

Some of those facing cancer find that the theological underpinnings of their lives suddenly need shoring up (see Chapter 10, "God"). Both those who are religiously observant and those who are not may find themselves making major new decisions—or reversing long-stated beliefs—in personal disease-treatment choices and maybe in a new will. There may be business decisions too.

As you, a critically ill person, make important new determinations at this time in your life, some may question the soundness of your mind. Expect this if your decisions give or take away things of significant value to other people. Expect it if you make an irrevocable health-care decision. It's logical to involve your attorney (or refer back to Chapter 15, "Public-Assistance Law") if you intend to make these resolutions stick.

26 Nine Easy Ways to Shoot Yourself in the Foot

Why live in fear, when you can live in denial?

Though the statistics are hardly ever mentioned, tens of thousands of adults who learn that they have cancer do absolutely nothing about it. Fear, in one form or another, just locks them up. Another large group responds to the news in bizarre ways that unnecessarily complicate the healing process or add to its cost. While there is no imagining all the ways that people fumble the ball, here are nine classics.

Way #1: "This thing overwhelms me."

The enormousness and the enormity of the cancer problem are more than some people can cope with. The threat, those masses of purposeful people in medical uniforms, the places to go, the things to be done—all these just blow the mind. Older patients are more apt to react this way. So may others who have settled into a life of limited intellectual exercise. People new to the

United States or to Western cultural ways can also be staggered by cancer's prospects. Like little stars at sunrise, they just wink out.

By contrast, most cancer patients quickly come to realize that they don't have to know everything. They listen, and learn, and go with the flow. They come to accept the guides who take them through strange experiences. They learn enough to be good patients and trust the experts to do their thing.

Way #2: "Deer in the Headlights" Paralysis

The early stages of analysis and treatment seem to be going fine. Then something about the situation mesmerizes the patient. Paralysis from analysis. The patient can't think of anything but fear of dying, fear of being very sick, fear of a radical treatment, fear of cancer's unknowns, of going to treatment centers, of nuclear medicine, of tests, of needles, of doctors, of crowds, of making decisions. The possibilities are endless. You've got a helpless deer, transfixed in the headlights.

The immediate need is to get the healing program back on track, but be aware that physical rescue may not solve the problem. A deer that recovers before the truck runs it down is apt to bolt, directionless, into the bushes and maybe headlong into a tree. Ditto our patient. A cancer-recovery care group or a psychiatrist may be needed to screw the patient's head back on straight.

Way #3: "I can beat this thing with mental toughness."

Some people decide that mental toughness will force their cancers to retreat. They cite notable cancer survivors who reportedly willed themselves back to health. What goes unrecognized until one checks the source is that those survivors also had the surgeries and took the medicines. They did the research. They thoroughly coped on every level.

Here is your core message: Meditation and visualization are highly recommended by the oncology community, as discussed elsewhere. But in every case, these powers of positive thinking are considered important *accompaniments* to physical treatment, not replacements for it.

It is also important for the patient to cope in a familiar way. A cheery disposition isn't a realistic goal if it's against the patient's nature. "Many pessimists cope well with cancer," says Jimmie Holland, MD, chair of psychiatric oncology at Memorial Sloan-Kettering Hospital, New York. "You can be as curmudgeonly or angry or whiny as you want—so long as it doesn't cause your doctor to throw you out of the office."

It is unwise to let a patient use "mental powers" to forgo, or even delay, every other avenue of treatment the oncologist recommends. Do it all. Victory goes, as Napoleon once noted, to the army with the most cannons.

Way #4: "I don't have the money" or "I object to the cost."

An attack by cancer used to produce an apparent quick win for the patient, as when the tumor was removed by surgery. Or things went downhill fairly rapidly. Either way, the tab was miniscule by today's standards. The health-insurance community used to joke that there was no reason to buy more than half a million dollars' worth of protection because nobody could survive that much doctoring. Today, there are ways of sailing past the $500,000 mark within weeks of diagnosis.

A newcomer to cancer who has little or no medical insurance is justified in looking at a possible six-figure bill and feeling defeated. How can you buy something that big with no resources? Even if you somehow got the care, bankruptcy would immediately follow.

The very poor have been conditioned to expect that some agency of government will step forward with care, if needed. Absolutely correct (see Chapter 22, "Public Assistance," and elsewhere in "Supporting Resources," Part IV).

Most of the rest of us—let's call ourselves the other than very rich—will also find that "Supporting Resources" (Part IV) offers financial support in many forms. Nobody loses to cancer because the help needed is beyond their means. They lose because of a lack of resourcefulness and persistence.

People also succumb to cancer by choosing not to incur treatment costs. Somehow death is necessary to protect the estate for children, causes, or even pets. If giving in to cancer rather than spending available resources is a serious question, discuss it with friends, family, and a spiritual advisor. Most people believe that it is better to deplete the kids' inheritance and that the kids would be the first to agree. (If they're not the first, hmmm . . .)

People also die mad at the system that has allowed people to charge obscene rates for cancer treatment. They grouse at the cost of medical care. They are appalled that a pill could cost more than a steak dinner, or that 24-7 home care by a team of RNs could cost $40,000 a month. Dear angry person: Dying of cancer is neither pleasant nor tidy. Get over the cost issue. Your insurance company and the hospital will do just fine with or without you. Pay the money. Get the miracle.

> Nobody loses to cancer because there was no help. But lots of people lose because they gave up trying.

Way #5: "The insurance company won't allow . . . "

Health-insurance rules and procedures frequently get in the way of timely tests and treatments for a major illness. It's a glaring weak spot in the system. Plan administrators know it. The nurse-advocate position within these companies is a reflection of the creativity they have applied to be more flexible and responsive. Even so, serious problems remain.

There are expensive, sophisticated tests that your oncologist may want to put you through right away. There are treatment choices that cost a bundle. There are people and places you may need to be moved to where capabilities or facilities are far better for your case. Your insurance company may object to all of it or demand delays of one sort or another.

Listen carefully to your oncologist and your insurance company. They may only appear to disagree. Or you may find that the insurance company's caution is perfectly reasonable.

But you may come to believe that your insurer's delays and foot-dragging are potentially life threatening. Discuss your concern with your oncologist. If the two of you side against the insurance company, you should become absolutely intolerant of further delay. Be particularly impatient with the insurance

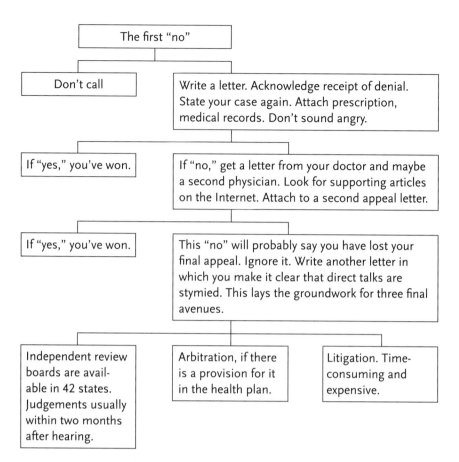

The first "no"

Don't call

Write a letter. Acknowledge receipt of denial. State your case again. Attach prescription, medical records. Don't sound angry.

If "yes," you've won.

If "no," get a letter from your doctor and maybe a second physician. Look for supporting articles on the Internet. Attach to a second appeal letter.

If "yes," you've won.

This "no" will probably say you have lost your final appeal. Ignore it. Write another letter in which you make it clear that direct talks are stymied. This lays the groundwork for three final avenues.

Independent review boards are available in 42 states. Judgements usually within two months after hearing.

Arbitration, if there is a provision for it in the health plan.

Litigation. Time-consuming and expensive.

26.1 The health-insurance / HMO appeals process—as close as most people ever want to get to genuine bureaucratic red tape. These are waters only lawyers and insurance administrators swim in. From "You Can Make Them Pay," *Wall Street Journal*, September 17, 2002.

company's appeals process. It is an ingenious contraption that only senior insurance executives should be required to experience. Suggestions for moving the process in the right direction, at top speed:

- Get a prescription for everything. A doctor's order for a complex treatment may also be called a "protocol." Paper the insurance company with these orders.
- Make certain the doctor's prescription or protocol demands treatment within a specific length of time. Terms applied to this time line, such as "life threatening" and "crucial to patient well-being," get rid of some of the fatuous objections of insurance clerks.
- Specific, serious consequences may come about because of a delay of the doctor's order. Be certain the written details go to the insurance company.
- Insurance companies and social services bureaucracies hate to be papered. It creates extra work. It implants the suspicion that you are laying the groundwork for effective legal action against them or a complaint

through political channels. Both are nightmares for them. When you paper, you become the proverbial squeaky wheel.

- If time is passing with no result, a phone call by the doctor, or by one of the staff in the name of the doctor, usually breaks the logjam.
- If a phone call doesn't work, refer to Chapter 15, "Public-Assistance Law." The issue we're discussing is an example of navigating managed care. An advocate experienced at negotiating with health-insurance companies at a very high level should get their attention.

At some point, you may have to grab the bull by the horns. If the debate rages interminably on, a time may come when there are only two alternatives left. You can wait for the process to come to a conclusion and take your chances on what cancer is doing to you in the meantime. Or you can go against the insurance company's instructions to you, and move on without approval with the course of treatment your doctor believes is important. Despite the best help of your advocates in medicine and in law, this may leave you exposed to a major financial obligation. It may also result in greater physical recovery, so that you have life left to worry about it.

Way #6: "God's will be done."

Cancer patients of religious persuasion—and some others who learn of the disease late in life—may honestly feel that "God is calling" the person to come "home." Significant numbers of people make this decision every year.

We do not know, of course, but God's wish could be that the patient take advantage of the resources massed to serve and save. There is the story of the fellow who was stranded by a flood. Three different boats spotted him and offered help, but he said, "No, thanks; God will provide." Finally, as the waters rose, a helicopter came to his rescue, but the fellow waved it off. Subsequently, he drowned. Upon meeting God later, he asked why a devout fellow like himself had been allowed to perish in that way. "I never wanted you to die," God told him. "I sent you three boats and a helicopter."

Way #7: "I am being punished."

You're not being punished. Just think of all the people who have committed unspeakable acts yet enjoy every privilege of health and wealth. Or think of all the people who are absolute saints and have miserable lives.

Way #8: "I'm not going to take chemo. It could damage my kidneys."

Most people who fear chemotherapy—or surgery or radiation—base their worry on hearsay rather than fact. Please do yourself the favor of consulting with your physician before making a decision. Chemo could in fact damage your kidneys or your hearing. Drugs used in chemotherapy may also damage other parts of the body. It depends entirely on which chemicals are used and how much, further mitigated by your physical condition. Today's improved drugs and practices often avoid causing the damaging side effects that were common a few years ago.

For more on medical aspects of this concern, see Chapter 27, "Treatments," and Chapter 33, "Things They May Forget to Tell You about Chemo." For more on the accompanying decision-making process, talk to your medical team, a spiritual advisor, or Reference Center resources and look into your heart.

Possible Reasons When Someone Says No

If you have come to this discussion because of concern for someone who has taken this stand, there are four issues relating to it for you to consider. The first is that maybe, just maybe, the patient hasn't figured out the life-threatening implication of this decision. The second possibility is that the patient is taking this stand to get attention. Lonely people do things like that. Third, people sometimes create this sort of crisis to test the love and loyalty of family and friends. Fourth, the patient may have had enough of the fight and this is your signal. Here the pain and the heartache and the apprehension end. There will be no more messing with this old bod. If death comes, so be it.

Way #9: "I am being sent to . . . "

You have not been hog-tied and shipped to some treatment gulag against your will. Nor are you under any other sort of binding obligation. Where you go and whom you see are decisions that you are responsible for.

You, as the patient, have a duty to pick the best people at the best sites to treat your illness. You. You. You. Not the HMO. Not the book they tell you to go by. Not a doctor. Any of these sources may suggest the perfect place. Matter of fact, one of these sources should provide the very best answer.

Detailed discussion about how to identify and explore options has preceded this chapter (see Chapter 7, "Deciding Where to Have Treatment"). The process and considerations explored there should govern your treatment decisions.

There is a second, rather delicate matter for you to be aware of. Business relationships exist between health centers and physicians, insurers, and other third parties. Recommendations you receive may be colored by agreements to share patients, when possible. The people and places in these exchanges are no doubt generally qualified. But they may not be the same choices that the doctor would make personally under the same circumstances. Don't blindly follow the business-card blitz, most particularly during the early, formative part of your treatment program. Closely examine all sides of your options. Ask pointed questions about experience with your specific kind of cancer. Go on the Internet to see if any of the leading lights you are being led to has special qualifications or has contributed to cancer treatment in any notable way. Take responsibility for the final decision. Then make a full commitment to it.

27 Treatments

Nothing is as easy as it seems.

When President Richard Nixon declared war on cancer in 1971, it seemed like a slam-dunk. Polio had just been defeated. Give a few million to the same bunch of scientists and this disease would be history in no time. Now, more than thirty years later, after an expenditure of resources greater than the United States needed for World War II, the struggle continues. Though the oncology community has a good deal of successful experience with your disease, it is still a fight. The outcome is not assured. But the remedies for your predicament are constantly improving.

As you may have already learned, your fight against your cancer is on several fronts at once. Your next trip to your doctor may be for any of five reasons, cancer treatment being only one of them. Cancer-fighting drugs, cancer surgery, and radiation produce side effects that are always monitored and frequently require a fix of some sort. Cancer, and damage to your body during treatment, will also make you susceptible to other, opportunistic ailments that must be attended to. Wasting diseases and lymphedema are important examples. Infections can be very serious. You may also have to deal with mental or physical debilitations from the cancer fight.

This is all highly confusing and more than a bit unfair. Your medical team goes after your cancer. The treatments you receive fix one thing, while they create new problems. All of this reduces your body's strength and stamina. These weaknesses bring on new diseases. Infections add to the misery, which makes you depressed. Your medical team, sorting through this mess, has to figure out what to do next.

In general, you can expect the doctor directing your recovery effort to be quite good at choosing the tools your body needs, at knowing when it needs them, and at dealing with consequent cause and effect. The more important point for you, the patient, is to understand that this is a complicated chess game, not the random confusion it may appear to be. Even some of the pauses between treatments are scripted parts of your journey back to health.

Surgery

Physicians have known for more than three thousand years that the first line of defense against a cancer tumor is to cut it out. Surgery remains the best way to counteract most cancers—if a surgeon can isolate the tumor.

The odds are that you will undergo at least one surgery. It may be a minor outpatient procedure. It may not. It may be to eradicate cancer. It may be for biopsy or another purpose. There may be more than one operation in your future.

Questions to Ask about Your Surgery

Why is surgery necessary? Cutting is a radical measure. It is probably the best next step when there is no less invasive way to achieve an absolutely necessary objective.

Please describe in detail. Many surgeries have a name. Learning it is the easiest way to answer the questions of friends and family. Surgeries with names also have drawings in books and on the Internet that show pretty much everything that will go on during the operation.

Should I bank blood beforehand? You may be able to bank your own blood, though having cancer makes it less likely. Others can certainly bank theirs in your name.

The blood donated creates a credit, like a dollar you put into a bank. You don't get that specific blood back, any more than the dollar bill you gave the teller is saved to return to you.

What form of anesthesia will I receive? How will it affect me? Will there be side effects? Your prime concern should be that postoperative effects, especially nausea and disorientation, are minimized.

Will I experience pain afterward? Yes. But there are great drugs. Be certain your anesthesiologist designs a postoperative program that minimizes discomfort and maximizes energy and the return of your mental acuity. There may be options that the doc can discuss with you.

Could surgery accidentally cause the cancer to spread? Cancer cells could be spread during the taking of biopsy samples and by surgical "accidents." Special, very successful precautions are taken to prevent this.

Could the surgeon cause the cancer to spread by exposing it to air? No. That is a myth.

Would a home nurse help me? If so, the surgeon's office will have names to suggest (also see the Reference Center "Yellow Pages" under "Nursing at Home"). Be sure you know how much it will cost, how long you will need nursing, and who will pay for it. Carefully consider your situation. Drop-in visits during the day usually suffice. Hope that you don't need 24-7 care. It gets very expensive, and financial help may be difficult.

How will my appearance change after the operation? If deformity will result, plastic surgery is often planned as part of the procedure. This is particularly true of surgery to the head or breast. It is not likely that you will have to ask this question. This is a very important issue that your surgeon probably wants to discuss with you in detail.

How long will I be hospitalized? Your hospital will give you a schedule from admission through release ahead of time, if at all possible. Patient rotation is a high priority. Rule of thumb: You will be out of there the moment it is safe.

Will I be sent home with tubes? With sacks? Could be. If so, the planning, training, and supplies necessary for you to recuperate at home with tubes or sacks attached will be carefully explained to those who will be caring for you. If you are going to have to buy supplies, see the Reference Center "Yellow Pages" under "Products and Supplies." Good prices. And they know how to pass on as much as possible to Medicare and insurance.

Will I have a scar? Yes. If it will be unsightly, expect that plastic surgery will be proposed.

Will a skin graft be necessary? Will this be done at the same time as the surgery? When skin grafts are necessary, the grafting is usually done as part of the surgery. The skin for grafting will probably be taken from your thigh or buttocks on the same side of your body as the surgery. For some reason, same-side skin is more apt to take. The site from which you lost the skin may bother you more than the surgery. It will feel much like the road burn you got when you fell off your bicycle. The itch may be exquisite. Get a lotion for it.

What are the likely complications? There are always a few things to watch out for. Infection is one. Expect the doc or a nurse to hand you a written list.

What postoperative symptoms should I report to my doc? This subject is sometimes simple, sometimes not. If there are major concerns, you will be advised.

Will I have to go through rehabilitation? There is often a rehab program after a major surgery. Ask about rehab if you are not given a sheet outlining a physical recovery program as part of a pre-op meeting. Normally, the surgical team or the hospital will treat rehab as a seamless part of your treatment. Be aware that you may save money or increase the allowed number of visits to the therapy center by leaving the hospital's rehab program for an equally capable third party. (If this is discussed up front and the hospital wants your business, it may make you a better offer than it otherwise would.)

When will I be able to go back to . . . ? Going back to work, flying or other high-altitude activities, returning to a favorite sport, housework, sex, and all those other parts of normal life need to be discussed. Take a list of all your concerns to a pre-op meeting.

Do I need a nutrition and exercise program? There are reasons to begin a special regimen as part of preparation for an operation. There are post-op activities and feeding programs. Your doc may recommend something, may send you to a staff nutritionist, or may see no need (also see Chapter 28, "Nutrition and Fitness").

Radiation

Cancer cells die when high-energy atomic particles strike them. So do normal cells. That is why the use of radiation is such an exacting occupation, with so many safety precautions. It is also a very safe way to treat many cancers, though it is usually not the only treatment.

Radiation therapy can be delivered by an outside source that beams these particles at the tumor area. It can also be delivered by a chemical cocktail that you drink, systemically by injection, or by seeds of radioactive material implanted near the cancer to shrink or annihilate it. After radiation, cancer cells are unable to replicate, or they die and are carried away by the bloodstream.

The process of attacking cancer with radiation is intentionally gradual. Delivering it in more than one session allows its effects to accumulate. This works much better than one massive shot, which, as you can imagine, would be traumatic and counterproductive.

Radiation itself is painless unless it involves the gastrointestinal tract, where discomfort can come from side effects. Radiation may also burn the skin or remove the hair from a site the beam passes through. Over the course of repeated treatments, radiation can decrease the blood's white-cell count, which increases susceptibility to infections and opportunistic diseases and saps energy.

Possible Permanent Changes to an Area of Skin

Repeated radiation may discolor or change the texture of the skin that the beam passes through on its way to the cancer site. The results may be permanent. Patients with breast, face, or neck cancers should be advised that this side effect is predictable, but sometimes the topic doesn't come up.

External Treatments

In general, patients receiving radiation treatments go in, get zapped, and leave without much fanfare. You don't confer with the doctor. You may not even see one. There is no result reported. You feel nothing during the treatment and generally no different afterward, though in some cases there is pain relief. You're not radioactive, so there's no reason to isolate you from others. (You may have to be isolated if you have radioactive seeds implanted, receive a systemic injection, or drink a chemical cocktail. None of those are parts of an external radiation treatment, however.)

Preparing for Radiation

Before your first treatment, you will visit the radiologist's clinic for a simulation. During this planning session, you will be fitted for any shield or special device that will be used. You may also have small aiming points tattooed on your body. (A tattoo is a permanent mark. When fresh, the ink may also permanently stain clothing.)

You can expect to receive blood tests every so often during radiation treatments. You will probably be weighed and have your temperature taken as part of every visit.

Matters to Cover before Receiving External Radiation

What kind of radiation will I receive? Do I have options? Different atomic particles may be options. X-ray, gamma, electron, and proton are the most common. These produce varied results. Your radiologist should be pleased to share this knowledge with you. Some forms of radiation therapy are not available everywhere. Travel and a stay away from home may be required. Your insurance company or HMO may have a restriction or cost ceiling that you will need to be aware of. If your doc recommends one thing and the insurer balks, details may have to be negotiated. Also, people will ask you what kind of radiation therapy you are receiving. If you don't know, you'll appear to be a ninny.

How many treatments? How often? Doctors sometimes forget to mention these details to patients. In other cases, the frequency and number of treatments depend on the cancer's reaction to a first program. Stay on top of this, making certain that your insurance provider is also supportive.

Will there be side effects? Sometimes there are. The most common are fatigue and "sunburn." Treatments to the abdomen may cause nausea and diarrhea. Chest radiation can cause shortness of breath, chronic coughing, or difficulty swallowing.

Will I be able to continue normal activities? Generally yes, but ask your doc to be sure. (Other peoples' opinions will be less reliable.)

Should I complete dental work first? Yes, if the radiation is to the head or neck area. (You should also complete dental work before chemo.)

Will radiation affect my sex life or fertility? Radiation to the pelvic area may have side effects you need to learn about from your oncologist or radiologist.

Are there eating restrictions? Ask your radiologist. When radiation is to a gastrointestinal area, restrictions may be necessary.

Any other precautions? Skin lotions, perfumes, deodorants, soaps, and shampoo residue may react angrily to radiation. The adhesive in bandage tape can boil. Discuss your situation with the tech or nurse before your treatment, to be safe.

Chemotherapy

When cancer is in the blood, bone, or lymphatic system, or in any inoperable form, chemotherapy becomes the oncologists' first line of response. Chemo is also a common follow-up to surgery and radiation. One drug, or a group of them, travels throughout the body, using any of several techniques to abate a cancer-based condition. Chemo is usually delivered on an outpatient basis. The time a treatment takes and the effects on the patient vary widely. Chemo may be no more than a pill or a shot, or it may require minutes to hours as the patient receives bags of fluids through an IV.

Chemotherapy delivers many of our most promising remedies for cancer. Though it is a complex subject, please take the time to understand what you are going to be treated for, and why the particular chemo drugs have been selected for you. The more you understand, the more you will be able to contribute to the management of your recovery.

Chemo's Bad Rep

When chemotherapy was developed in the 1940s, it was a monster. Patients were often hospitalized before treatments. The things pumped into their veins were so harsh that patients were sometimes given last rites before going into treatment. People vomited for days afterward. Dehydration was so severe that it was life threatening. Even with all of that, chemo saved lives when nothing else had helped.

Patients still feel nauseous or sick after some treatments. But the experience is far more tolerable. Sometimes patients lose hair, which your medical team should bring up at the time chemo is prescribed. Overall, chemo drugs are much more targeted at the cancer than in the early days and easier on the rest of the body. The techniques for delivery of treatments are better. Pre-meds—things that ease the body's acceptance of the treatment, steady the stomach, and calm the soul—also remove much of the dread from the event. But it remains something you will remember. See Chapter 33, "Things They May Forget to Tell You about Chemo," before embarking.

How Chemo Is Delivered

A chemo treatment can be a shot or just a pill. But it is best known in the form of one or more bags of liquid dripped into a vein over a period ranging from minutes to several hours. The medication is usually repeated over a period of days, weeks, or even months.

Most times, chemo is delivered in an infusion room, usually called the Chemo Room, in a hospital or clinic. Each visit begins with a weigh-in and at least a cursory exam by a nurse, perhaps including a blood test, blood pressure, and temperature. This checkup is to make sure that you are well enough to cope with the physical impact that comes with treatment, and to see that you are not going to carry any obviously infectious symptoms into an area frequented by people with lowered immune systems.

The place of treatment is often a communal room that features beds or reclining chairs, with monitors, intravenous fluid pumps, and the stands, or "trees," used to hang IV bags scattered about. Things are relaxed. There may be a table of salty munchies, fruit, and candy, often stocked by patients. There are books and magazines to read and pillows for those who want them.

You settle in. A nurse may offer you a warmed blanket to counteract the chilling effect of the cold fluids you will receive.

If you are going through relatively frequent treatments, you may have a catheter, sometimes called a "port," installed. This is a semi-permanent connection to a major vein, usually on your upper chest, where an intravenous line can be plugged in. If you are more typical and receive a treatment once a week or less frequently, a nurse or tech will install an IV port for each chemo session. The top of a hand is a convenient site, as are the pits of elbows and wrists.

You begin with pills and injected pre-meds to reduce nausea and other discomforts. You may receive a bit of Valium or another "happy pill" to make the experience relaxed. After an allotted time for these first medications to kick in, along comes the main course. Typically, the chemo is in one or more bags that are hooked onto your tree. Tubes are connected that run through an IV pump down to you. A drip is started. The pump regulates the flow. You sit back, perhaps contemplating a piece of chocolate or a bag of potato chips from the goodie bar.

Sometimes people receive chemo privately. Most of the time, the dosing is in view of other patients, some of whom may chat while others read or doze. The dose and the nature of the chemo influence these inclinations.

Chemotherapies and peoples' reactions to them vary all over the lot. Moreover, a person's reaction to a first or second dose may be quite different from the same person's reaction to later doses. There is only one general guideline:

Ask the nurse running the show to estimate the length of time a specific chemo treatment is apt to take and what kind of condition you are going to be in afterward. You can bet that he or she will know.

A typical chemo treatment will wipe you out, along with at least half the day. Someone should drive you home afterward. That's home. Don't plan to go back to work or shopping or to some social outing. Nor can you allow yourself to go into a situation that may require an important decision. You will not be as lucid or as sober as you may think you are.

Collateral Consequences

If you are going to lose your hair, you will be told so at the time chemo is prescribed for you. Other side effects will also be known. In general, it is best to listen carefully and to ask as many questions as come to mind. You should also be given the same information in writing.

You will be at a distinct disadvantage at this meeting. You will be shocked and confused. You will be apprehensive, if not scared silly. So do your best. But before the meeting breaks up, make sure you get the name and phone number of someone you can call who can answer all the questions that come up later.

This is also a good time to go back to the Reference Center. Find some people who have gone through what's ahead for you and get acquainted.

More thoughts, mostly about hair:

- You will get over the shock, but you will never forget the experience.
- You will get through it, and life will go on.
- If your hair is long and you are going to lose it, you may sell or donate it.
- A good way to deal with the hair-shedding process is to have it cut short before you begin chemo. Then shampoo it off in the shower after it loosens.
- Women: If you're lucky, you won't have to shave your legs or under your arms or to accommodate a bikini for months. (You may not lose your eyebrows, but they may turn gray.)
- Women usually buy wigs. Men usually don't. Growing numbers of women stick with scarves and hats, which are more comfortable than hairpieces.
- Hair often comes back thicker and curlier than it was. Sometimes it comes back grayer than you remembered. The curl and body will gradually revert to their usual condition. The gray will only increase, but your stylist will have some good ideas for taking care of that, if you choose to.
- Don't permit the sun to tan you for at least one year after chemo is over. Sun can do some really nasty things to your chemo-induced extra-photosensitive skin.

Matters to Cover before Receiving Chemo

What drugs will I be given? People will ask you the names of your chemo drugs, the dose amounts, frequencies, what pre- and post-meds you take.

Each chemo has a short type descriptor, such as "small B-cell inhibitor." You need to know that, too. It is not the grasp of medicine so much as the gee-whiz sound of the words that lends magic to the telling. If you doubt it, explain why Techron sells gasoline.

Is my treatment precleared by my insurer? The stuff you are about to be given costs a fortune—possibly several thousand dollars a dose, plus a (usually buried) Chemo Room corkage fee. There are so many therapies that even well-established drugs may become a subject of argument. Make sure your insurer accepts the protocol your doctor has prescribed for you. The safest way to do that is to have your medical team call the insurer.

What about scheduling? Get all the details of your chemo program on a calendar: what, where, when. This is your first priority until it's over and you're recovering.

What side effects can I expect? Presuming your chemo is not wildly esoteric, you will receive a written list of possible and probable side effects. (Also see Chapter 33, "Things They May Forget to Tell You about Chemo" and "Collateral Consequences" earlier in this chapter.)

Will I be able to continue normal activities? Probably, sort of. Expect more fatigue than usual. Evaluate side effects. Do not promise to head the new division at work or even accept the nomination for office at the PTA. Chemo is your number-one job. Discuss your personal limitations with your doctor. Things like sense of taste or sex may not go so well for a while.

Will diet and exercise help? Ask your doc or the staff nutritionist. There are two parts to the answer. First, a nutritious diet and exercise help maintain healthy reserves but may be optional, so far as your medical team is concerned. Second, there may be substances, including herbs, that you mustn't eat because they could effect the chemo.

What conditions will my medical team want to know about? Make notes as they discuss this with you. Carefully report. In general, if you feel better, you probably are. Don't get a cold or flu. Take infections seriously. Follow the directions on each of those pill bottles.

Can chemo cause mood swings? Yep. If you get seriously blue, tell your doctor.

When will we know if it's working? An improving pattern of test results is always a good sign. If you feel better, you probably are. These positives can be temporary. Think healing thoughts and stay on your toes. Never miss a checkup. As your good health continues, don't allow your insurance company to delay you more than one year between checkups, even after five or ten cancer-free years.

Hormone Therapy

Hormones, the body's chemical transmitters, travel through the bloodstream to moderate or accelerate vital processes such as growth, metabolism, and sexual development. Certain hormones also stimulate tumor growth, most commonly in the breast, endometrium, and prostate. Drugs that lower or stop the activity can at least discourage cancers that respond aggressively to these body functions. It may be better to think of this as antihormone therapy.

Some drugs used in this way also attack malignant blood cells associated with lymphoma, leukemia, and myeloma.

Potential side effects:

- Men lose sex drive, and impotence follows, which can be temporary or permanent.
- Women may experience disruption of the menstrual cycle and vaginal dryness. Temporary or permanent infertility may also occur.
- Some hormone therapies cause nausea, vomiting, swelling, or weight gain. Interestingly, other hormone therapies are sometimes used to treat these symptoms.

Immunotherapy

Cancer succeeds by fooling the body's immune system into believing that a cancer cell is normal. So the immune system leaves the cancer alone and may even protect it from some cancer medications. Immunotherapy uses several amazing and complicated strategies to help the immune system recognize and attack cancer cells. Immunotherapy is also an important part of successful transplant operations (see Chapter 31, "Vaccines," for more).

Bioimmunotherapy

Physicians are intrigued by cases in which bacterial infections such as malaria and typhoid appear to make cancer vanish. This discovery is credited to observations by William B. Coley, MD, in the 1890s. Patients may come across references in current literature to success using "Coley toxins."

Other research looks at the differences in people of regions where cancer is rare.

Those with some unusual genetic conditions are also studied. A person with Down syndrome, for example, is less apt to contract certain cancers and will respond better than the rest of us do to treatment for others. These clues lead scientists to magnificently inventive strategies that give new hope to patients with certain inoperable cancers and offer possible prevention strategies for future generations

Gene Therapy

Gene therapy alters the genetic makeup of the cancer tumor, or of the patient, to upset the passive environment the cancer enjoys. When it succeeds, the cancer may simply disappear, or the immune system may strike it down.

Bone-Marrow and Stem-Cell Transplants

Leukemia, lymphoma, multiple myeloma, and certain cancers of the testicles, ovary, and brain have been successfully treated by marrow- or stem-cell-transplant operations. There are hospitals with entire transplant wings, so that this specialty can be offered to more patients. You also need to know that transplants are not successful for every sort of these cancers or for all patients.

The process of transplant begins by wiping out all the patient's bone marrow, malignant or not. This is accomplished by chemotherapy drugs and whole-body radiation. The cancer is theoretically obliterated. The patient is also left without much defense against disease or infection. Red blood cells, which transport the body's oxygen; white cells, the body's first defense against infection; and blood platelets, which stop bleeding, are all dangerously depleted.

The patient is admitted to a special, highly antiseptic section of a hospital for this procedure. Disease-free marrow or stem cells are infused into the patient's blood. New, cancer-free bone marrow develops, along with a rejuvenated immune system. Direct contact with the patient is carefully controlled until a new immune system has kicked in.

Finding a donor for a bone-marrow or stem-cell transplant is a major obstacle. Acceptable matches between people with no blood relationship are at least 7,000-to-1 shots. The most likely donor candidate is a brother or sister. One in four siblings is compatible. Parents and children are also good possibilities. Some developments in the production of specialized stem cells make more transplants possible now than in the past. To find experts for further discussion, see the Reference Center "Yellow Pages" under "Transplants."

Questions to Ask about Your Transplant

How do I prepare for this hospitalization? Take care of any family, business, or school matters before you arrive. You will not handle any of them effectively once inside and under way. Have your protocol approved by the insurance company, or by whoever will be paying for this, in advance. Get a second opinion that completely concurs with this transplant plan. Make sure your personal affairs are in order. Assign a durable power of attorney. Make a living will.

Where will I be staying? You will live in a small private room designed to make you comfortable for a long stay. Pictures of this place are probably available.

What clothes should I bring? A coordinator is assigned to help with all questions of this sort. You will also receive extensive written instructions. All that said, you will be allowed to make your space in isolation as personal and comfortable as possible. Anything that can arrive nonallergenic, disease free, and clean should be fine.

Can I have visitors? Once the process begins, you will be able to see and hear but not touch visitors. After initial recovery, you will be allowed visitors who are healthy and reasonably germfree. Pets may qualify.

Can I eat normally? No. A controlled diet will be served, nuked as thoroughly as you have been. In fairness, most hospitals try hard to provide interesting and varied fare.

Can I eat normally after I go home? Depends on what you normally eat, of course. As your body recovers its immunity, raw foods and certain things that are more prone to contain live microbes will be permitted.

When will I be able to return to . . . ? Return to home, work, school, church, public transportation, and other locations that are part of your normal life will be permitted on a schedule that should be roughly known before you begin this adventure. Delays are predictable if your recovery is more complicated than is anticipated. Be safe. Don't schedule anything important until your doc allows you to.

What precautions against disease and infection will be necessary beforehand? A program to wipe out any colds, flu, or other diseases before you begin the transplant will be instigated. This care will continue after you are released.

How long will the bone-marrow team follow my case after I am released? This varies. It may be five years or longer.

Home-Care Dos and Don'ts for Recovering Transplant Patients

It has taken an army of people and a truckload of time and money to get you through the transplant process, out of the hospital, and home to continue your recovery. If you screw up now and the mistake doesn't kill you, your medical team may want to.

This is not a complete list of precautionary measures. You know not to do or eat things in obviously unsanitary ways. This is a list of other stuff that might not be as obvious.

- Do not allow the sun to tan any part of your head, arms, or body for at least a year. Your skin is extra-photosensitive. Burns and other effects from the sun offer multiple ways to get you into deep, serious trouble.
- Learn and practice sterile procedures in the kitchen.
- Don't eat anything raw that you didn't peel just beforehand.
- Don't eat anything spoiled.
- Don't eat raw shellfish or other uncooked seafood.
- Don't eat alfalfa sprouts.
- Don't consume unpasteurized dairy products.
- Slice prepared foods at home. Don't buy them cut up, such as sliced meats in a deli.
- Wear latex gloves to protect your hands from touching possible contaminants.
- Use a hand can opener. Keep it very clean.
- Defrost foods in the refrigerator or microwave. Never allow them to thaw on the counter.
- Set the refrigerator temperature at 40° F, or colder. Set the freezer temp at 0° F.
- There may be vaccinations or shots to take before beginning the treatment process. Check with the head of your transplant team.
- Consider the possible problems of having an unhealthy pet.
- Don't clean up pet urine or feces.
- Don't change baby diapers, wipe noses, or touch vomit.
- An air purifier is a good idea.

- If you garden, wear gloves. Don't inhale garden sprays of any kind.
- Clean your teeth with a soft-bristle brush and nonabrasive toothpaste.
- Don't be near a vacuum cleaner in operation for at least three months after returning home.

Other Treatments

If a treatment of interest to you has not been mentioned in this chapter, do not be surprised. The intent here is to cover the subject broadly. Ask your medical team for more information and look the treatment up on the Internet.

28 Nutrition and Fitness

Diet and exercise may make a higher level of recovery possible for you. They will also help you battle serious side effects.

The vast majority of us don't exercise, much less do it regularly. Nor do we pay much attention to proper diet—whatever that is. So what?

So this: You now have a disease that will make a serious effort to kill you. Two of its attack strategies will be to reduce your ability to refuel your body effectively and to degrade your physical stamina. If your cancer can succeed at one or both of these objectives, you will have lost at least a major battle, and maybe the game.

About ten million Americans are cancer survivors. They represent the first reversal in the attack of cancer on humanity since the dawn of time. You have a terrific chance to join them and refer to cancer in the past tense if you take a better-prepared body to your oncologist.

After studying the literature and other available information, the American Cancer Society has found no evidence that any specific dietary regimen is useful as a cure for cancer. Lacking such evidence, the American Cancer Society strongly urges individuals with cancer not to use dietary programs as an exclusive or primary means of treatment.

American Cancer Society Web site advisory

Too Overweight, Too Out of Shape, Too Old, Too Sick

Most of us are overweight, which may rival tobacco use as a cause of cancer. One-third of U.S. adults are clinically obese. The average American exercises most between the ages of eighteen and twenty-four. After the midtwenties, the amount and the quality of physical exertion decline dramatically. Four of ten adult men and women are totally sedentary. If you are part of this great gelatinous mass, you need to do something about it.

Believe it or not, the most difficult thing about shaping up is persistence. The taste of food in a good diet is not bad. The exercise is at least easy, if not fun. You may think that you are too overweight, too out of shape, too old, or too sick. But you are not too late to put meaningful roadblocks in the way of this thing that's coming after you.

Vital Conditions, Not Cures

As you begin learning more about fighting cancer through proper eating and exercise, you are apt to see or hear the word "cure" bandied about. Cure is a completely different matter (also see Chapters 5 and 38). The core values of good nutrition and decent physical fitness are that they improve your effectiveness as a cancer fighter and reduce the side effects, including pain.

Five Enemies to Fight

Proper nutrition for your exact circumstance and the best possible physical fitness will make it more likely that you will survive five enemies that you now face. They are: (1) your cancer, (2) your cancer treatments, (3) the opportunistic additional diseases that look for openings, (4) the infections, and (5) the physical and mental debilitations that accompany cancer and its treatments.

Yes, you are at risk from your treatments and other diseases, infections, debilitations, and the wounds you get in the fight, as well as from your cancer. Patients succumb to all of them. Nutrition and fitness, even if they mean coming from a long way back, give you something more to fight with on every front.

A Realistic Take on Nutrition and Exercise

You cannot jog far enough or spend sufficient time in the gym to defeat cancer. You can't eat enough of any food or take enough of any food supplement to cure it. While the cancer-fighting properties of certain foods and food supplements are recognized, it is a mistake to confuse the improved conditions that good nutrition and fitness make possible with the radiation, surgery, and powerful medicines that do the heavy lifting.

No Panaceas

Please do not infer that surgery or prescribed medications are cure-alls either. These are steps taken after careful consideration and medical team consensus. As Dr. Daniel J. Lieber, oncologist and assistant clinical professor at the USC School of Medicine, points out, effective treatments may also be complex and dangerous, with emotion-laden consequences.

Misleading Generalizations

Many, many cancer patients are successfully using diet and exercise regimes under the direction of highly experienced oncology teams. The temptation is to generalize the details of all these other peoples' good experiences, then oversimplify them to apply to ourselves. It doesn't work.

When you use proper diet and exercise to fight cancer:

- The advance of the disease may slow.
- Surgical recovery time is less.
- Problems with infections and opportunistic illnesses are reduced.
- Aging signs are fewer.
- You have more energy.
- Your physical flexibility is greater.
- It's better for your sex life.
- Your pain meds are more effective.
- You sleep better.
- You are mentally sharper.
- Your outlook is brighter.

Sally has a broken bone. I have a broken bone.
Sally got along without having her broken bone splinted. Therefore I can, too. Right?
Wrong. Way too simple.
Which bone did Sally break? Did you break the same bone?
If no, there's no real comparison, is there?
If yes, is it broken in the same place? To the same extent?
Are your bones and Sally's of the same health and age?
Maybe Sally's bone had no hope of being healed, so the doctors chose not to treat her . . .
Maybe you are different.

Do you see where we're going here? Are you beginning to appreciate the dangers that oversimplifying complex issues may hold for you?

The point, which is vitally important if you are to make the most of this chapter, is that you will need the people on your medical team to design diet and exercise programs specifically tailored to your individual needs. Filter all the other voices you may hear and all the other data you discover through your oncology doc or the designated expert on your medical team.

Other Voices

Armies of health-through-nutrition advocates will encourage you to make broken bone–type mistakes in thinking about your disease. They will claim that the vitamin, the enzyme, the oil, the electrical stimulation, the tree-bark tea, the eating of two pounds of raw spinach a day, or whatever they have chosen to advocate will improve your situation, whatever it is. No physical exam or lab work required, so far as they're concerned. In other words, no responsible, scientifically based examination of the circumstances. One size fits all.

This oversimplification, this ignoring of the medical treatment process, is one of the prime reasons that mainline oncology teams cringe when patients ask them about these claims. What can they say to a serious questioner who is coming from such a shattered base of misinformation and ignorance?

The National Institutes of Health began an evaluation of alternative medical treatments in the early nineties that evolved into the National Center for Complementary and Alternative Medicine. The center's activities and grant money earn it at least partial credit for new courses in alternative therapies now found at most medical and nursing schools.

At least eight new medical journals devoted to alternative medicine were also launched in the nineties. Other established professional journals also report on the subject regularly.

Medical insurance and managed-care companies have started to pay for some alternative therapies. These include an estimated 65 percent of major health-maintenance organizations.

The further frustration is that the vitamins, oils, stimulation, or spinach may turn out to have healing powers.

Some of those with the greatest optimism in this area are on staff at oncology centers, attempting to apply science to the study of these assertions in hopes of proving them. Emotion, business interests, politics, lack of intellectual rigor, and the occasional proclivity to seek mysticism in the battle against evil masks the issue so completely that we search for truth in very murky depths.

Therapeutic Diets

The National Cancer Institute says that 20 to 40 percent of cancer-related deaths "may result from nutritional status rather than the disease itself." While all the ways nutrition contributes to cancer development and treatment are not entirely understood, the NCI says that good nutrition helps a patient maintain weight and soundness of body, improving one's sense of wellness while reducing nausea and constipation. Poor nutrition may increase the nasty side effects of treatments and increase the risk of infection, says the NCI, "thereby reducing chances for survival."

Obviously, the type of cancer, the damage it does to your body, and the treatments you receive to combat it are major variables, as are the physical differences among patients. Close direction and monitoring by an oncology nutritionist are necessary to allow diet and food supplementation to make the greatest positive contribution to your recovery.

Diet Guidelines for Cancer Patients

Caution: Even these broad, generally agreed-upon standards have exceptions and provisos. Your doc or nutritionist must approve all aspects of your diet.

1. Get between 15 and 30 percent of your calories from fat, and two-thirds of that from nonanimal sources.

And God populated the earth with broccoli and cauliflower and spinach and green and yellow vegetables of all kinds, so that man and woman would live long and healthy lives.

And Satan created fast food. And fast food brought forth the 99-cent double cheeseburger with secret sauce. And Satan said, "You want fries with that?" And man said, "Supersize it."

But God said, "Try my crispy fresh salad."

And Satan brought forth creamy dressings, bacon bits, and shredded cheese. And there was ice cream and cake for dessert.

And God created the healthful yogurt.

And Satan froze the yogurt, and brought forth chocolate, nuts, and brightly colored sprinkles.

And God brought forth running shoes.

And Satan brought forth cable TV with remote control.

God sighed, and created all manner of food supplements, diagnostics, medication, radiation, and surgery.

And Satan created the HMO.

Author unknown

---

2. Increase soy protein, which appears to play a particularly important role in cancer prevention (soy, red kidney beans, garbanzo beans, green beans, peas).
3. Increase foods from the cruciferous family: broccoli, cauliflower, cabbage, brussels sprouts. These contain plant-protective factors shown to be anticarcinogenic in animal and tissue-culture studies.
4. Eat fruit, vegetables, and whole grains with meals and as snacks every day.
5. Protect yourself from the sun.

Nutrition Buildup Before and During Treatment

There is no need to worry about a specialized nutritional buildup before or during treatment unless your doctor tells you so. In that case, you will be introduced to a specialty within oncology nutrition that will help.

The nutritionist will address evidence that your cancer has damaged your body's ability to put food to its best uses, or that the treatment you will receive may damage food processing. The anger, fear, and confusion you have felt since learning that you have cancer may also be getting in the way of normal eating and drinking. Protein-calorie malnutrition (PCM), which can result from any of these conditions, is the most common secondary problem in cancer patients.

In addition to loss of appetite, you may not find the foods you try to eat tasty. You may have trouble swallowing or keeping food down. You may also develop allergies to certain foods. Glucose and dairy-product intolerance are common. Resistance to insulin and changes in the ways the body manages fats and proteins can also take place.

The nutritionist who helps you with these matters will be part of a team assigned to this specific problem. The team may also include physical therapists and physicians with new specialties, including psychiatry. There will be testing, imaging, and more. In addition to food and food supplements, pharmaceuticals will be used. The superior balance of many specialties and remedies together is the key to success, not the performance of any one factor.

Managing Weight Loss, Insomnia, and Malaise

During the active phase of treating your condition, you can expect to experience at least two, if not all, of three common side effects of cancer: weight loss, sleeplessness, and ill-being. Each is apt to require the support of experts on your medical team. Each results from a complex interaction of factors that may include the two others.

Cachexia, a progressive wasting away of both fat and muscle, is one of the worst of the opportunistic conditions that may accompany weight loss. It is not well understood. Some patients come to it through anorexia, which 15 to 25 percent of all cancer patients experience. Others who get it appear to have been eating normally. Some patients come to this condition early in their cancer treatments. For others, wasting away accompanies late-stage cancer. For some, but not all, significant weight loss follows chemotherapy or radiation treatments.

Your oncologist and your nutritionist team up with your psychologist or psychiatrist and your pharmacist to help you with weight conditions. Early warning of these conditions is one reason you are weighed before every doctor visit.

Insomnia and malaise are predictable side effects of chemotherapy. They are also byproducts of weight loss and cancer progression. You are apt to experience sleepless nights, bad dreams, and periods of feeling a vague disassociation from your normal world anyway. They come with the anger and grave concerns of being very ill. The same team, using the same types of tools, can help. But unlike the weight scale, which can't be fooled, insomnia and malaise have to be reported and discussed. Don't be embarrassed by these feelings. Your medical team expects you to have them at some point because everybody does. Serious consequences may result unless these feelings are treated.

Specialized Feeding

Tubes

People with cancers in the path that food takes, from lips to tail, frequently can't eat or drink normally because of their disease or treatment. When that happens, an enteral feeding tube is necessary to deliver nutrition directly to the stomach. Sometimes these tubes are installed shortly after hospital admission, before any other treatment. This is particularly the case for people with cancers in the head or neck area. Poor nourishment is one of the common early symptoms of these cancers, so it is the first matter the medical team takes care of.

Historically, about 60 percent of all cancer patients have some sort of surgery performed during their treatment. The possible uses of oral nutritional supplements or enteral and parenteral (a drip into a vein or under the skin) nutritional support are also standard tools of the trade.

Sometimes a feeding tube is used to help a patient recover from chemotherapy. Tube feeding can help alleviate taste changes and "early satiety," a feeling of fullness after just a bite or two. This is also a successful strategy when nausea and vomiting after eating are problems.

Radiation of tumors in the gastrointestinal track may also create a situation that requires tube feeding. Recovery from radiation treatments of cancers in or of the head, neck, lungs, esophagus, cervix, uterus, colon, rectum, and pancreas may cause you to have a tube installed.

In some cases, tube feeding becomes a long-term nutritional strategy. Patients who can be discharged into a clean, safe environment with someone judged competent to take care of them may use a feeding tube at home. Should that become something you would like to know more about, your oncology team may have helpful pamphlets or a video. If not, contact the Oley Foundation, listed in the Reference Center. You may also want to check out "Products and Supplies" in the "Yellow Pages" section of the Reference Center.

Dietary Modification

Dry mouth, loss of feeling in your mouth, sensitivity to heat or cold, temporary severe reactions to certain foods, conditions that make everything taste bad, inability to swallow, and feeding strategies that allow food to bypass a point of surgery or a sore will require your medical team to conjure up something on your behalf. The conditions that lead to this situation are predictable. The only one who may be surprised is the patient.

It is usual for one of the supervising doctors or a nurse to prepare the patient carefully for this experience and to explain the strategy. For some patients, these feeding procedures last only a short time. For others, they could last months. You may not mind this feeding ordeal very much. But if it is uncomfortable for you, your nurse may be able to help.

Nutrition Education for Partners and Friends

You need to have your partners and friends on the same nutritional wavelength as your doc and your oncology nutritionist. That way, they will better understand the thinking behind the nutrition program that your medical team has developed for you.

You and your friends are beginning this study of nutrition to get educated, not to make a scientific breakthrough. You realize that folks with a few hours of study under their belts do not have one one-hundredth of the capability or background that an accomplished oncology nutritionist can bring to your needs. Nutrition education for the patient and loved ones is for the purpose of getting up to speed with the experts. If this were football, it would be like learning the plays so you can join the team.

This brings up two points:

1. Give careful thought to just how you will deal with conflicting nutritional advice you may receive from unqualified sources. Unless your self-anointed expert has the same level of academic preparation as your medical team, the advice is apt to be wrong—maybe even dangerous.

2. If you have not received nutritional advice from your medical team, you need to know why. It is usually because your situation does not require a nutritional component right now. But there is a possibility that nutrition is being neglected for a nonhealth reason. (Examples: "We don't offer that" or "It isn't covered under your health plan.") If you suspect that you are not receiving comprehensive health care, get a second opinion at another, wholly independent cancer center. If you find that better health care is available somewhere else, you have cause for major alarm. Act. Don't put this off. Also be certain that the next steps you take are sober and prudent.

Good Sources for General Nutrition Education

If you are a patient at an oncology center of any size, it will have staff and a library to help you. There will be brochures in the waiting room. Videos, audiotapes, and CDs will probably also be available. Ask your doc or nurse.

If you prefer, go to the Internet. Check out "nutrition" and "fitness" at the Web sites of any major oncology center (M. D. Anderson, Mayo Clinics, Dana-Farber, USC/Norris Comprehensive Cancer Center—there are literally thousands, including your favorite university medical school or teaching hospital). You can also find a highly rated nutrition guide at www .thewellnesscommunity.org. In all cases, please explore with the help of a guide from your oncology team.

Remember that there is no Web sheriff. The Internet features absolute freedom of speech. High-quality information appears side-by-side with a lot of other stuff. Do not trust information from a commercial bookstore or a health-food store either, unless you can separate the excellent information on some shelves from the wholly unsubstantiated blather on others. Be wary in a public library for the same reason.

The Internet is not the only repository of unsubstantiated advice. Many radio and TV programs that air at off-peak hours are apt to feature some amazing potion, exercise product, healing place to visit, or therapy. There are reasons this information is presented to you on a Saturday morning, not during prime time. Perhaps the explanations are credible. Perhaps not.

More broadly, and as a general rule of thumb, something new that you discover has probably been thoroughly explored in literature available to your medical team. But don't let that deter you from learning all you can.

One place to begin is Chapter 32, "Nontraditional Healing Practices." The chapter features some of the most prominent modes and manners, in hopes of helping you direct your examination more quickly to the heart of the matter.

Exercise

If you have led a vigorous, athletic life to this point, you are part of a small minority. If you are typical, with love handles and a fondness for relaxing, this is probably not the time to get serious about that marathon you always thought about running. Your physical sickness, compounded by treatments that give you even less time or will to exercise, have you boxed in. But don't give up. Determine to exercise regularly in some way.

Your medical team should be thrilled to know that you are committed to doing something physical on a regular basis. Over the years, it has become increasingly evident that lack of exercise creates the right set of circumstances for unnecessary cancer complications and for the appearance of other opportunistic diseases. The patient gets sicker. Fatigue and ennui take away the will to fight. Body systems shut down. Bingo.

Cachexia and protein-calorie malnutrition, two of the fancy terms that have been tossed at you since this chapter opened, are terrible illnesses that directly contribute to the deaths of more than one hundred thousand cancer patients per year. The screaming frustration is that they could be pretty much avoided, except in very late-stage cancer, if patients would take care of diet and exercise.

The Need for Physical Activity during Treatment

If you can't deal with the damage done by your disease, or if you can't recover from treatment ordeals, you cannot be a happy camper. Scar tissue formed because of radiation or surgery needs to be gently stretched to keep it malleable and minimized. Muscles have to regain tone. Cardiovascular stamina needs rebuilding. That time in bed has to be counteracted by time out of bed. Decide—now—to start doing something physical. Get your medical staff to work with you.

If you are recovering from a procedure that has you stuck in bed, set a walk to the bathroom as a goal. Next, go stand at the window for one minute. Enjoy the sunshine. Walk all the way to the end of the hall and back, even if you have to push an IV stand or use a walker. Get permission to take an unassisted shower.

Physical Therapies

It is the responsibility of your medical team to direct you, at the proper time and place, into the exercise program that is best for you. But you share this responsibility. You may realize that you are ready before your medical team does—in which case, let them know.

Running and Walking

If you were a runner or a walker before this cancer thing came along, you will probably want to go back to running or walking as soon as you can. Your doc and your physical therapist will want to help, unless there is a medical condition that gets in the way. Bring up the issue. Set modest goals at first.

If you have not run in the past, walking is a more reasonable goal. Get the right kind of shoes. Consult your physical therapist or an orthopedist.

Yoga, Qigong, Pilates, and Tai Chi

If you have observed others stretching in bed, moving in slow motion, or assuming ridiculous poses, all with looks of serious purpose, this is your chance to be like them. As a bonus for electing to use one of these programs, your coach may regale you with stories about how you are really practicing a martial art that the peasants used to beat the king's warriors by posing as waterbirds or gargoyles. And you may come to believe it—because these programs work, and you may feel physical and mental improvements in an astonishingly short time.

Massage

Heaven is probably a place where everyone you know knows massage. In addition to providing a great deal of pleasure and some pain, massage manipulates muscles and increases oxygen levels in the body's soft tissues.

Massages of various kinds are common remedial treatments. But ask a therapist to recommend the correct massage in your case and to demonstrate the best technique. Don't permit manipulations that have not been specifically prescribed by your medical team.

Sports

Physical contact sports are for people prepared for both hitting and its consequences. Baseball, swimming, tennis, bowling, and golf also have various energy and physical conditioning thresholds. They can be healthful activities if you take them as such. Avoid exercise-reducing amenities such as golf carts, as you can.

Gym Exercises

Dancing, lifting weights, doing aerobics—all wonderful. Have your physical therapy guru get you started with things appropriate for your time and place.

Family or Friends Activities

Ride a bicycle. Go for a walk—take a picnic to add to the enjoyment. Toss a football or a Frisbee. Fly a kite. Go fishing. Go to a movie. Play a lawn game with your grandparents or your grandchildren.

Other Supporting Activities

There are things that you can do even before many physical activities are practical.

Distraction

Believe it or not, they've found a way to bill your insurance carrier for the time you watch television. It is called "distraction therapy." Going out with friends, reading this book, and doing art and crafts are also "distractions." Insofar as reading this book is concerned, we observe the honor system. You can pay the author when you see him.

Biofeedback

In biofeedback, a machine retrains your mind and body to work together. Electrodes are attached that measure changes in breathing, temperature, muscle tension, and heart rate. The unit beeps when a desired state is reached. Biofeedback also helps some people control pain.

Meditation

Sometimes thought of as more than an art, methods of focus and quiet contemplation achieve significant goals for some people. Almost every successful athlete uses visualization or some other form of meditation to enhance performance. Someone proficient in meditation may be a good coach. There are also many, many self-help books on this subject.

Visualization

While all kinds of actions are important, I would rate at the top getting the patient to practice relaxation and visual imagery three times a day for 15 minutes each. It has powerful potential to help and no possibility of hurting if done properly.

In 1976, a clinic admitted 150 cancer patients that were considered past the point that any treatment for their cancers might save their lives. Specialists taught the group deep relaxation techniques and helped them visualize improvement in their conditions.

Two years later, 10 percent were completely free of cancer. Another 10 percent were dramatically improved. A third 10 percent had their cancer stabilized.

This study came to our attention at the time that I had just been told that my lung cancer was terminal; that I should not expect to live more than a few more months. My wife and I made up our minds that if visualization gave me a 30 percent chance of staying alive instead of none, we were going to go there.

I cannot say that visualization is what cured me, but I can recommend it—in addition to everything else the physician wants to do.

Richard Bloch

Hypnosis

Hypnosis is a common component of some palliative cancer treatments. It helps reduce physical discomfort and stress, which promotes healing. There may be additional benefits.

29 Implants and Replacement Parts

An introduction to subjects that cancer patients can be forced to consider because of radical surgery.

The presumption of this chapter is that you need to know more about radical surgery. You have gone through or will soon go through the process of diagnosis, recommendation, second opinion, concurrence, discussion, and decision. And then you will face the loss of a body part and its aftermath. It's a lousy deal and an added challenge you didn't need.

The Loss

Whether your loss is a breast, eye, nose, ear, hand, arm, foot, leg, or something else, you will go through profound shock, followed by a period of adjustment. A substitution may be possible to restore appearance or some measure of capability. This can require further adjustment.

Your surgical team or hospital staff may introduce you to people with similar losses. Those who work in this environment know that you need to be as well prepared as possible to cope in this new place. If introductions don't happen, go to the Reference Center. Contact the organizations listed under "amputee" and one or more of the groups listed under your specific disease heading. Ask to speak to someone who has completed the process you are facing. As with the selection of other kinds of partners in this ordeal, the same sex, approximate age, range of interests, and family status may matter to you. You will benefit from the lessons they have for you and the encouragement of the example they set for you.

What Everybody Knows

From this point forward, don't be surprised to hear references to things that "everybody knows" about what's happening to you that you don't know anything about. Some of this supposed knowledge is fable, coming from people who don't know any more than you did before all this became up close and personal. Sometimes medical staff and third parties like insurance companies forget that you don't spend every minute of every day immersed in the detail of this stuff the way they do. They presume everybody knows.

Either way, stop the proceedings. Find out the details of the matter being discussed. Don't allow the doc or anyone else to ramble on. To the question, "Don't you know what I'm talking about?" answer, "No. And I need to. Please explain."

Other Things to Know About

Phantom Pain

After the amputation, you will probably experience discomfort that feels as if it is coming from the part of you that's been removed. This is known as "phantom pain" and is quite normal. People on your healing team may make references to it and to measures that minimize it. Or you may just wake up in the middle of the night, certain that someone's stuck a knife into a foot that's no longer there. Nobody can predict who will experience phantom pain, how severe it will be, or for how long – days, months, years – it will recur.

Physical Therapy

You will also face physical therapy to help surrounding muscles readjust to new demands. For example, it may puzzle you to learn that after breast surgery, time in a pool is necessary. Swimming to help damaged chest muscles is a normal part of recovery from some mastectomy procedures.

Prostheses

Recovery

There will be both professional and recreational activities that you will want to continue as an amputee. You will be amazed to discover how many newsletters and magazines out there support and help with whatever your interests are.

If you have lost a hand, arm, foot, or leg, you will probably decide to be equipped with a replacement part called a "prosthesis." This will be a surprisingly time-consuming and expensive experience, involving a specialist called a prosthetist. Go to the amputation listings in the Reference Center for all sorts of further information on this subject.

Your residual limb, often crudely and somewhat cruelly called your "stump," will be carefully treated to make sure it is healing properly and to prepare it for the stresses and strains of a prosthesis. Improper care, infection, or damage to it can lead to more surgery and perhaps even greater incapacitation.

If you lose some or all of an arm or leg, you will be using the services of a prosthetist for the rest of your life. Get a good one. For specific help in this important task, visit www.americanamputee.org. In the Web site's "Library," click on "National Resource Directory." Read the article on choosing a prosthetist. Then discuss your needs and situation with someone you trust who has been through this process ahead of you (see resources listed in the Reference Center).

You should probably end up with multiple prostheses. You may need one type for everyday activities. You may need another for a sport or for other reasons. If you have lost an arm, you may need multiple tool attachments for the mechanical replacement. "Young people often need sports limbs," Catherine J. Walden, executive director of the American Amputee Foundation, advises. "Older leg amputees are most likely to have swim legs prescribed . . . [but] many amputees do not have multiple prostheses because they can't afford it."

Demand funding for the full outfit, if you can. You will need the financial support and program continuity, if at all possible.

Your first prosthesis, or group of them, will probably not be your last. The industry standard is that an artificial limb wears out in three to five years.

After an initial period of adaptation, your body changes. The "socket" end of your prostheses will need to be adjusted as your stump changes. The adjustments may be less frequent after the first year or two but will never truly end.

The advance of prosthesis development will continue to be rapid. There will probably be advances that you want by the time your current tools wear out. Unless you are independently wealthy, keep financial support in your corner. All prostheses are expensive. The really great ones with electronics and high-tech materials may top $50,000. Sports equipment, such as an arm designed for golf or a special leg for running, can be equally expensive.

Work and Lifestyle Changes

Perhaps you plan to return to the job or type of work you had before the loss. Your prosthetist and your health insurer will expect to work on this with you. But maybe you feel that your life has been changed in a way that points you toward a new line of work or a new lifestyle.

Give this question careful thought. Leave room for options in your program and in the financial plan that supports it. Years ago, for example, a fellow who had lost a leg heard about an opening at a theme restaurant for a peg-legged ship's captain. He got an old-fashioned wooden "peg" and wore it to the interview. It led to a satisfying career with Chicken of the Sea tuna. There was also a fellow born without toes on his right foot who held the long-distance field-goal-kicking record in the NFL for several years.

Self-Help Groups

It has already been suggested that you consider joining a cancer-patient support group. Amputees are apt to benefit from the specialized wisdom of a second support group made up of other amputees who are not necessarily cancer patients. You have new issues and skills that will go down a whole lot easier with some informed help and the encouragement of people who have struggled with these problems ahead of you.

There are many support groups for amputees. The staff of your orthopedic surgeon probably invited you to one. Unless you live in a sparsely populated place, more are close by. You can also join virtual support groups on the Internet. The publications discussed in the section that immediately follows have helpful articles and organizational listings.

Information for Limb Amputees

If you are faced with the loss of a limb, have recently become an amputee, or have a child, parent, or other loved one facing this additional complication to life, order and review these invaluable resources. Between them, most questions are answered:

- The American Amputee Foundation offers a national resource directory that lists self-help, advocacy, and assistance groups. It contains basic advice on joining a support group, choosing and working with a prosthetist, prosthetic and orthotic products, residual-limb care, special needs of children, sports equipment, associations and organizations, publications, sports, and physical therapy. Call 501/666-2523 or visit www.americanamputee.org.

- The most comprehensive information for limb amputees is probably in *First Step, A Guide for Adapting to Limb Loss,* published by the Amputee Coalition of America. 126 pages. It also publishes a good bimonthly magazine, *In Motion.* Call 888/267-5669 or visit www.amputee-coalition.org.
- Join organizations. Learn about special people and places. Check out www.pvamagazines.com for sports and leisure opportunities. At www.activelivingmagazine.com, subscribe to *Active Living,* published quarterly in Canada. For a terrific place to shop, visit www.abledata.com.

Breast Reconstruction

Seventy-five percent of women who have a tumor removed from a breast also have reconstructive surgery. About half of these patients decide on a procedure called a TRAM flap, which takes the necessary building materials from elsewhere on the body, usually from the tummy, to reshape the breast. The other half choose artificial implants.

The woman who designed Barbie, Ruth Handler, pioneered the gel prosthetic in the 1970s and named it Nearly Me. It evolved into a family of products worn in bras, swimsuits, and other garments. Early implants followed. The resulting appearance of patients was often extremely pleasing, both to themselves and others. But the integrity of the implants and related health issues sometimes became problems later. Breast-implant technology is now far safer. For details, see your oncology team or the specialists it refers you to. Other resources are available under "Breast" in the "Yellow Pages" of the Reference Center.

The two ladies lounged and chatted in the assured manner of successful young professionals. It was somehow unremarkable that their heads were starkly hairless or that IV bags hung above them, dripping fluids. The topic was new breasts. "John really went for the way pregnancy changed me," the first one confided. "So I decided to go with a larger, fuller shape." "Well, I expect to get back to running. And Steve has always liked me skinny," the second one said. "I'm going for a high, perky look. My doctor calls them my 'sports boobs.'" They laughed.

Eyes and Other Cosmetic Parts

There are remarkably lifelike eyes, noses, ears, and other cosmetic parts that a patient can choose to wear. Plastic surgeons have methods of further improving their lifelike appearance. Some can be implanted.

In that regard, let's be candid. These sorts of reproductions are never perfect. Don't let that deter you from improving your appearance. For a great deal more on this, see the references under your cancer in the "Yellow Pages" of the Reference Center.

Cosmetic Surgery Package Deals

It is often wise to negotiate the processes of surgery and reconstruction as one package to make sure that everything is properly completed and paid for. If that fails and new costs come along, they may be quite substantial. Go for it anyway. You've only got one body. Repair of battle damage is essential. Financial help may materialize, even when it seems there is no hope. Just be sure you thoroughly explore the Resources Section. Let everybody know what your problem is so that help can find you.

Electronics

The science of myoelectronics now makes it possible for an artificial hand to tell the wearer that something is hot or cold, or to indicate the amount of pressure being put on something by the hand. There is an experimental chip implant that replaces functions lost after brain surgery. Much more is coming. Be certain you ask for the state-of-the-art when appliance shopping.

Orthotics

The manufacture and fitting of braces is known as the field of orthotics. Amazing feats of engineering help the spine, arms, legs, and joints. Some of this equipment has "smart" electronic components. An orthotics technician joins the orthopedic surgeon's team when needs in this field show up. One wag has suggested that the presence of an orthotics team at your bedside is a hopeful sign, indicating that there's still lots and lots of money in your health-insurance account. Humor aside, particularly for children and young adults, orthotics makes an important contribution to improved physical development. And if you don't have the money, see "Amputee" in the Reference Center "Yellow Pages" for leads.

Training in Using Replacement Parts

Learning to use replacement parts is not easy. Listen to your medical team and partners in this process. Believe it when you hear, "No pain, no gain." Moreover, you will experience failure before you reach success, and you will probably be depressed at times during the process. It may help to tack up a picture of a person you know who has gone through this ahead of you and made it out the other side into the sunshine.

Old age is no excuse. People in life's later years are the second-most-likely bunch to face this problem. (The largest group is kids aged ten to twenty.) Many programs are specifically designed for success with the geriatrically challenged.

You do what you gotta do.

Unlikely Heroes

Strange as it may seem, you will come to appreciate the ministrations of your trainers—Lash, Helga, and the Marquis.

30 Transplants

The transplant process includes complexities that your medical team must explain. Other subtleties, notably economic ones, are also important to know about.

For a quick overview of the subject, see "Transplants" in Chapter 27, "Treatments." Those few pages will do fine as a short course that explains the general topic and its implications. Furthermore, this chapter presumes that you have read them.

Your Medical Team's Transplant Literature

At the time your condition causes your oncologist to begin considering transplant therapy, you can expect to receive a ton of printed material on just what it's all about. Your doc specifically selected this info to explain the particular path your treatment will take. This will probably include an introduction to the place your medical team recommends that you go for the procedure. If you do not receive either the transplant explanation or the location recommendation at the time of your first transplant conference, it's probably an oversight. Mention it. You may also be shown a video or invited to a class or seminar on the subject. Patients who feel up to it should definitely attend the meeting. Those that don't should send a partner. These are helpful sessions.

The Lengthy Transplant Process

A transplant process dominates the patient's life for the first several months after it begins. It will continue to be a major health consideration for at least two years. It will affect your vigor. For women, conception during this time would be a very poor idea. See the list of questions to ask and "dos and don'ts" in the transplant section of Chapter 27.

Financing Your Transplant

Please be certain that all parties are in agreement on a full payment plan *before* you begin the transplant process, or be prepared to pick up a six-figure tab.

Hospitals have distinct business styles. Some don't mention payment before treatment begins. If the medical team doesn't make the bill an early order of business, you must. Transplant procedures cost hundreds of thousands of dollars, which could end up as your debt.

Once your medical team has arrived at a specific program recommendation, you must take this matter to your health insurer. Transplants are a common exclusion from medical insurance programs. If you're covered, fine. Get all the details in writing. If you're only partly covered, or if "transplant" is an exclusion, *do not go forward without a financial solution*. This forces everybody to address the problem at a time when all sides are strongly motivated to solve it. In this atmosphere, any number of creative alternatives can work. Nor should you worry that it will take very long.

Your medical team's administrator may help. Seek the financial advice of organizations listed under "Transplants" in the Reference Center's "Yellow Pages." You'll find more possibilities in the chapters in "Supporting Resources," Part IV.

Donor Searches and Other Loopholes

Some of the less obvious costs associated with transplantation are often not covered by the health insurance provider, even when the procedure itself is supposed to be. One of the potentially most ruinous is the search for a donor. When a sibling or other blood relative fails to produce a match, large pools of candidates must be searched. This is typically done on an open-ended hourly-fee basis. A bill in excess of $10,000 is not unusual.

Before you agree to finance such a search, talk to experts you can find in organizations listed under "Donor-Patient Matching Programs" and "Transplants" in the "Yellow Pages" of the Reference Center.

If you know you are going to need a donor and none of your blood relatives are possible candidates, you may be able to donate blood or bone marrow to yourself. Your doc knows all about this. Ask if you can donate before chemo or some other treatment makes it impossible.

Check for other loopholes within loopholes. Your health insurer may not cover costs of treating diseases caused by the transplant process, prosthetic devices, hearing aids, physical therapy, dentistry, ophthalmology, and extended home care. If these discrepancies are discovered ahead of time and negotiated, the financial impact may be at least manageable.

The Patient's Typical Experience

The information that your medical team gives you will cover the details of the transplant experience in as positive a way as possible. Sometimes it smoothes things over a bit too much. Patients miss the point that this isn't going to be all sunshine and flowers.

You need to know that you're going to feel sick during at least a portion of the time you are undergoing the chemo preliminaries, and again during early weeks of recovery in isolation. Another low point of your isolation is usually at least one bout with serious infection—which can be life threatening. It may help to remember that you're going through all this because, if you don't, your cancer's going to kill you. You've got to go forward. And you can expect your medical team to minimize your discomfort.

It won't be all that bad. The more important point is that you must not be deluded into supposing that you'll have the inclination to catch up on your reading or the mental acuity to make good business decisions. You're going to be a blob dozing through daytime TV at least some of the time. Particularly given your alternative, that's okay, isn't it?

A New Birthday

Growing numbers of transplant patients consider the day they got new marrow or stem cells to mark a rebirth. You will see references to birthdays in the literature. If you join a support group, you may even get a cake on your transplant anniversary. Your transplant will have rules for maintenance and intervals at which it must be checked, but it is a gift from the magi, well worth celebrating.

A Fragile and Perishable Opportunity

Your medical team thinks a transplant is the proper treatment for your form and stage of cancer, or they would not have proposed it to you. What you may not realize is that a transplant proposal also implies that your general health permits it. You have a window of opportunity that may not remain open. In some cases, transplants can be performed only once. Ask your doctor about both these general conditions.

If a transplant has been suggested to you, move forward with all deliberate haste. You obviously need to finish your qualification tests. You must know about the side effects, both temporary and permanent. You need to decide on the place to receive treatment and on the terms of payment. There's a group of doctors sitting on a supervisory tumor board that will probably have to approve plans for your transplant. Then accept this offer or at least make certain that you are not sealing a door you may want to open later.

Extra Goodies

If you are receiving financial aid, the provider may specify where you will receive the procedure. If not, spend a little time exploring your options. There are more available spaces at transplant facilities than there are patients. And so, insofar as they can, some of these places will compete for your business. Look at the offers. Maybe "Ask Jeeves" on the Internet. Discuss choices with your medical team. There may be costs that can be waived, a nicer place to stay, free accommodations for family nearby, better food, a better library, cable TV, activities, a pet-visitation center, or some other extra goodie to cash in on.

If an insurance company—or an HMO or government-plan administrator—is directing you to a treatment facility and you discover that you won't be admitted immediately, discuss the delay with your doctor. Any wait, when prompt medical attention is prudent, is sufficient reason for you to be allowed some alternate choices. The quality of your treatment should be the paramount concern, of course. Maybe the outfit with the crowded calendar has the best staff or the most complete facility. Then again, maybe not. If there is no compelling medical or economic reason to go there, you may be able to use the delay as an excuse to transfer your case elsewhere.

31 Vaccines

This chapter should have been called "Immunotherapies." But who'd have understood what we were going to discuss? (Come back in ten years, and everybody will.)

People generally expect a cure for cancer to be found one day. They envision a vaccine along the lines of what we have now for measles, mumps, smallpox, tetanus, and polio. There is no such general prevention for cancer on the horizon. But the vaccine concept—that effective fighters made from parts of the problem can be used to defeat it—has been producing encouraging results. Cancer assailants made from cells of the disease, human genetic material, and elements of the body's immune system are now in use, with many more coming. These are parts of a treatment concept broadly referred to as "immunotherapy." One or more of its products may become very important to your recovery.

Immunotherapy Q&A

Might one of these new medicines be ready for me now? Yes. The FDA has approved several immunotherapies for use against specific cancers. This has been mighty important to patients with certain inoperable conditions and for others whose cases did not respond to the drugs that normally work.

Many additional immunotherapies are moving through the clinical trial process. Some play new, sophisticated roles. Others replace chemotherapies. The chemo-replacement role has been particularly good news in situations where the old treatment was stressful to patients, or when the patient's system would not tolerate further chemo.

Custom immunotherapies are also being used with great success. Made from the patient's own cancer, genetic material, or blood cells, these are known as "autologous vaccines." Just imagine. Your own custom medicine. Vaccine for an army of one.

Should I want immunotherapy? This is a complex question. It may help if we think through some aspects of your circumstance.

The ideal course would be for you to receive the tried-and-true treatment for your type of cancer and to have it do the trick. That's likely to be some mix of surgery, radiation, and chemo. Immunotherapies are reserved for cases in which the cancer is a tougher opponent. So in the sense that you'd rather have your case be cut and dried, it's not particularly good news to have an immunotherapy recommended to you.

If an immunotherapy is proposed that is still in clinical trial, you face an even less conservative treatment path. This is noteworthy but not necessarily alarming. One of the terrific benefits of these new strategies is that they can be effective when the patient's condition discourages the use of chemo or surgery.

Two more reasons to avoid immunotherapy are cost and time. Some of these medicines have to be ordered or require the patient to travel somewhere. The autologous ones take time to manufacture. In all cases, the costs of treatment go up—sometimes way, way up. No point in wasting money, even if your insurance company has you covered.

Table 31.1 Types of Vaccines (Also Known as Specific Immunotherapies) Available in 2005

Vaccine Type	How It Works	Current Applications (mostly in clinical trials)
Tumor cell	Dead or neutered cancer cells in the vaccine create antigens, substances that provoke attack on the patient's disease by the immune system.	Breast Colorectal Kidney (renal) Leukemia Lung Melanoma Ovary
Dendritic cell	A type of white blood cell that is "taught" to spot the antigens of the patient's cancer and to point them out to the immune system for attack.	Colorectal Kidney Lung Melanoma Non-Hodgkin's lymphoma Prostate
Antigen	A specific antigen or group of them are used to encourage the immune system to search out and destroy a cancer that it might not otherwise recognize as a threat.	Breast Colorectal Melanoma Ovary Pancreas Prostate
Anti-Idiotype	Antibodies are soldiers the immune system sends to fight disease. Each type of antibody has its own weapon, called an idiotype. Sometimes a vaccine that dumps a lot of weapons into the body stimulates the immune systemto send out more antibodies. In the process, cancer cells are discovered and destroyed.	Breast Colorectal Lung Lymphoma Melanoma Multiple myeloma
DNA	Bits of DNA are used to stimulate production of cancer-fighting antibodies when vaccines become less effective.	Head and neck Leukemia Melanoma Prostate
Cachexia (generic name)	Helps block the onset of a disease of the same name, an opportunistic affliction that wastes away the bodily resources of cancer patients.	Cachexia (not a form of cancer)

Are there immunotherapies I can take to prevent cancer? No. All immuno-therapies are parts of the defense against a present enemy.

There is quite a lot one can do to avoid cancer, however. Of the cancer deaths in 2004, "about one-third [187,900 were] related to [poor] nutrition, physical inactivity, overweight, and other lifestyle factors," the American Cancer Society reports in its annual summary of cancer facts and figures. Smoking, heavy drinking, and irresponsible sex were the three most danger-ous "other lifestyle factors." (The current edition of this document is avail-able at www.cancer.org.)

What kinds of immunotherapy are available? Here are some generally rec-ognized kinds of treatment that fall under the heading of immunotherapy. Though the listing was complete at the time of this writing, science in this area changes rapidly. Check "immunotherapies" at www.aboutmycancer.com if your interest is casual. But if your need pertains to a current illness, the oncologist in charge—or the resource that the oncology team directs you to—is the place to go.

1. Vaccines: These are also called "active specific immunotherapies" (see the nearby table, "Types of Vaccines").
2. Cytokine therapy: Two cytokines, interferon-alpha and interleukin-2, are impressive for the way they help the body attack advanced melanoma. The strategies for fighting other advanced-stage cancers—notably meta-static renal (kidney), leukemias, lymphomas, breast, prostate, and myelo-mas—sometimes include cytokines. Oncologists aren't fond of cytokine therapy because it makes patients sick and encourages fluid retention.
3. Monoclonal antibodies: Antibodies that specifically attack some non-Hodgkin's lymphomas, leukemias, and breast, colorectal, prostate, and multiple myelomas are being manufactured in laboratories. The FDA has approved several of these. More are in clinical trial. A few are radio-active or contain radioactive particles.

Volunteer with Caution

There is a saying among test pilots that you can tell the pioneers by the arrows in their backsides. The implication holds true for the sometimes unpredictable results of experimental medicine. Don't go there without a persuasive reason—and watch out for consequences.

In current medical literature, "traditional" healing practices are those that meet the standards of modern science. A "nontraditional" one is anything—drug, treatment, device—that has not met those standards.

The pace of medical science is much faster today than ever. We have learned more about cancer in the past three years than in all the centuries before.

Things to do or wear or eat—without the benefit of scientific proof—make up the vast majority of all medical treatments that have ever existed. Humankind has been dosing itself for this or that medicinal purpose for more than 10,000 years. By some accounts, not until 1910 did good health and healing practices begin the steep climb to today's scientific heights. So you have 9,900 years of rattles, chants, poultices, herbs, and eye of newt on one side of the dateline, and 100 years of fancy chemistry and statistical analysis on the other.

In our mind's eye, people seem to have done all right in the good old days. We need to be reminded that, in 1900, the average man in the United States stood five feet, four inches tall and at birth could expect to live to age forty-seven. That was not very long ago. Healing traditions persist concerning all the thousands of things that people consumed, wore, imbedded in each other, cut off, bled, purged, put into their water, gave to their livestock, sacrificed, buried, dug up, bathed in, and burned. We have, after all, evolved—not cast all aside.

When the truth comes out, that most alternative therapies have little or no compelling clinical evidence to support their effectiveness or safety, most people we talk to are stunned. . . .

Perhaps even worse is the way the popular media introduce alternative medicine concepts; . . . reports promote it as if it has been proven.

Dónal O'Mathúna, PhD, and Walt Larimore, MD, Alternative Medicine *(HarperCollins, 2001)*

Many things that people took medicinally a hundred years ago worked. Some have met the standards of scientific examination and continue in general use. Others have remained as folk remedies. More have been improved upon or discredited.

Respect for Those Who Want to Help

This seems a good place to point out that, while you may not share their conviction, there are likely to be people around you who believe in various home remedies for your cancer. They may beg you to do or not do something because of your condition. They may have a stone that you should keep in special "medicinal" drinking water, a copper bracelet, herb tea, a rabbit's foot. Be sure to thank them. Check with your doc if there is any chance that something from their remedy may enter your system. But try to honor the giver by going along with the intent of the gift. Friends shouldn't be dismissed.

Nontraditional Cancer Medicine's Success Record

A person diagnosed with active cancer who does nothing or takes an exclusively nontraditional treatment path will die either of the disease or of any of many ailments that ensue during development of the disease about ninety-six times out of a hundred. This figure is based on repeated studies by the National Cancer Institute and the America Cancer Society.

Maybe ninety-six out of a hundred is harsh. There is justifiable debate over whether a whole list of effective treatments such as blood products, Cooley toxins, and gamma globulin are traditional or nontraditional. Let's further acknowledge that the statistics could be prejudiced by other factors. Now, ladies and gentlemen of the jury, what do you think? Could you imagine that all that quibbling could bring the ratio down to 90 percent—nine out of ten? Maybe eight out of ten? Do I hear seven? If so, would that encourage you to go against the best advice of your oncologist?

With that exact objective in mind, a plaintive murmur of argument comes from the people and remarkably large industries that dwell on the fringes of this subject.

Family custom, values, emotions, money, fear, and disappointment further confuse treatment issues. But after the talking's done, it always comes back to a personal decision that can have an irrevocable result.

We have seen popular public figures like Steve McQueen fight cancer with every resource wealth and science can marshal—and fail. The last things that McQueen tried before he died were nontraditional treatments. Both sides in the dispute have cited his example. The nontraditionalists use it to point to the less than perfect record of oncology medicine. Traditionalists say he should have stayed in the hospital program. It strips down to this: Each side is trying to make debating points and perhaps a profit. You have cancer. You don't want to make points or money. You want to be healed. Choose the treatment path most likely to be in your best interest.

Some Nontraditional Methods in Perspective

If you are a hunter, you know that you have a better chance of dropping a bear with a large-bore rifle than with a .22. The little gun works. But it's foolish. In the same way, everyone acknowledges that some teas, poultices, vitamins, and other "natural" products are healthful. The argument for the pharmaceuticals used in oncology is that they multiply whatever healing power these products have by manyfold and may focus more precisely on the trouble spot. You shouldn't trust something out of a health-food store to remediate cancer anymore than you would trust a .22 to stop a bear.

Now, if it's your last chance before the bear eats you, you'll try whatever's handy. That's probably what Steve McQueen figured.

The 2 Percent Exemption

In about 2 percent of cases, cancer goes away. There does not seem to be any pattern, any necessary correlation between type of patient, cancer, stage, and the occasional miracle cure. It just happens.

You must keep this pattern of happenstance in mind when you are confronted by a tale of some amazing cure. It may have happened exactly the way the teller explains it: The 5 mg dose turned the cancer green and the

Nearly half of all U.S. adults now go outside the health system for some of their care, . . . 600 million visits a year . . . [for] practices ranging from acupuncture and chiropractic, to . . . coffee enemas.

Geoffery Cowley, "Now, 'Integrative' Care" (Newsweek, December 2, 2002)

REPORT FROM THE COMEBACK TRAIL *The Lowly, Disgusting Leech: Credited, Discredited, Then Credited Again . . .*

One of the presences in the operating room during your next surgery may have five pairs of eyes, thirty-two brains, and three hundred teeth. The FDA now approves the use of leeches to avoid toxic blood clotting. A medical tradition dating back to Greece, fifth century BC, slithers on.

20 mg dose sent it packing. Or it could be that something else contributed, or it could have been coincidence.

A tale of amazing cure is called "anecdotal." While true, there is no proof as to why it happened. Medicine cannot repeat the success. Much worse, this sort of isolated good news does not escape the possibility of being part of the completely baffling 2 percent exemption.

Books and Country-Club Clinics

A not-uncommon scenario: The posh clinic that looks like a country club invites you to spend an afternoon with its founder. The first ten people through the gate will receive a free copy of the founder's book.

Some patients who experience wonderful responses to exotic treatments, or who escape from their cancer altogether, form organizations to tout the miracle. They also write books. They are sincere, one hopes. But unless the experience or treatment has passed through scientific study and can now be repeated at will to the benefit of similar cancer patients, the proof is anecdotal and the process is experimental. You get no promises, much less guarantees. You get no money back, and you get no sympathy if all was not as it seemed.

Please keep the 2 percent exemption in mind when you contemplate the vast array of nontraditional helps and solutions offered to cancer patients and their families. Look them up on the Internet. Ask your oncologist about them. Bring caution and skepticism to the evaluation process.

Palliative Contributions of Nontraditional Therapies

There is no question that at least some of the "natural foods" and other plant products that have helped humankind for thousands of years can make us feel better. When Marco Polo visited China, he discovered a culture with sixteen thousand herbal remedies in use. His own country knew of a few hundred of them. Herbal compounds he brought back to Italy were far more important to the advancement of European civilization than the pasta was.

Booze is another great example. If you're Italian, you may put anisette on the sore gums of your teething toddler. If you're Irish, it may be whiskey. The active ingredient remains the same. It can relieve tensions after a bad day. It can promote romance. It won't cure cancer, but it may be just the thing you need after a cancer treatment.

Costs of Nontraditional Healing

If you are weighing alternatives to mainline cancer treatment because you think it may be a cheaper or faster way to go, here are some considerations to keep in mind.

1. Limited health-insurance coverage: Physicians worked with actuaries to design health insurance in all its forms. Health insurance mirrors the standards and practices that docs learned about in med school. Litigation

Beware of any alternative treatments marketed in TV, radio, Internet, and print ads without scientific evidence to back them up, or requiring travel to another country. Other warning signs include therapies that claim to cure all forms of cancer, or those that urge you to avoid other treatments. Ask your cancer specialist for an opinion on alternative therapies.

M. D. Anderson Cancer Center Web site bulletin

The FDA reports that 1,400 plants are used to make 20,000 herbal remedies in the United States. Few have been tested in controlled studies.

has further shaped these plans to discourage you from treatment areas that lawyers think may result in lawsuits later.

2. Longer active suffering: Most of the tools of nontraditional medicine are not as sharp as those of the mainstream oncologist. Though it is dangerous to generalize, your cancer probably won't respond as quickly, and natural pain relievers are less effective.

3. Travel: Clinics that offer nontraditional medicine are nowhere near as numerous as mainstream treatment centers. It is likely that you will need to travel and stay to receive the full benefit of the program at such a place.

4. Loss of employer confidence: There is a general belief in the United States that the oncology community has it more right than wrong. Patients who trust another path may find their judgment questioned.

Alternative and Complementary Therapies

Some important therapies reside in a place between today's nontraditional and traditional brands of medicine. They are generally believed to have

Table 32.1 Alternative and Complementary Therapies

Type	Description
Acupressure	Finger pressure that accomplishes much the same result as acupuncture needles, with an accompanying often luxurious massage
Acupuncture	Asian practice of inserting fine needles into the body to stop pain and promote healing
Aromatherapy	The scent of plant extracts used to reduce pain and promote relaxation
Chi Kung (one of several names)	Oriental exercise program that helps some people, particularly seniors, improve vitality
Chiropractic	Adjustments in the alignment of the spine that promote healing and mobility
Guided imagery (also called visualization)	Mental focus on dreams and goals, sometimes with pictorial and verbal aids, that reduces stress and promotes healing (a notable element of sports psychology)
Herbs	Teas, poultices, potions, and pills that may be available under the supervision of your oncologist
Massage	When the form of cancer permits it, relaxes muscles and stimulates circulation
Other touch therapies	Asian and Native American therapies involving touch, and often heat, that can improve the sense of well-being and may have other benefits
Vitamins	Food supplements that promote good nutritional balance in the body
Yoga	Exercises that promote healing, mobility, and sometimes tranquility

merit, but the degree of their value and related questions have not been fully answered, so far as oncology is concerned. Even so, it is not unusual to find practitioners of these arts available in the clinic, if not actively serving on oncology teams. If any of the many benefits of these therapies appeals to you, please make certain that your oncologist approves it in advance. In the case of substances you are expected to ingest, your pharmacist also needs to know.

An Old Story

I first became involved with Brenda's care after she was brought to the emergency room while having a seizure. The MRI showed cancer had spread to the brain and bones. Brenda told how for more than a year she had worried about a growing lump in one breast. She had thought it merely part of her fibrocystic breast condition, an annoying ailment though not dangerous.

Brenda had gone to her local health food store where the well-intended owner recommended a number of nutritional therapies and dietary supplements. Brenda also saw a local alternative medicine practitioner who, without even examining her, recommended other alternative therapies.

Days passed, then weeks. The lump continued to grow. By the time I saw Brenda, a young woman in her twenties, there would be no cure, no happy ending. I could only try to relieve her pain, guilt and suffering.

Walt Larimore, MD (in Alternative Medicine, *by Dónal O'Mathúna, PhD, and Walt Larimore, MD [HarperCollins, 2001])*

33 Things They May Forget to Tell You about Chemo

Forgetfulness has always been with us. "Oops" is an excuse most of us learn around age two.

Some people never forget anything that they'll need on a trip. If you're one of them, that's just disgusting. Most of us forget something. Some of us have left children.

This chapter is a collective lost-and-found of issues medical teams have forgotten to tell patients about upcoming chemo treatments. Read the section on chemotherapy in Chapter 27, "Treatments," if you haven't already. Some of the information in this chapter duplicates it, to provide context. Please read both chapters to get the whole picture.

If you are headed for chemo and you find something noted here that your medical team has not discussed with you, ask about it. The most likely explanation is that what you found here does not apply in your case. But ask. Preparing for chemo is an important and complex process. Doctors and chemo nurses sometimes forget things, too.

Orientation

Chemotherapy is the generic name for a type of systematic administration of drugs to treat, or to prevent, some condition in your body. Your chemotherapy drugs may attack your cancer directly or treat some related thing, some unrelated thing, or a group of things. Your chemo may come in the form of shots or pills. It comes most famously as a series of infusions that you receive intravenously from bags over minutes to hours, during sessions in an infusion room. Being "systematic," these sessions may occur daily, weekly, or monthly.

While not meaning to slight pills or shots, this chapter focuses on the sort of chemo that comes from bags, in Infusion or Chemo Rooms.

Fear

Chemo isn't going to be the most difficult thing you have ever gone through—not even close. If you have broken a bone, you have been through a far more difficult experience and much greater pain. If you have been seasick, it is likely that you have endured more severe nausea than will come from the chemo experience. If you've ever had a bit too much to drink, you've experienced greater disorientation. Everyone loses sleep from time to time. Everyone has had a day when a nap in the afternoon was nice. That leaves maybe losing your hair as a new experience, though most patients don't.

Millions of people—literally millions—have gone through these chemo experiences ahead of you. Some of them are standing by right now, hoping you will phone them. Go to the Reference Center. Look in the "Yellow Pages" under "Counseling" or the listing for your type of disease.

On a Chemo Day

What to Wear

A physical examination before or after chemo may require that you disrobe. Not chemo. Most patients receive it in street clothes. If a catheter has been installed, wear a shirt that allows easy access to the port, of course.

Most patients receive chemo in a semi-reclining position. Women may find pants more comfortable than a skirt. Jewelry and makeup are optional.

Chemo is often administered in a room with other patients. If that is a possibility, perfume and shaving lotion are apt to distress others—most certainly those with respiratory difficulties. On general principle, arrive clean and unscented.

What to Bring

(This section presumes that your destination is a Chemo Room bed or over-stuffed chair from which you will receive chemo by intravenous drip over a period of perhaps an hour or more.)

Bring a companion if at all possible. If you will be leaving the clinic by car, it is advisable to bring a person with a driver's license. You probably shouldn't drive right after a treatment. The chemo will inhibit your reflexes, depth perception, and judgment to some extent.

A cell phone that goes off in a Chemo Room is going to disturb other patients. Your conversation with the caller will further annoy. If you must be inconsiderate, be brief, and remember to apologize to those around you afterward.

Knitting, quilting, and other personal projects are fine distractions to bring. Game Boy and other toys help pass the time. There are usually people trying to read. The subject had better be a good one. Some of the drugs can make you sleepy. A laptop computer may be fine, though you may find it difficult to use with one hand or arm hooked into an IV.

Bring extra socks so you can kick off your shoes and still keep your feet warm.

Salty snacks are particularly satisfying to some people during chemo. Bring a bag of your favorite potato chips, nuts, crackers, or some such.

Many Chemo Rooms have a communal table for goodies. People bring fruit, cookies, candy, popcorn—whatever snack they want to share. You may see expensive chocolate next to homemade s'mores. There's no general rule about what to bring, and no stigma to those who don't contribute.

Every Chemo Room has its own personality. It would be wise not to bring anything for sharing on your first visit. Make note of how things are organized. If there is a goodies table, you will get a good sense of what to bring next time—if, and only if, you are inclined to.

Your Activity Schedule

Before you go to chemo, finish whatever needs to be accomplished that day. Until you know better, plan nothing after you get home from chemo except a nap.

A percentage of those receiving chemo return to work or to some other productive activity later in the day. This is more apt to happen following later treatments than after the first one or two. The body becomes more accustomed to the drugs. If you have things you must do, and if the effects of chemo can be overcome, your doctor probably won't object. As a general principle, pushing yourself is not a good idea. There may be health, stress, misjudgment, and other unfortunate consequences, such as vomiting.

During Chemo Treatment

Drink lots of water. With all the liquid going in from the bag over your head, the suggestion that you drink lots of water during chemo may seem strange.

Believe it or not, chemo patients may become dehydrated during treatment. Also, you will have fewer side effects if you drink several glasses of water. The nurses love to see patients make trips to the bathroom during treatment. It means their chemo session is being hydrated and toxins are being flushed to the place they belong.

Coffee, tea, soft drinks, and other beverages that are mostly water are not as effective in this role as plain water. The temperature of your drink does not matter.

Keep your head well above your waist. Sometimes, patients who receive chemo while lying down leave with "puffy face." It won't last long, and it doesn't cause any medical concern, but you look like you've been rode hard and put away wet.

Make a friend. Learn a name. Get a life story. Compare photos. Never, never, never just sit there. Friendship and laughter are healers. Fears go away. Friends also provide wisdom and new knowledge. You may look back on your chemo experience as rewarding because of the new acquaintances or advice that came out of it.

After a Chemo Treatment

Keep a couple of airsickness bags and a box of tissues handy when you pack up to go home after treatment. You may be exceptionally prone to motion sickness during the ride. Those plastic bags that the clinic provides to patients who need to store street clothes may be an excellent substitute for airsickness bags. The opening is bigger. You can stick your whole head in to be sure you're hitting the mark. Just be certain the bag is waterproof and sturdy.

Chemo and Self-Medication

Alcohol

Sometimes an oncologist will suggest a glass of wine or a beer in the evening, following chemo. The doc means one or, at the very most, two glasses. If a bit of the grape appeals to you, ask your doc. You can expect to get the nod unless your chemo or one of the accompanying drugs reacts negatively to it.

It is definitely unwise to drink more than that after chemo—or at any other time during the weeks to months of your treatment program. It is crazy to drink before going to chemo: Alcohol may not sit well; it may disrupt the treatment's effects; it could embarrass you.

Drugs

If you habitually take a controlled substance that your doc does not know about, you are in big trouble, as you know. Talk to a drug-addiction counselor immediately. If you don't know one, look up Alcoholics Anonymous in your phone book's white pages. They can help, even if you are not an alcoholic or addict.

Health Tips

You need to stay healthy. Avoid people with colds and flu. Don't give infection an opening. Some general lifestyle practices that will help during the time you are receiving chemotherapy and immediately afterward appear in the "Health Tips" table.

Table 33.1 Health Tips

Recommendation	Comment
Wash your hands after exposure to germs or infection.	Wash with warm water and soap for at least twenty seconds. Waterless antibacterial lotions also work.
Use air purifiers at home and at work.	Explain your need to have safe air to the manufacturer. Get a recommendation.
Aspirin may have serious side effects.	Ask your doctor to recommend an over-the-counter pain remedy.
Insist on clean, healthy friends.	Demand that they have clean hands and no communicable diseases or stay away.
No manicures, pedicures, or similar procedures that may cut or abrade.	Exceptionally serious infection may result.
Get dental work done first.	Complete dental surgery and teeth cleaning. Consult with your oncologist before dental work during chemo.
Avoid physical contact with the general public that may transmit a cold or flu bug.	At work, church, and sports stadiums. Professions such as teaching pose extra risks. Discuss a facemask or, much better, take leave or a sabbatical.
Play only with healthy children.	No diaper changing. Don't wipe noses. Don't touch vomit.
Reduce stress at work.	Little or no overtime. No high-pressure environments.
Avoid travel; visiting a third-world country would be insane.	Applies to all public conveyances—busses, ships, trains, planes. Commuting included.
Vaccinations, flu, and pneumonia shots may be reasonable safety measures.	Discuss with your oncologist first.
Don't put off or interrupt treatments.	Get chemo started right away. If you delay, a condition may evolve that is no longer responsive. At that point, your remaining options can be limited.
Stay out of the sun.	Do not allow any part of your body to become suntanned for at least a year after completing chemo. Your skin is extra photosensitive. Burns, infections, and other nasty side effects can be serious. Should someone suggest a ride in a convertible with the top down, recognize their thoughtfulness, then decline. The breeze and sunshine are too much of a good thing for you.
If you garden . . .	Wear gloves. Don't inhale garden sprays. Beware of biting bugs.
Learn and practice sterile procedures in the kitchen.	Keep dishes, work surfaces, walls, and floors extra clean. Empty trash. Keep the disposal clear. Clean the refrigerator. No insects, especially winged ones.

(Continued)

Table 33.1 (Continued)

Recommendation	Comment
Avoid raw fruits and vegetables.	Don't eat anything you didn't just pick up and peel yourself. (All must be peeled.)
Don't eat raw shellfish or other uncooked seafood.	Exclude even the temptations of a sushi chief.
Don't eat alfalfa sprouts.	This is an ingeniously eclectic plant.
Don't consume unpasteurized dairy products.	Few are available. Some markets and delis carry unpasteurized cheese products.
Slice prepared foods at home.	Don't let the butcher or deli person cut up chickens, cheeses, or deli meats for you. Take them home whole.
Wear latex gloves when around dirt and grease.	If a glove tears, remove it, wash the hand carefully, then put on a new glove.
Use a hand can opener.	Keep its cutting area very clean. Put it through the dishwasher frequently.
Defrost foods in the refrigerator or microwave.	Never allow thawing on a counter.
Set the temperature of your refrigerator at 40°F or less. Set the freezer temp at zero.	The area of your refrigerator nearest the freezer may freeze foods stored there. Consider those acceptable losses.
Be aware that pets can be a health problem.	Consider the possible problems of an unhealthy pet. Don't clean up pet urine or feces. Don't change the birdcage liner.
Keep your teeth clean.	Use a soft-bristle brush and nonabrasive cleaner.
Don't vacuum.	Don't enter a room in which a vacuum is in operation for at least three months after completing chemo.

Don't Hide If You Don't Have To

You may be avoiding friends and family for fear of contagion when your immune system is in fact working fine and you are not particularly susceptible to infectious diseases. If you are short of white blood cells or a white-cell constituent called neutrophil, your hazards are greater. You can stay abreast of this condition by checking blood-test results. Learn the numeric ranges of normal and abnormal, and what each portends. Discuss this with your doctor.

The Long-Term Effects of Chemo

Some chemotherapy can have a lasting effect on organs and the immune system. During the weeks to months it may take for you to recover fully, the opportunities for various complications are great. Get your oncologist to discuss these with you. You will need to know what to do and when. You may also experience less ability to concentrate, to remember, or to perform other acts of mental agility that were normal for you before you were affected by what your med team casually calls "chemo brain."

Often-Used Chemotherapy Drugs

About thirty pharmaceuticals plus "investigational" drugs are used in cancer chemotherapy. It's a dynamic list. Compounds are added. Others drop out of use. Dosages change. So it is not wise to question anyone other than your doctor or a Chemo Room nurse about the specific effects of the treatment prescribed for you.

You may be in regular contact with people you've met at a charity or at a support-group meeting who have disturbing things to say about the chemo drugs prescribed for you. Before you take their words to heart, be sure they have specific knowledge of your exact protocol. For example, some established drug may have caused nausea or hair loss in the past. But used differently today, it is less likely to produce these side effects.

Key People to Tell about Your Chemo

Your Dentist

Chemo can cause gum disease and tooth decay. Have a copy of your oncologist's treatment protocol sent to your dentist. Then consult. Your dentist may want to schedule examinations during or following chemo or prescribe a special regimen of oral hygiene for you. This tip is of particular importance to children and teenagers.

Your Ophthalmologist

Another copy of your treatment protocol should go to your eye doctor. Cataracts and other eye disease may be side effects of chemo. The American Ophthalmological Society advises even people with 20/20 vision to have eye examinations after chemo.

We are specifically talking about a medical doctor who specializes in diseases of the eye who can examine you with more than an eye chart and write you a prescription. Some of these doctors even have oncology specialties. We are not talking about a person who may have a title that sounds much the same—and may be called "doctor" by the staff—but who does not have a medical degree and who is limited to selling you glasses and contacts.

Side Effects That May Confound Your Health Insurer

Medical insurance often slights coverage for dentistry and eye disease. So be prepared for an automatic rejection when you open the subject of coverage for special examinations and treatments after chemo. This would be a good time to call your case nurse, if your health-insurance provider has assigned one to you. Your oncologist may also be needed to differentiate these dental and ophthalmologic needs from the routine visits of the past.

The manufacturer of your chemo drugs may also have an interest in seeing that you have these expenses covered. To solicit the company's help, go to its Web site and explain your situation in an e-mail.

Supplemental Internet Research

Your chemotherapy-drug manufacturer's Web site will include a carefully crafted statement about results and side effects. It may or may not detail everything of interest to you. These blurbs have been so thoroughly masticated by the lawyers that some of them are no longer specific enough to be helpful. If you are given to this sort of investigation, you'll most likely consider your visit to this Web site to be a net plus, anyway.

If you "Google" the names, you will find newspaper articles and scientific papers about your chemo drugs. They may inform. There may be statements that disturb or depress you. And you will likely come across information that is totally pointless. It is still worth your while to be as informed as you can be. Then take your questions and concerns to your oncologist.

34 Taking Your Medicine

> You've got a lot of people prescribing things for you. Make sure somebody who understands the implications is keeping track of them all.

The law requires that only doctors write prescriptions because of the dangers. Controlled substances can be very sharp tools. So you are specifically instructed what to take, how big a dose, how often, and for how long. You may also be told about side effects, especially hazards like sleepiness or euphoria. So pause when the pharmacist smiles at you and asks, "Have you taken this medicine before? Do you have any further questions?" Think carefully. You're talking to a health expert who specializes in medicinal compounds. If it's your neighborhood pharmacy where you've been buying medicine for a while, the professionals behind this counter know quite a bit about your medical history and present condition. Probably more than you think. Behind that smile is an invitation to a valuable free consultation.

Asking Questions

Doctors who prescribe a medicine are responsible for telling you a bit about it and what it is expected to do for you. They may forgo these bases if you have taken the medicine before. Or the circumstances may be such that you missed key parts of a rapid-fire delivery. But if you don't understand— fully—why you are being given a medicine, you are expected to stop the process. Ask. This is a job that only you can take care of, and it is critical to your recovery. Make it a habit to know the name and the benefit of every drug the doc orders for you. Given the number of medicines you may be taking and all the tongue-twisting nomenclature, it is a good idea to write the information down.

So now you have returned home from the doctor's, clutching your new prescription paperwork. It was a bad day at the clinic. Everything was rushed, and you were not feeling very well to begin with. Maybe you remember your new drug's name. Maybe not. You probably remember what it's supposed to do for you. Maybe the warning of side effects is still vivid. Anyway, now you've got questions. What do you do? Relax. Make a list if you have several, so that you remember to ask them all. When you go to the drugstore to fill your prescription, ask your pharmacist.

Your Go-To Person

Your neighborhood pharmacist will follow all the instructions from all the doctors you see and jump through whatever hoops are necessary to get you the meds they order for you. This is an important person to you, from the beginning of your treatment program through that moment, perhaps years from now, when your oncologist tells you that you are officially a cancer survivor.

"Maybe we're a little more approachable than doctors," says M. T. Hanson, a man widowed by cancer and a pharmacist for thirty-five years. "More and more cancer patients come up to me with prescriptions and ask, 'What's this for?' I think it also has to do with confusion." Pharmacists, he says, "often have to repeat what the doctor has said and maybe explain things in words the person is more familiar with. This frequently brings up new questions, which we're very glad to answer. The more a patient knows about a drug, the better." Cancer is a strange and frightening experience. Patients deserve to hear explanations repeated and to ask new questions.

Your Medication Manager

Medication reactions are the fourth-leading cause of death in the United States, linked with more than a hundred thousand deaths, a million hospitalizations, and two million severe or permanently disabling reactions annually (*JAMA* 1998).

Jay Cohen, MD, Over Dose: The Case against Drug Companies (Tarcher/Putnam, 2001)

Note: These statistics are for all drugs used in all procedures in the United States during 1997. The portion ascribable to cancer treatments is a fraction of the whole.

During your battle with cancer, the responsibilities of your pharmacist are obviously important to you. If it is possible, you need to pick one pharmacist to coordinate all your drug needs or, at the very least, to know about them. The nature of your experience, which is apt to include treatments by multiple teams, is also apt to involve multiple pharmacies—the clinic's, the pharmacy in another specialist's building, perhaps several more—plus whatever medications the doctor gives you during treatments. But you can keep records of all of them and let your primary pharmacist know, and you should.

How to Get Started

Consider starting a better relationship with a central coordinating pharmacist by tossing all the medications you currently take into a paper bag, plus those old bottles still on a shelf, and going to see your pharmacist. "There's so much helpful information in a complete drug inventory," Hanson says. "Things the patient wouldn't know to tell me that are very important to the patient's recovery." For example: "You also have dental visits and reasons for seeing other doctors—more prescriptions and over-the-counter drugs can come from them." The number of pill bottles in the medicine cabinet becomes excessive and even dangerous. The result could be that you lose track of which you're taking for what, while a nascent chemical brew churns. With uppers working against downers and the green pills canceling out the blue ones, you need intervention by a central coordinating pharmacist just to keep the hair from growing on your forehead during full moons.

"I have to deal with conflicting medications every day," Hanson says. Different doctors treat patients for different things. On top of that, patients occasionally fib to get something with an extra, uh, appealing result. While this sort of thing is not a good idea during better times, promiscuous drugging during cancer treatment is like a person with the hiccups taking up sword swallowing.

Herbs, Tobacco, and Alcohol

Make sure your pharmacist knows about the nonprescribed things you put into your system. Herbs and vitamins from the health-food store, the little bit of wine you chase the pills with in the evening, the cigarettes you're supposed to have given up, the over-the-counter painkiller, analgesic, antacid—any of these may impact your recovery.

Feeling Worse

Until the science of medicine becomes as precise as, say, mathematics, there will be times when everything is done right and things still go wrong. Standard doses of medicines that usually do the job sometimes fail or do damage. If a new medicine you are taking does not produce the result you were told to expect or if it makes you ill, call your pharmacist.

Your doctor will also need to know about this. Discuss the best means of keeping your entire medical team, or teams, informed. In some cases, your pharmacist, as a medical professional, is better equipped to explain the circumstances to the others than you are. You just need to make certain that it happens.

No Quitting

It is fairly common for a patient to simply stop taking a drug because of some unpleasant experience: diarrhea, dizziness, insomnia—something like that. Don't just quit. Call your pharmacist and explain the problem. "Patients sometimes forget some of the instructions the pharmacist has given them," Hanson says. "They often don't read the complete instruction that comes with the prescription. Or they forget to take it in the way it was prescribed, such as with food. A quick phone call will usually help the patient use the drug in the way it was intended."

Sometimes there are side effects that can't be avoided, Hanson adds. Then pharmacist and doctor can consult. Solutions such as switching to another drug or adding a second compound to counter a side effect may solve the problem. "So long as the patient works with us, we'll usually find a way to achieve the treatment objective," says Hanson. "What scares us is when the patient makes decisions unilaterally."

Saving on Drugs

The fact that a first-class airline passenger who pays $2,000 for a seat and a coach passenger who pays $200 arrive at the destination at precisely the same moment has an analogy in the drugstore business. Tom Hanson: "Let us compare Nexium, a new stomach-acid controller, to Prilosec. The two compounds are quite similar. Prilosec, having been on the market longer, costs less. More important to patients on a budget, there's a Prilosec generic at a fraction of Prilosec's price." Hanson is always pleased to show patients the differences. In many cases, the prescribing doctor has no idea how much can be saved by substituting one drug for another. Many of the pharmaceuticals a cancer patient needs, including supplies, have options and price competitors.

Some things you can shop for and some you can't. If the co-pay on a prescription at one drugstore is twenty dollars, it will be the same everywhere you go.

The Forgotten Art of Compounding

Some of the more capable pharmacists can make up custom compounds. Radiation patients with skin burns may benefit from a special salve. You may need something out of the ordinary for a surgical wound or sores. A custom compound can relieve persistent pain in a particular muscle or joint. Your medicine can be reformulated minus the food dye you're allergic to. Your doc and your pharmacist can work together on distinctive solutions, if you ask them to.

But can pharmacists just make up a medicine? Isn't that illegal? Yes, they can, and no, it isn't. Pharmacists, particularly those who work in hospitals, frequently make custom compounds, usually because of the special needs of the patient. This was the normal procedure for all pharmacists until the 1960s, when the manufacture of drugs became much more strictly regulated by the Food and Drug Administration. Today, custom compounding is closely watched but remains essential and legal, despite reports to the contrary. "Compounding pharmacists fill at least 30 million prescriptions a year, or one percent of the three-billion-plus prescriptions dispensed in the U.S. annually," according to the *Wall Street Journal*.

Topics to Discuss with Your Pharmacist

Your pharmacist is accustomed to working with your medical team on specific solutions to problems that result from the disease, surgery, or medications and that relate to:

nausea	"dry eyes" (artificial tears)
pain	infections
sleep	fevers
nutrition	regularity
weight gain or loss	diarrhea

vitality
vitamins
sexual matters
radiation side effects
"dry mouth" (shortage of saliva)

organ damage
osteoporosis
digestive problems
anxieties of all sorts

Your pharmacist can help you with matters having to do with medical equipment and supplies or direct you to local resources. You can also discuss with a pharmacist the difficult and perhaps embarrassing aspects of incontinence, ostomy, and other procedures that require special care and consumable products.

35 Watching and Waiting

Is sitting on your hands ever a productive cancer strategy?

John and Marsha Dagenti have shared their lives for more than sixty years. Now, as cancer patients, it seems certain that they will share the same final illness. Though both are rapidly failing and John is no longer certain of his surroundings, their daughter, Barbette, regularly drives them to the St. Joseph's Cancer Treatment Center, where they receive chemotherapy and radiation.

Among the two hundred other cancer cases at the clinic are several apparently healthy patients who have been told that the therapy they need must be delayed. Some blood test shows an insufficiency, or the doctor thinks it would be "best" if "we put off further radiation for a while." Come back in a month. We'll check you again.

Isn't waiting dangerous? Cancer is a progressive disease. And why continue giving treatments to the Dagentis, who are not responding, and deny help to more vigorous patients who appear to be so needy?

This chapter is here because newly diagnosed patients and those close to them need to be aware in advance of the whats and whys of these sorts of events. It helps patients understand two of oncology's common tactical decisions. This background also helps partners be the supporting teammates patients need. And close observers cope better, with less need to be critical.

Watching and waiting are vital to good oncology, even though they don't appear to be moving the recovery process forward. The Dagentis are receiving this treatment. So are the patients told to come back in a month.

If this were a medical journal, there would be multiple chapters on each example. Fortunately, all we need to understand is that what appear to be wasteful treatments and maddening delays are neither.

The oncologist smiled at his patient. "You know, I don't find any change in your condition. We ought to wait a bit more before deciding on a next treatment step."

"I don't think so, doctor," the patient replied. "Something's not right."

With just an edge of exasperation: "Well, what do you want, another CT scan?"

"Yes," replied the patient thoughtfully, "I think so."

The result of this exchange revealed cancer progression that required immediate action.

Palliative Watching and Waiting

Palliative care is the type of treatment John and Marsha Dagenti are receiving. Its only objective is to ease suffering. It doesn't remediate their cancers. This type of medicine is part of many treatment programs that lead to recovery, though in the Dagentis' example it is part of preparation for a hospice program.

"Palliative care" is the general term for any medicine, radiation, or surgery whose foremost aim is to bring comfort to a cancer patient. The same term describes supporting measures such as hypnotism and positive mental imaging. In hundreds of thousands of cases a year, palliative care permits better rest and recuperation, and it gives the patient a much brighter outlook on life in general.

Palliative care can be part of an aggressive treatment program that includes measures that attack cancer. For example, patients about to receive anticancer drugs intravenously (chemo) will often first receive palliative meds to combat flulike symptoms and nausea. "Palliative" also describes the drugs patients receive to fight all sorts of cancer pains and to rest more comfortably after surgery. It is the sole form of treatment in other cases, such as the Dagentis'.

Timed and Measured Response

The docs know that watching and waiting is best in several sorts of situations.

- Sometimes a pause in treatment is necessary to allow recovery after chemo or radiation.
- After remission has begun, everybody waits to see what the cancer may do next.
- It may be necessary to allow time for damaged organs or the immune system to recover from events.
- Time may be needed to get over surgery.
- A delay in cancer treatment could be necessary to work on some other medical or physical need.

Observing from the wings, we don't know. And that's the point: A case comes to a treatment plateau for many reasons. You need to pay attention to what's going on in your case to avoid a misunderstanding.

What to Do While Watching and Waiting

Even though the big moves against your cancer have been made and everybody feels that things are going well, your doc may have a few chores for you.

Body Rejuvenation

Nutrition, exercise, and body-replenishing drugs may become main parts of your recovery process at this point. Periodic tests can accompany these. The purpose of such a program is to help your body build up its stamina and defenses and perhaps to combat some secondary, totally unrelated condition that you have. This is not a period of active cancer fighting. It is a time to replenish and rejuvenate, to be quietly vigilant.

Extra Treatments

Plateaus in disease treatment may call for chemo, even though cancer is no longer detectable. There's been a great deal of success recently using chemotherapy to extend the periods of remission from some cancers in this way.

System Overload

Your body's reaction to toxins may reach a point where the doc must stop using some medication, even though the cancer remains. The usual practice is to use another strategy to continue the battle, while an environmental cleanup of some sort has time to work.

These situations can also come along when damage to a natural serum, such as a blood product, forces a halt or slowdown. There are usually ways to help a situation in which, for example, an anemic patient can no longer receive blood transfusions.

Other Conditions That Change Treatment Patterns

Patient's Will to Live

The will to live has prolonged the life of many, many cancer patients beyond the point where the oncology community felt any optimism. Children will live out of obedience to their parents. Elders will live for children. Parents will hang on to see a graduation or to meet a newborn grandchild. Dogged determination, a respected part of the cancer-care equation, may bring on treatment changes.

Doctor's Sworn Oath and Legal Issues

In any case where there is doubt as to what to do, the doctors and lawyers force the battle to continue through any means available. The patient may be only technically alive, but some treatment continues because of an unresolved medical or legal issue. One of the justifications, the so-called miracle recovery, is a particularly tough thing for next of kin and those who watch

It is not uncommon for cancer patients to suffer heart attacks or to face second long-term illnesses like diabetes.

from the sidelines to deal with unless the patient has made wishes known in writing, ahead of time.

Hospice Care

Palliative care—which aims to relieve symptoms, not to cure—can be extremely valuable at the end of life. It permits lucidity and promotes dignity. Close observers such as Claire Tehan, president of a large Southern California hospice provider and a respected authority, generally agree that patients should choose the transition to hospice care when it is recommended to them. Remedial treatment can be resumed if there is the slightest indication of a change in condition. Meanwhile, hospice status allows very liberal use of palliative drugs and physical therapies. Hospice status also transfers any remaining costs relating to care to insurance carriers and Medicare.

36 Always Wear Your Game Face

Actively, constructively fight your cancer every day.

Chances are you've visited someone who was gravely ill, perhaps stricken by cancer. You could tell that things were not going well. The patient was unkempt and unclean. The room was disorganized. Things smelled. You kept the visit short. The patient was preoccupied. The entire conversation revolved around how bad the patient felt and how poor the situation was. The sickness was pervasive.

You left with a sigh of relief. Even though the patient was a person you cared for, it was an unpleasant experience that you did not want to repeat. Perhaps you returned. Perhaps you thoughtfully brought pictures or some other diversion. But your visits felt more like labor than love.

Experience is a great teacher. Is there a lesson here?

The Head Game

Appearance matters. If you answer the door in a frowsy kimono, unclean, hair askew, the visual message is not positive. People know you are sick, but you get no free pass. Instead, the run-down appearance reinforces the fear that the cancer is winning. You are headed south. People around you, including your partner and your medical team, unconsciously revise their expectations accordingly.

Living without courage is toxic.

You will make a bad impression on yourself, too. That day when you lay around until two in the afternoon, then looked in the mirror, the eyes that stared back reinforced every negative suspicion about your prospects for recovery.

There is a head game you need to practice, which is the point of this chapter. Always have your game face on. Be clean and groomed. Wear fresh, attractive clothing. If odors are a possible problem, keep an air freshener going in the room. If you're bedridden, put out pictures of the family. Put up get-well cards and children's art. When visitors arrive, turn the TV off. Don't let something on the tube dominate the attention of those in the room. A visit is your show and you are its centerpiece.

These are indications that you are living your life to the fullest extent possible. These touches contribute to healing and happiness. You deserve them. Don't settle for less, no matter how badly you may feel, or why.

Your partner, your family, and your medical staff need to understand that your game face is as important to you as any other part of your care. They must immediately attend to any part of your bathing, changing, or room ambience that you cannot.

Visitors can be asked to bring flowers. A single rosebud or a carnation will do. It is attitude that sustains your game face, not ostentation. Always replace flowers before the petals fall or wilt. Change vase water daily.

If you should ever have one of those bouts with sickness or because of treatment when all the world turns cold and ugly, your game face will fuel a sustaining fire to warm and comfort you a little. Your medical team and partner will feel it, too. And visitors will sense your determination. Your room will emanate positive vibes: The lights are still on and there's fire in the boiler.

The Difference between Crazy and Stupid

The United States is an asylum run by the inmates. It considers its pleasures and its wealth, its wholesomeness and its beauty, to be rights. That is, of course, insane. These are only opportunities, which people fumble away every day. Moreover, there is unequal distribution. You, for example, have the added burden of cancer to get in the way of your fair share of the good life.

Peel off the expectation that you have a right to health, as if it were the warm-up suit you wear before a race. You're going to have to win your health back. Look down the track ahead. That is where you will be pursuing your future. You will not do this to escape the asylum, because you can't. You will do this because it is your key to survival on life's best terms. You know this because there's a difference between being crazy (which we all are) and stupid.

Reasonable Goals

Medical science tells us that every day you continue to battle your cancer is a victory day. The damage this experience may do to you today is less than it could have done to you yesterday. Your comfort is better, your prospects for longevity improved.

There are three facts of cancer survivorship that you can hold high on even the darkest moment of your bout with this thing:

1. These days, more people beat cancer, or at least fight it to a draw, than ever before. Because of better technology, ten million more Americans are alive today than would have survived in your parents' day. This trend will carry on and accelerate, and you will continue to benefit.

2. Do not presume that because others have succumbed to your particular cancer, it will take you. Even the deadliest varieties are now being beaten. Talk to the survivors of your cancer at toll-free phone numbers you can find in the Reference Center. Stack a few of their names, like firewood at the side of the house, for the time when you may need the warmth of their wisdom and assurance.

3. "Incurable" does not mean "doomed." People live long happy lives despite having deadly, incurable afflictions such as heart disease, HIV, stroke, Parkinson's, diabetes, and many others.

The Dulling and Lulling of Cancer

Cancer patients and those close to them go through phases of more and less enthusiasm for the fight. In the beginning, fear and resolve predominate. Later, the patient falls into a test-and-treatment regimen. Things become better understood, more routine. The fortunate ones begin the road to improvement and don't look back. At least until a relapse occurs, which is always a possibility, these folks have their normal lives back.

Others must take a longer, more circuitous route. Should you become one of these, fatigue and anger and frustration may begin to color your view of life. If you don't watch out, these bad vibes soon evolve into dull acceptance of being sick. This is a dangerous place to go for both patients and their support teams. Actively, constructively fight your cancer every day.

Get your game face on. If possible, set a goal or start an important undertaking. Is there a garden or renovation project you can discuss with a contractor? Is there a church project to finish? Is there a grandchild to recover for, so that the two of you can go fishing? Are there fences to mend? Beat back the dulling and the lulling that cancer tries to use against you by reaffirming the things you have to live for.

The years 1956 and 1957 were terrible ones for Kyle and Andy Anderson. Their beloved son, Jerry, died in an automobile accident. Six months later, Kyle underwent cancer surgery. Then another tumor was discovered. A far more radical procedure was necessary. Then came radiation, a new and imperfect weapon in those days. A third operation followed.

Through it all, Kyle remained a devoted wife and adoring mother to her remaining children, Dana and Sally. She resumed golf, which, given the extent of the damage surgery had done to key muscle structure, required heroic determination. Her strength and unselfish love brought her especially close to her niece, Karen, who has coped—somehow—with the loss of our teenage son, Scott, and the onslaughts of cancer.

Forty-eight cancer-free years later, the children, grandchildren, great-grands, and hosts of family and friends celebrated Kyle's memory after her death at the age of ninety-four. She loved life and she loved mischief, and you would have loved her, too.

Dave Visel

---

37 Getting "Better"

Reports of your progress are apt to be mixed.

The question that perpetually hangs front and center for any cancer patient is How am I doing? Am I getting better, or worse? It seems simple. It isn't.

Step one in the search for the answer is to get close to your oncologist and stay there. Patients are often assailed by the opinions of others, including some others who provide medical services. Take these opinions, most particularly those that cause you concern, directly back to your team leader for sorting out.

Step two is not to take too much to heart anything that your oncologist isn't worried about. But be sure you understand why the doc is or is not concerned by something. Otherwise you could miss the real point.

No Simple Answer

As we saw in Chapter 28, "Nutrition and Fitness," a cancer patient's health is threatened on five fronts: the cancer's direct attacks, the results of drastic treatments, other opportunistic diseases that come along, infections, and the mental wear and tear from all of this. Here your doc is, with all these balls in the air, and you expect a simple answer to "How am I doing?"

Suppose your tumors are receding but damage from a treatment was worse than the doc thought it would be. You may need minor surgery to repair something. On top of that, there are signs that you have contracted a wasting disease. An underweight condition may be a problem soon, contributing to a further loss of energy. But the severe depression you have experienced in the past is gone, which greatly increases your overall chances for recovery. So what does the doc say in answer to "How am I doing?"

Doctors have individual styles. Some try to color everything to imply good news. Some prefer conservative, even negative, assessments. Sometimes a patient gets a "good cop–bad cop" routine from the medical team. One says, "You're doing great." The other says, "I'm concerned about . . . " This offers you a kind of information-cafeteria plan with an optional reassurance station. You take the combination of dishes that strikes you as right.

You can also expect the answer to be couched in terms your doc thinks you can deal with. If the conversation moves into specifics like platelet counts and the possibility of the latest big-deal wonder drug, your doc is honoring the time and attention you are paying to the details of your illness. If the doc tells you, "Things look pretty good today" and then starts mumbling instructions to a nurse, you may have just learned that you got a failing grade for Chapter 5, "Know the Illness," and Chapter 6, "Learn the Lingo." Better go back and review.

Rose-Colored-Glasses Syndrome

Patients and those who love them are eager to feel good about the course of events. So eager in fact, that they may twist bad news into good and convert evidence of poor progress into something hopeful through amazing leaps of illogic. The fantasies they create can take on lives of their own, becoming fact for the patient or friends. If you decide you have gotten better and no longer need the medicine, tests, or therapy, ask your doctor specifically about it before you take any action on your own. To put things into computerese, the logic for your operating system may need a reboot.

Dangers of the Syndrome

Rose-colored-glasses syndrome is dangerous for two groups: patients themselves, and friends and relatives.

Members of the patient's medical team, possibly led by a psychiatrist, must decide how to counter flights of fancy. Support groups (Chapter 19) can sometimes do the best job of keeping the patient's feet planted in the here and now. Patients and former patients, in the privacy of care-group settings, have special believability.

Sometimes conditions are such that the professionals decide to permit irrational good cheer and baseless optimism, as long as somebody close to the patient keeps in touch with the real world. Motives for this decision may vary, but the reasons for allowing excessive optimism are seldom part of a recovery plan.

People want to hear good news about the patient largely because they do not want to deal with the alternative. Some real or imagined scrap of hope mushrooms. The next thing you know, myth is born and has puppies. The first and best control over this behavior by friends is in the hands of the patient, if he or she is able. "I'm really pleased to hear that I look well, but no, I'm not around the corner with this thing just yet. As a matter of fact, I have some treatments coming up that I'm not looking forward to." On behalf of the patient, the partner can also help squelch rose-colored comments. So can friends who are close to the process.

What about bending the truth a little so that Grandma doesn't have a heart attack? Or coloring the picture for children to shelter them? First of all, it probably won't work. Word will get out. Grandma will figure it out for herself, or the kids will. And once the lie has been caught, future credibility suffers big-time.

You are new to this problem, so it was not unreasonable for you to hope that this solution would work, but it won't. The chance that Grandma or the kids will be better off living in a fantasy world is remote. Most of the impetus behind this rationalization comes from the person who must be the bearer of the bad news—a person who will do anything, believe any rationalization, to be excused from truth telling. The escape routes, this person hopes, are either to say nothing or to be fanciful. Sorry. This is a skunk you've got to skin.

A Penalty for Denial

One of the very cruelest and most unnecessary results of wishful thinking comes as the "surprise" that happened because no one took to heart what the doctor had been saying for months or years. This form of denial can also account for poor treatment choices and for neglecting testing or therapy. Sure, it's important for the patient and partner to feel that there is hope. But they must not neglect prudent means and measures, for any reason.

Ways the Docs Handle Progress Reports

Most oncologists believe that one should tell a patient as much truth as the patient can deal with. At the same time, cancer poses so many unknowns and surprises that it is unprofessional to forecast many coming events or to make outcome promises. A doctor's way around these issues is to sprinkle reports to patients with as many caveats as necessary. Listen carefully to your doctor to learn which are favorites and what these code words may indicate.

Here are two examples, taken from an almost endless supply.

"You are in clinical remission." Caveat word count, two: "clinical" and "remission." Since "clinical" obviously modifies "remission," it must mean that cancer is still detectable. "Remission" also implies down but not out.

Having thought this through, you reply: "So I take it that my cancer has reduced in size and does not appear to be aggressive at the moment. Correct?" Your doctor's affirmation or further explanation gives you the balanced detail you wanted.

"You are looking very well today." Possible caveats, three: "looking," "well," and "today." Maybe "looking very well" is the best that the doc can think of by way of saying hi. Or you may have remembered to brush your wig this morning, for which you are being complimented. Or today is better than the last time the doc saw you, when you entertained the clinic with that grand mal seizure.

Every condition is different. Every medical team has its own makeup. Every case develops its own caveats. Look for them. Point them out, so that everyone has a chuckle. "Am I looking good again today, doc?" Better communications and greater honesty are team builders and life givers.

Medical Terms That Relate

Spontaneous Remission

As we have already learned (Chapter 32, "Nontraditional Healing Practices"), the disease just goes away in a small percent of cancer cases. No correlation can be proven between this spontaneous remission of the disease and any treatment the patient may have received. It is also true that a few patients, aware of this rare occurrence, bank on it. This is not wise unless you like the idea of betting your life on a fifty-to-one shot.

Complete Remission

A victorious round over cancer is like a knockdown in boxing, except that the referee's ten-count takes five years. Meanwhile, keep an eye on your opponent. Keep your Sunday punch ready in case cancer tries to get up. Don't even think about using the "cure" word until after the ref has raised your arm.

The term "complete remission" may be the one most commonly used to describe success to a patient. It means that the recent treatment program has caused the cancer to disappear completely or, more accurately, to become undetectable. Maybe gone. Maybe not. It does not follow that your treatments are over. Oncologists have learned that it is prudent to continue on a prescribed course to be as certain as possible that undetectable levels of cancer are also wiped out.

As was just implied, "complete remission" is like the "bumper-to-bumper, unconditional guarantee" on a Cadillac. This isn't a promise you can rely on. There are plenty of hidden agendas, conditions, and caveats.

The oncologists' ability to detect cancer has limitations. Tumors below about one centimeter in diameter may be very hard to spot, even with the latest imaging equipment. Cancers of the blood may require testing at or near the cellular level. In other cases, science relies on a tumor marker, like the prostate-specific antigen (PSA) test that announces a likelihood of that cancer.

Some "complete remissions" are permanent. In cases where a certain tumor is known to be responsive to a type of treatment, the oncologist is apt to be very encouraging. But note that the word "remission" is used, not "cure." Treatment may continue. Periodic testing most certainly will. There is a point between one and three years after the last detection when most of these cancers come back, if they are going to. There is a second point at the five-year anniversary when your doctor may express "high confidence." Savvy cancer survivors continue annual checkups forever.

Cure

"Cure" is an accounting artifice applied to a patient who has been free of cancer for five years. Past this mark, cancer can no longer be used as a reason to restrict your professional progress at work. The life- and health-insurance agents may begin calling again. Statistically, it's a pretty good bet that the cancer won't return. There are exceptions that your oncologist will tell you about if you ask. It is less likely you will learn this detail if you do not ask.

Don't bet the farm on a clean five-year record, or after ten years, or twenty. Continue regular checkups by a doctor who demands state-of-the-art testing. If the supervising physician, or more likely the third party bearing the brunt of the cost, says it's okay to slack off, carefully consider the source and its possible motivations. Annual checkups for life are as important for those declared "cured" as they are for those who have been "in remission."

Partial Remission

"Partial remission" has come to mean that the tumor or the general population of blood cancer cells has been reduced by more than 50 percent but is still there. This is decidedly better news than you might have had. It is still worth no more than a crouching ovation.

Sometimes the term is used when the effectiveness of the present course of treatment has reached a plateau. A new strategy will be needed to continue reducing the presence of the cancer. Listen very carefully. The doc may be indicating that the medical team has done all it can do. You may need to accept a status quo or move your case to another treatment team. Don't presume any of this. Ask pointed, specific questions. Keep in mind the possibility that HMO resources or health-insurance limits may be influencing the situation.

Stabilization

The term "stabilization" is used to indicate that the condition is getting neither better nor worse. It's great news if "stabilized" indicates that a raging attack has been turned back. It is less than great new when used month after month to indicate that all is still quiet on the Western Front. You and the doc know the bad guys are still out there, and you should both be puckering.

Cancer "Progression" or "Aggression"

Things are going badly when either "progression" or "aggression" comes up. You need to start the treatment program that has been recommended. Or you need to get a better one started. Second opinions may be needed, too. Focus. This is not the time to let anything take higher priority than your cancer treatment.

No Change

When cancer is fought to a draw and remains in that state—unchanged for an extended period of time—"stabilized" may be replaced by "no change" to describe it. Events in the cancer-fighting process, whatever the medical team calls them, are taking place less frequently and usually with less urgency. The patient is exhausted and functioning at well below normal. Issues like sleeplessness and inability to perform at work are of greatest concern to both doc and patient.

The oncologist may have announced the arrival of this time in your struggle by explaining that recent tests indicate that your body needs to recuperate from treatments. Perhaps your bone-marrow system is "exhausted" and must rest. Healing from a major operation or extensive radiation may be called for. These kinds of things demand a cessation of aggressive treatment. To continue on the offensive could have serious consequences. It might even be life threatening.

There are also treatment protocols that prescribe periods of quiet, during which the oncologist carefully watches the cancer's response to drugs, radiation, or surgery. This process is usually explained before the treatment starts, but not always.

There are also cases when a treatment program has run out of gas. The medical team has no new ideas. Your cancer is not being attacked as successfully as it once was. Carefully consider the possibility that a second opinion may be helpful to everyone.

It is also possible that you have been pushing yourself in some way that is unrealistic. Be prepared to accept the second opinion that you need to listen more carefully to your doc or to back away from unrealistic goals you had set for yourself.

Agents of "No Change"

Your insurance company may have deliberately slowed down your treatment program. The normal profile of services and medications for your type of case has been delivered. Based on the insurance company's ever-present standards, you're supposed to be either cured or dead. Now that you have outlasted its precedents, it hesitates to authorize further treatments or tests.

If you suspect that there is a need, get your oncologist or your partner to review what other people with your cancer are doing about it at this present stage of conflict. Get a new PDQ from the National Cancer Institute (see Chapter 4, "The Patient's New World"). Go back to your support group or find a new one to discuss this with. Do something to refresh your healing program—or get very positive assurance that "no change" is a status you can live with. (Double meaning intended.)

Inactive, Passive, Slow-Growing, Et Cetera Cancers

Some cancers never bother the patient. For example, some prostate cancers in older men and some forms of leukemia in adults may never really threaten the patient. Even so, a conservative checkup schedule must be observed. Recommended blood and other tests must continue. Complacency can never be permitted. Stable conditions can suddenly change into very aggressive ones without any apparent cause or warning.

The Preemptive-Strike Strategy

Sometimes the patient or the oncology team may consider treating a cancer that is merely present—not affecting health, and not on the attack. If you are part of such a debate now, very seriously consider the age-old question, If it ain't broke, why fix it? It can make great sense to take care of a problem before it becomes a bigger one. But preventive strikes have sometimes turned inoffensive cancers into nasty ones. Be certain to get second opinions that agree with both the decision to treat a somnolent cancer, and the form that the treatment will take. Consider adding your requirement that medical case histories be cited that further testify to the wisdom of teasing this sleeping dog.

There are kinds of cancer that usually don't kill people.
Treatment at the earliest stage of many other cancers is often
successful too.

The NBD Impression

Sometimes patients get the impression that, because the doctor says it is
curable, their cancer is NBD, no big deal. That is a perilous mindset. Easy
cancer will never get any easier, but it almost assuredly can get harder if you
wait or take ineffective countermeasures. At a minimum, a cancer should be
given the same respect one gives a poisonous snake. Don't mess around with
it. Make sure the experts are in agreement as to exactly what you have. Listen
carefully to the course of treatment prescribed. Get the second opinion of a
specialist if you feel there is the slightest need, or if someone on the medical
team—or your employer or health insurer—thinks it might be a good idea.
Then get "it" done—whatever the doc has told you is necessary to do to be
rid of the thing.

The treatment may be as simple as having liquid nitrogen sponged onto
the spot. It might be outpatient surgery or something more extensive. You
may have to take some pills or visit a radiologist. You may have to take time
off from work or postpone a vacation—that part, in fact, is NBD, though you
may not agree.

Plot the course. Set the sail. Get it done. Now.

Skin Cancers

Cancers on the surface of the skin are generally of three sorts. The most
common are called basal cell and squamous cell. About 1.1 million people
will be treated for them this year, according to the American Cancer Society.
Properly dealt with, they rarely threaten. That's why their numbers are not
included in the oft-quoted statistic of 1.3 million cases of cancer diagnosed
annually in the United States. Even so, improperly dealt with or ignored,
either of them may eventually get a patient into a good deal of trouble.

The third form of skin cancer, melanoma, is the least common but very
dangerous. It is among the most malignant of all cancers, demanding treatment without delay. Once the tumor has penetrated the second layer of skin,
the dermis, cure is in doubt.

The lightest-skinned people get more of these cancers than others. Those
who work or play in the sun get more of them. Men are two or three times
more likely to get them than women. They become more common as we
age. Skin cancers sometimes occur on the eye or on outer layers we don't
normally think of as "outer," such as in the mouth or anus.

Precancers

One common outcome of a colon examination is the discovery and removal of precancerous polyps. "Precancer" is the doc's term for any abnormal cellular change or condition—in the colon or elsewhere—that is known to produce malignancy at least some of the time. Once a precancerous condition is discovered, the usual action is to remove it surgically and then to test it for malignancy through the biopsy process, just to be sure. Depending on what the test shows, further examinations may be scheduled.

Early-Childhood Leukemia

Many leukemias discovered in children are considered curable, even though the same diseases in older patients may not be. A combination of how a young body responds, the form that these diseases take in children, and the treatment techniques known to work instills great confidence among pediatric oncologists.

Prostate Cancer

Specialists treat earliest-stage prostate tumors with high confidence in the patient's complete recovery. Men past middle age with prostate cancer may be advised to consider a no-treatment option. Should you be so advised, make sure you know exactly why your doc suggests this approach and then find another equally well qualified oncologist who agrees. All decisions regarding this and every other cancer are apt to be based on a complex set of circumstances. If an answer sounds too simple, respect your inner doubting voice.

Early-Stage Cancers Generally

"Stage zero" and "stage I" are terms given to some precancers and malignancies that are discovered at their place of origin in your body. The tumor or tumors are quite small and have not spread to other sites. These cancers can likely be successfully treated.

Recurring Cancers

Listen carefully to your oncologist's evaluation of a cancer that appears to have returned. Even if it is discovered at stage I and meets other conditions of an "easy" cancer, it may not be. Your most important clue is that cancer, which had been dealt with, is back. It could be new, a recurrence, or metastatic, meaning it traveled from somewhere else in your body. Discuss all the implications of the situation with your oncologist, including the best strategy for covering treatment through your health-insurance company.

In the grand scope of things, whether your insurance covers the cost or not is definitely of secondary importance. But the recurrence of a cancer happens to be one of the most common exclusions from coverage in many policies. If you and the doc know about this loophole from the beginning, your medical team is apt to find a positive way to document your case.

Botching Easy Cancer

Medical science offers us precautions. Periodic physical examinations take most of them into account. There are exam add-ons that we are expected to endure as we grow older. Women need mammograms. Men need PSA tests. The indignity of a periodic colonoscopy comes along, usually after age forty. Sores that don't heal, bleeding from various places, skin blemishes that change and grow, and anything else that worries your doctor is worth a check.

If blood relatives of yours have experienced cancer, you will need to be checked for the same disease even if "everyone" says that environmental conditions or bad habits caused it. Speak to your relative's oncologist. Get a recommendation as to when to be checked—and then how frequently to be checked after that.

Many types of cancer are believed to travel along hereditary lines or to favor certain genetic makeups. Perhaps none are more common than breast cancers. Daughters of mothers with breast cancers may be advised to begin annual mammograms as early as their teens or twenties.

When cancer is discovered, do what your doctor says. Sure, you've got tests and second opinions and maybe other things to go through, but once all that is done, take orders and follow them. If you feel that a religious solution or some alternative to the medical protocol of your oncologist is a more attractive choice, the chance that you are turning easy cancer into tough cancer increases.

Excuses for Not Dealing with Easy Cancer

Here are some dandy excuses. If you are impressed by the implacability of cancer, don't use any of them.

I don't have time. / This is inconvenient.
I'm worried about physical loss (breast, face, limbs, sight, hearing,
    speech, etc.)
I'm afraid I'll lose sexual ability.
I dislike the indignity of physical explorations down the nose or throat,
    or up either of the passageways from the other end.
It costs too much.
It's against my religion.
How about we skip the exam this year?
It makes me sick.
My insurance won't cover it.
My insurance company and my doctor don't agree on the best procedure.
    (Suggestion: Make sure your doctor wins this debate, and quickly.)
My insurance company hasn't gotten back to me / is still deciding.

39 Tough Cancer

The downside of today's advanced state of medicine is that oncologists sometimes have the tools and experience to predict the time and means of our demise with some assurance.

Getting "the Word"

"On March 28, 1978, the doctor told me that I had a malignancy. My lung cancer was inoperable. I should get my estate in order." So begins Richard Bloch's narrative from *Cancer . . . There's Hope,* a book the Bloch Cancer Foundation gives to anyone who requests it. (If you'd like a copy, call 800/433-0464. For more, look under "Bloch Cancer Foundation" in the Reference Center.)

Bloch applied his money and his wits to the problem before him. Looking back on those frightening days, he lists five key factors in his recovery. Variations of Bloch's message are repeated in the recovery stories of many other men and women who were told that their battles against cancers were hopeless. An oncologist, recalling the typical responses of patients to news of tough-cancer diagnoses, summarized: "Some give up, and some don't." Some, he said, have already sensed that death is near. Many are sick, tired, and ready for the release. Even so, he said, in agreement with Bloch, a patient does no service to himself or his family by not continuing an aggressive, imaginative, positive fight.

Table 39.1 *Estimated Cancer Deaths in the United States, 2004*

Male		Female	
Lung and bronchus	91,930	Lung and bronchus	68,510
Prostate	29,500	Breast	40,110
Colon and rectum	28,320	Colon and rectum	28,410
Pancreas	15,440	Ovary	16,090
Leukemia	12,990	Pancreas	15,830
Non-Hodgkin lymphoma	10,390	Leukemia	10,310
Esophagus	10,250	Non-Hodgkin lymphoma	9,020
Liver	9,450	Uterine corpus	7,090
Urinary bladder	8,780	Multiple myeloma	5,640
Kidney	7,870	Brain	5,490
All others	65,970	All others	66,310
	290,890		272,810

Source: *American Cancer Society, Inc., "Surveillance Research," 2004.*

After "the Word" and before Anything Else . . .

Hearing It Right

When somebody tells you that you are going to die, it is highly unlikely that they composed the message in haste or delivered it to you before all doubt was gone. But it is not inconceivable that there was more to it. Yes, cancer is considered incurable. Yes, contracting it is a sort of death sentence. But perhaps not for a while. People manage to hold many incurable diseases at bay for long lifetimes—heart disease, diabetes, HIV, Parkinson's, . . . cancer.

The real point of the gloomy message may be that you should (1) take it more seriously, (2) follow the doctor's instructions more faithfully, (3) stop some unhealthful habit, (4) begin a treatment that you've been putting off, or (5) consider this fair warning to get your affairs in order.

Hearing It All

Cancer is evaluated in two ways—medically and statistically. The medical outlook may not appear alarming. You may not look or feel very ill. Your doc knows that nevertheless—according to the National Cancer Institute's current mortality tables—your sort of cancer is rarely stopped. In that case, you may be told to expect no more than a certain number of months or years to live.

If that is your situation or if you think it might be, you must go back and confirm it. Statistical probability is nothing to be ignored. It keeps Las Vegas in business. But odds can be beaten. There is room for hope and special reason for further examination of your prospects.

There is also good incentive to begin an evaluation of your life's loose ends and the things you should do out of love for family, friends, and the institutions you value. You may want to chat with your family, a religious advisor, a business advisor, and a lawyer.

Checking with Your Partner

People often confuse what they want to hear or what they expect to hear with what was actually said. If it's bad news, the very important information that followed it may be blocked out by the "Oh-my-God, oh-my-God, oh-my-God" screaming in your head.

Later, when you regain some semblance of your senses, ask the partner who was in the meeting with you to summarize the message. See how closely it matches your recollection. Carefully rerun the entire scene.

Getting More Information

Ask your doc for an appointment to come back. Then ask the questions you didn't think of the first time. Let your partner ask all the other questions that have come up since that meeting.

Getting a Second Opinion

Continue this thorough diagnostic procedure at the second and every subsequent, equally well-qualified cancer center until at least two agree completely to the patient's satisfaction. Repeating for emphasis: You, the *patient*, are the person who needs to be satisfied—not your family, not your doctor, not your boss at work, not your insurance company or your friend with all the answers. If you are unsure, you have an obligation to keep asking questions and to keep searching. When you are certain you are right, assert that certainty.

Getting a PDQ

Chapter 4, "The Patient's New World," tells how to perform a Physicians Data Query, an up-to-the-moment survey of every treatment protocol under way in the United States for any patient with your form of cancer. Might it be helpful to look at the current report?

Considering the Long Shots

Lori Monroe was diagnosed with inoperable, terminal cancer at age forty-two. She went to Vanderbilt University, where she received a second opinion that agreed with the first. She argued that, being young with no other health problems, she could survive a very high-risk operation. The doctors who had first examined her had "already condemned me to death," she wrote in a diary.

She found an oncologist on staff at Vanderbilt who performed the surgery and subsequent procedures. At the time of this writing, she had survived long past the most optimistic date her doctors gave her. She is in pain and physically incapacitated. But she is alive for her daughters and available for promising new drugs and procedures if any become available.

In 2001, the National Cancer Institute sponsored a study that looked at cases like Lori Monroe's. It concluded, in part, that cancers such as hers are viewed by the medical community with "a pervasive sense of therapeutic nihilism . . . to create a medical environment in which many patients with advanced cancer are not even offered treatment."

At what point do you draw the line? "Would you operate on someone to get three more weeks of life? Three more months? Two more years?" asks David P. Carbone, MD, Monroe's current oncologist. The answer seems to be that it is the patient's decision whether or not to buy the time, while taking the risks and enduring the consequences.

Making Life Decisions

Those facing tough cancer feel an almost irresistible need to speak bravely about miracles. Unfortunately, after the opinion, second opinion, further information gathering, and all the rest that we have discussed, the consensus is almost always right. At some place in all this, the patient comes to understand the implacability of the coming transition. It isn't what one wants or welcomes. But it becomes unavoidable. At that point, patients who have not lost clarity and wits to the advancements of the disease have new sets of issues to consider.

Instructions to Doctors

There may be medical measures that you oppose on personal, philosophical, or religious grounds. Transfusions, amputations, and transplants are among the most common of these. You can insure that your medical team stops short of any of these measures, but you must do so with a legally acceptable recording or document.

If you want your medical team to continue fighting for your life past a point when you could recover even partial sentience, do nothing. If you want to be permitted to pass without further heroic measures, after all hope is gone but you remain alive, you must make specific arrangements. Your family lawyer, religious advisor, or doctor can help. An arrangement of this kind usually kicks in at a time when resuscitation is necessary to delay death.

We are not discussing euthanasia, nor will we. Like suicide, euthanasia is a subject that in this book is out of bounds.

Instructions to Family Members

You know your family. If there are things that your serious illness or death may cause someone to do—and that you can prevent by leaving an instruction—now's the time to get it done. If you are leaving dependents behind and you have a plan for their well-being, now's the time to be sure it's in place.

Instructions to Your Partner

During the final stages of your illness, your partner may face unhappy, awkward choices. You can make those choices now.

For example, you can make your own funeral arrangements. The funeral industry is well prepared to work with you on this. By making the choices now and paying for them, you lift a huge burden from the shoulders of family and friends.

There are alternatives to some or all funeral services to be aware of. A donation of "remains" to a scientific project or medical school can be made. Cremation and private disposal of the ashes are also possible.

You can pick a church. You can ask the person you have in mind to sing or to deliver the eulogy. You may want to leave general guidelines that eliminate choices that you don't want considered.

Instructions to Executor and Attorney

If you have changes that should be made to real estate or other holdings that you do not feel comfortable leaving to someone else's discretion, you must act. If you have been working on a major transition from a portfolio that requires active, informed management to an estate that pretty much runs itself, throw the switch now or forever hold your peace.

Get out your will and powers documents. Review them. Make sure that obsolete versions are destroyed and that your attorney has bulletproofed the versions that should be in place. Also take care to put them into the right hands for safekeeping.

Have your business plans been brought to a place that you are comfortable leaving them if you have to? Have your business promises been kept? Have you looked out for the best interests of those whose careers and incomes are in your hands?

Time-Capsule Messages

There are several schools of thought regarding the advisability of planning to leave a voice from the grave. If you are interested in help deciding this issue, now's a pretty good time to seek it.

Possibilities include a parent who wants to leave a message for a child on an occasion such as bar mitzvah, graduation from college, marriage or a message to accompany a bequeathal, to right a wrong, to release a spouse.

An unsolicited observation: Most people who give this idea careful consideration don't leave messages.

The Most Fatal Forms of Cancer

Cancer Facts and Figures 2004, from the American Cancer Society, makes it clear that some general types of cancer are far more survivable than others. The report explains that some cancers kill because they are difficult to treat. Other cancers are usually detected at too late a stage. But no form of cancer is hopeless.

Every type of cancer has points at which it can be attacked. Every one has inspired a team of top-ranked researchers at a major U.S. research organization to find the chinks in its armor. Every team has made important recent progress.

You should be able to name at least one major medical institute that is performing cutting-edge research on behalf of all those with your specific affliction. If you care at all about possible advances, please return to Chapter 7, "Deciding Where to Have Treatment," for help identifying your champions and the things that they are working on.

40 Dealing with Pain and Nausea

You can—and should—keep control of these troublemakers.

Causes of Pain and Nausea

Tumors and the secondary effects of advancing cancer can cause pains of many sorts, both at the cancer's site and elsewhere in the body. Pain also accompanies some surgery and some radiation treatments to the gastrointestinal tract. Also understand that headaches can increase in both severity and duration due to cancer and its treatments.

Nausea is most commonly experienced during recovery from anesthesia and as a reaction to chemotherapy. One of its forms that you might not expect, carsickness, can hit unexpectedly if the patient has recently received chemo or anesthesia.

Cancer-Pain Philosophy

Everyone in oncology agrees that no patient should suffer pain. "First of all, only 20 to 30 percent of cancers patients get severe pain," says Vincent T. DeVita Jr., MD, former director of the National Cancer Institute. "For those who have pain, there are plenty of drugs [and] neurosurgical procedures."

Pain inhibits recovery. Your doc wants it eliminated.

The Patient's Role in Pain Management

The medical community generally agrees that pain relief is an area of oncology best managed by a physician who specializes in it. If you have persistent pain, and if your medical team has not introduced you to a pain physician—usually an anesthesiologist—ask about it.

"Even my hair hurts" or "Agggh!" is not enough information for your doctor to work from. There is a series of questions that you must answer. Listen carefully and follow along. You may think that your pain is in your big toe. But after the doc has worked with you, it could turn out to be a nerve in your leg, a back problem, or something else.

As you work with your painmeister, you will learn how to analyze your condition, which is all you need to bother with. If you would like to open an interesting short book on the larger subject, try *The Cancer Pain Sourcebook* by Roger Cicala.

The Danger of Silent Suffering

There is no reason to suffer. You won't recover better or faster. Living with pain won't help your doctor. It doesn't save money or time.

Pain is a primary fear of 72 percent of new cancer patients, only slightly less than the percentage that fear dying. More than half of those surveyed believe that dying of cancer means dying in pain.

Institute of Medicine, Approaching Death (1997)

By knowing what bodily structure or structures cause a pain and what type of pain it is, a doctor can treat it more effectively; . . . it will not only be less frightening, but you can do a better job of explaining your pain to your doctor.

David van Alstine, MD, The Cancer Pain Sourcebook, assembled, edited, and largely written by Roger S. Cicala, MD (Contemporary Books, 2001)

Suffering doesn't save you from the risk of addiction to pain medicine. The sorts of pain that require the help of major-league medicine will block out your other senses and your ability to think clearly until you get relief. Don't challenge this notion. Accept the meds. See more under "Addiction," later in this chapter; also see the several discussions of palliative care in Chapter 35, "Watching and Waiting."

Planning for Pain and Nausea

Your medical team will probably be able to warn you in advance when you will face either pain or nausea. Nevertheless, effective relief can be a complicated place to get to. A bit of trial with various drugs may be necessary before they learn which remedies are best for you.

Expect your doc to bring up issues of pain and nausea before the problem occurs. As a part of your medical team's preparations to thwart them, expect questions about your physical health and lifestyle. Be as accurate as possible when describing your body's allergies. Never shade the truth if you drink alcohol, smoke, or chew. Carefully disclose every sort of drug, vitamin, food supplement, herb, and tea that you have taken recently.

Early Defenses

You will probably start a nausea med before taking the drug or beginning the procedure that could make you sick. The hope is that you never experience nausea, much less vomit.

You may also start taking pain meds before any pain could start. Your diet may be altered or restricted too. Sometimes the side effects include drowsiness or difficulty sleeping. Take any warnings such as "Don't drive" to heart.

Regularity

Prescribing physicians and pharmacists may fail to mention that the patient may also need a laxative, stool softener, or vitamins as part of a pain-relief plan. If you don't see such an instruction, ask. It can't hurt. But three days without a bowel movement can.

Aftereffects

Reactions and Discomfort

If the drugs you get for pain or nausea don't work, immediately tell your doc or pharmacist—whoever is closest. (The one you tell will immediately contact the other one through channels that are faster than those available to patients.) The need to make adjustments to what you take and how you take it at this point in your cancer battle is common. And, to repeat, it is important that you be comfortable and pain free.

By the way, your body and its disease may change in reaction to the drugs you take. This will probably make it necessary for changes to be made in your pain and nausea protocols from time to time.

The Dialing-In Process

Sometimes the complexities of pain or nausea defy early attempts at solution. There are other circumstances in which the right drug for one thing gets in the way of something else. So patient and doctor have to work through a series of variables and alternative meds.

In one recent case, the patient did not react well to any of the usual drug solutions for nausea relief before chemo. Finally, the patient suggested sea-sickness tablets. It was a bit off the wall but the doc thought it was worth a try, and it worked. The only trick was that the patient had to learn to continue taking it for two days after each treatment was over.

Pharmaceuticals are not the only path. Look into psychological therapy, bio-feedback, hypnosis, physical therapy, and massage. Perhaps there are more (see Chapter 32, "Nontraditional Healing Practices"). Generally, it is possible to use several methods simultaneously.

Addiction

Most oncologists probably downplay the possibility of addiction to pain medications. They don't want the patient to feel that taking the pain remedy is optional. Addiction, they believe, isn't a threat during the time that great pain is being alleviated. Or, worst case, addiction can be dealt with through a tapering-off process in conjunction with other drugs.

But if you have been addicted to tobacco, alcohol, or a legal or illegal drug and had difficulty overcoming it, you should have a healthy respect for the consequences of taking addictive pain medications. You should discuss with your doc or with a recommended pain-medication specialist a specific plan for using—and then recovery from using—high-octane painkillers.

Recovering addicts can also discuss this with an advisor in a support-group setting. This problem becomes serious only if you take it lightly.

Finishing the Drugs

Take the drugs, exactly as prescribed. Take them all. If you have an unpleasant side effect—say, cramps or diarrhea—report it to your doc or pharmacist. They'll consult and fix the situation. Never, never just stop taking the prescription.

Auntie Em's Secret Sauce

This is self-evident, but it needs stating anyway: Don't take leftovers out of the medicine cabinet or some friend's "try this" remedy. Don't try a nickel bag from the projects or somebody's weed. Stay with the pain and nausea meds your medical team has recommended. They are more effective and cheaper.

There is no chance of a side effect such as food poisoning or infection. If you must experiment, do it in full view. You will find your doc a knowledgeable, sympathetic soul mate.

Finding Sanctuary When Needed

Pain can take a person to a point where the prospect of going immediately to hell is appealing. Drugs, and perhaps pain-relieving radiation or surgery, must be the first and foremost counteractions. But don't neglect these additional ways to greater comfort.

1. The arms of someone who loves you. Cuddle. Hold on. Love and be loved.
2. The closest place of prayer (in a storm, any port). Chapter 10, "God," will be important to go back to at a time like this if you do not have an active faith. If you do, you did not need this reminder. One related point: You will find that you can take your faith into the nondenominational religious sanctuary in your hospital or someplace down the street where the form of worship is unfamiliar. God will be fine with any setting you choose.
3. A quiet walk or a sunny perch. If you have the energy to walk, you will receive the double blessing of pleasant distraction and good exercise. When walking is difficult, hitch a ride in a wheelchair or find a sunny perch. The point is to get out of yourself and the gloom of the moment. Be reminded that there is a greater place to savor. Contemplate it and the things you plan to do in it later.

Staying Sober

Do not try to escape through unprescribed drugs or alcohol. It's dangerous under normal circumstances. In your present condition, it's an absolute peril. And it doesn't work.

Depression

Physicians and psychologists teach us that depression is an opportunistic disease that often attacks cancer patients. Sickness can cause it. This is a serious condition that clouds thinking and delivers anguish. It can lead to any of many poor decisions regarding selection of treatment options, family, home, and work. For the severely depressed who are not treated for it, it can lead to suicide.

Depression is anger without enthusiasm.

Sick and Tired of Being Sick and Tired

Between the malaise and the never-ending rounds of things to be done, a time may come when the patient has no fight left. Those around the patient may realize that their loved one is too drained to answer the bell for the start of the next round. The patient is completely dependent on others to continue. This is the beginning of the end for many cancer patients, unless the medical team, *led and encouraged by the partner and other loved ones*, carries on successfully.

41 Recovering from Surgery

I'm black and blue and stapled and glued. I look like Eddie Munster's third-grade art project. Just like they promised, if everything went well.

The "Sort of Want to Know" Conundrum

No surgery is fun. Logic and the medical staff tell us to actively prepare. The more serious the operation, the more important getting ready for it is. We know this. We sort of want to hear about what's coming. And we don't. It's like getting ready to jump into an icy lake with everybody watching and your good hat floating just out of reach from shore. You've got to go for it. But please, dear God, help me stand the shock.

Under the best of circumstances, things will turn out far better than you were told they might. No complications. Recovery ahead of schedule. You still need to know what might happen. If you go in unprepared, you're set up for a sucker punch.

What You Will Go Through

No one can guarantee your surgery's outcome. A great many factors contribute. Your doc or another member of the team will give you the most likely range of outcomes. You may be able to find people who have recovered from the same general type of surgery you are about to have by calling one of the toll-free phone numbers in the Reference Center "Yellow Pages" under the general name for your disease. Former patients in particular will remember the things they wish they had prepared for.

The Recovery Process

Every operation has specific components. The outcome of each part of the surgery and recovery process will have many variables. That is why the instructions given to you before surgery are so important. You must listen and read, and you must take all your questions back to your surgical team for answers.

Here are some general comments regarding this process, condensed from information provided by the National Cancer Institute, the American College of Surgeons, and the American Cancer Society.

Anesthesia

Anesthesia, normally in the form of drugs, sometimes assisted by unconsciousness, relieves the patient of discomfort during an operation. When the

---

Surgery offers the greatest chance for cure for many types of cancer, especially those that have not yet spread to other parts of the body. Most people with cancer will have some type of surgery.

American Cancer Society's introduction to surgery (cancer.org)

Communicate!

. . . because it's compassionate.

Those who love the patient—spouse, parents, children, good friends—are apt to be very worried about surgery's outcome. Co-workers and others with ties to the patient will also anxiously await news . . . . and because it's necessary.

In case after case, someone who didn't know assumed the worst and made a decision that everyone regretted later.

patient undergoes a surgical procedure while awake, aided by local anesthesia, recovery is faster and less complicated.

The first hurdle a patient faces after awakening from general anesthesia is a return to sobriety, which may take hours or overnight. At a minimum, a patient recovering from general anesthesia should not drive or participate in any important decision making until the next day.

Another problem, nausea, is more apt to be experienced after general anesthesia. Trying to do too much at the beginning of the recovery process may lead to vomiting.

Sore Throat, Squeaky Voice

Once you are asleep under general anesthesia, an endotracheal tube, referred to as an ET, may be slipped down your throat. It carries air to your lungs. The net result is that you will wake up with a sore throat and you may not have much voice for a while.

Intravenous Connections—

Linda Goldston, a reporter for the *San Jose Mercury News*, collected comments from those whose pets helped them recover from operations. "I had major surgery five years ago, and he was by my side all the time," began one. "Whenever I don't feel well, he looks after me," began another. For more, go to the Internet archives of the newspaper, www .mercurynews.com. Goldston's article was posted February 18, 2004 (also see Chapter 13, "Friends").

When you wake up after general anesthesia, IV tubes that lead from bags hung above the bed through a little pump that regulates flow into a vein will be part of the scene. Painkillers, nourishment, antibiotics, hydration solutions, and all sorts of other liquids are administered in this way to improve your recovery. You may have to drag the whole apparatus everywhere you go for a few days.

Catheter(s)

Sometimes a catheter tube is run up the urethra into the bladder to assist urination. Plumbing problems for the first week or two after surgery are common parts of recovery. Sometimes the tube is removed and then reinstalled, much to the mortification of the patient.

Tubes into the incision are also common. They drain away fluids that collect after the operation is complete. These are usually removed in a day or two.

Eating

Most patients are given something to eat shortly after awakening from surgery. It may be just ice chips or a sponge on a stick that you dip into something and suck, but it heals and encourages your body's recovery process. From these, you graduate to Jell-O, custards, and things that sound better than they taste. (What did you expect for $2,500 a day, cruise cuisine?)

Breathing Exercises

One of the earliest therapies after surgery is breathing exercise. You get to float a ball over a tube by blowing into it or something equally entertaining. Restorative breathing exercises are a vital part of getting the recovery process underway.

Relief

The functioning of the stomach and lower tract are often the last parts of the body to restart after major surgery and general anesthetic. In addition to checking on your repair work, your doc will listen with a stethoscope for bowel sounds and will ask if you have passed gas. You will remain on clear liquids until you have "cleared the air," so to speak.

Getting out of Bed

Your recovery team wants you out of bed. Even a few steps will help restart bodily functions that contribute to healing. Walking also reduces the danger of blood clots forming. If you can't get up, a physical therapist will help you with alternative exercises.

Pain

You will have bouts of discomfort during recovery, sometimes for days or weeks after surgery. In the hospital, a nurse will help you. But if the pain persists, you must ask your surgeon or your anesthesiologist for the remedy. If the doc isn't around, ask your nurse to take a message for you.

A related point: Changes in pain medication are common during convalescence. When pain returns, the doctor expects the patient to report it. Adjustments in the treatment regime follow as necessary.

Ostomy

In this process, rare except following lower GI surgery, an exit for your colon is made in the abdominal area. A bag is attached, which is changed as necessary. This may be either a brief or a longer duration accommodation for the conflicting needs of healing and the demands of bodily function. Ostomy patients and their caregivers must manage this situation with great care (see "Ostomy" in the Reference Center "Yellow Pages").

Infection

Infection is possible during both the hospital recuperation and later in a recovery center, nursing home, or your home. At the time of the patient's discharge from the surgical center, the patient's caregiver should be given specific instructions as to how to identify and report infection. If this does not happen, get this information and follow its instructions carefully.

Depression, Discouragement, Sadness

Bouts of gloominess are part of recovery from major surgery. Your disease and the repair work have taken a toll on you. Discomfort, weakness, worry, and maybe sleep deprivation can combine to make you feel this way. These

At the time of discharge from the hospital, the physician in charge of pain management sometimes gives surgery patients or their partners a kit of alternative supplies. The rules for the kit are that nothing from it is to be given to the patient unless the caregiver observes a specific set of circumstances or the doc gives further instructions. The goal is to have the right meds immediately available for any of the more predictable sets of circumstances.

emotions are genuine. Well earned. But they are part of your illness. Getting over them is part of recovery.

Perhaps a funny video, your spouse, or your pet will help. Perhaps your doc or a friend. Perhaps a hobby or some light work from your employer will pull you out of it. If not, get the help of a psychiatrist, psychologist, church leader, or someone else recommended by your medical team.

Pneumonia

If you learn that pneumonia, an infamous type of lung infection, has been detected, be concerned. If not dealt with, it is potentially fatal.

Pneumonia is not uncommon following surgery in lung-cancer patients and in other patients who smoked. It is sometimes the last disease of the elderly, particularly those weakened by the fight against cancer.

Digestive Tract Infection

If the digestive tract was opened during surgery, the patient will be given powerful antibiotics, some with important side effects. Recovery may be slower than one might expect.

Bleeding

Even after discharge from the hospital, internal or visible bleeding may begin. Attend to it carefully. If you have the slightest doubt that the bleeding has been stopped, get back to your doc ASAP. More surgery is sometimes needed to fix the problem.

Home Emergencies

Discuss with your doc in advance the possibility that you may have a home emergency. Decide whom you will telephone if a medical situation demands it. If the patient must be seen by a physician, decide who and where. You may also need to keep emergency medical supplies at home. Your doc will know if this is a good idea and will help you decide what you should stock.

Steps you can take ahead of a home emergency:

1. Preplan the means of getting the patient to the right door at the right clinic.
2. Get the best phone number to call at the emergency medical treatment center you will use. Plan to call it just before you head out. Put the phone number on speed dial or on the wall near your phone. Stipulations: You need a (1) direct phone number that is (2) answered by a doctor or a nurse (3) before the third or fourth ring (4) around the clock, seven days a week. Your doc will probably have to get this phone number for you. A general hospital line that puts the caller through an interrogation by a telephone-answering computer will not do.
3. Ask your doc if you should say anything in particular when making the notification phone call. If so, write it down. Keep it near the emergency

phone number. You will also need a list of all the patient's current medications and allergies.

4. If you will be taking a cab, put the fare in an envelope. Keep it with that emergency medical stash of yours.

Recovery-Team Support and Training

Your medical team will want you out of your hospital recovery setting as quickly as possible, and so should you. But this process may have mixed consequences if careful preparations aren't made.

Will you be going home to bed? Will someone in the family need medical care training? Will your home need supporting medical equipment? Supplies? Ask your surgical team and your oncologist (also see Chapter 43, "Care at Home").

Will you need medical outpatient services—radiation, chemo, imaging, testing, pharmacology, other surgeries, or treatment for other maladies? Will these services be readily available to you? Are financial arrangements made?

Will you need professional home nursing? Reserve the service ahead of time and get the cost approved by your insurance carrier, Medicare, or whomever.

Will you need physical therapy? The details can be complex. Get the overall purpose and process description from your surgical team. Get the details from the rehab unit it recommends. Learn by discussing the experience with others who have been through it. Get a time schedule and a budget. Have both approved by your insurance carrier (also review Chapter 28, "Nutrition and Fitness," and, if necessary, Chapter 29, "Implants and Replacement Parts").

Is "discomfort" going to be a part of recovery? Get a pain specialist on your team ahead of time. This is usually an anesthesiologist specializing in the treatment consequences of cancers of your sort. Get a program going so you stay ahead of the worst of what you might otherwise have encountered. Be very pleased that you will not have to endure things that a patient might have faced as recently as ten years ago.

Will plastic surgery or some other form of bodywork be necessary? It is often best to seamlessly integrate this restoration into your recovery process. Once again, pay attention to cost, who will pay and when, any necessary pre-clearances, the notable exclusions and exceptions of your health-insurance policy, and the rest of that stuff (you may need to review "Supporting Resources," Part IV, and Chapter 14, "Health Insurance," in particular).

Amputees and those who will lose their hearing, sight, or voice face the same issues of preparation, planning, programming, physical therapies, costs, and so on (see Chapter 29, "Implants and Replacement Parts").

How to Make Recovery Easier

Those close to the patient can take steps that improve both the quality and the speed of recovery after surgery.

Should your insurance company or Medicare reject funding for part of your recovery plan, the head of your surgical team may need to reword the surgical protocol. Or different billing codes may be necessary.
These steps have nothing to do with recovery. They have to do with computers and claim forms.

Stress-Free Environment

Don't allow smoking in the patient's house, much less in the recovery room.

Do not bring arguments or crises to the patient's bedside for solution. Don't bring anger. Don't scold the children, scream at the dog, berate the postman, or argue on the phone within earshot of your sick loved one. Don't whisper, either. Make the patient's room Disneyland, the happiest place on earth. Even patients who are professional worriers and alpha-type family managers will rest better and recuperate faster.

Fresh Air and Light

Daytime television can get as stale as a tray of dirty dishes. Freshen the fare with movies, travelogues, home-study courses, Internet exploration, a CD of family pictures.

Even then, the time will probably come when looking at anything off the screen will become preferable to looking at anything on it.

No less an authority than the National Institutes of Health prescribes a recovery room with a view—not looking out on a brick wall, in other words. Weather and the patient's condition permitting, it is nice to have a window that opens, admitting fresh air. Put an air freshener in the room to keep out unpleasant odors. Keep the room picked up and clean. Provide light so the patient isn't a cave dweller. Many patients like music, as well as TV. And your sick person gets to choose the station, all the time.

These are ideal conditions, of course. Rooms without a window or a view can still be made inviting. See Chapter 43 for more tips to improve the healing powers of a recovery room.

Surgery-Recovery Group

Major surgeries require major recoveries. In some cases, this process is more easily managed by the patient with the help of people who have already been down this road. A patient with a little energy can find people to chat with by phone or computer. Don't be offended if the patient prefers privacy during these conferences.

Mobility

You may be introduced to crutches, a walker, or a wheelchair during convalescence. You may need more—an orthotic or some other sort of brace. These things are not supposed to be surprises. Normally—but not always—your surgical team prepares you. If, in discussing your surgical plan with a veteran, you learn that help getting around is sometimes necessary after the sort of operation planned for you, go back to your surgical team to see if it is a possibility in your case. If so, ask to be prepared, and be sure your insurance coverage is ready.

Consulting on the Internet

More and more people put their faith in the Internet. While you may find lots of information that pertains to your procedure, your hospital, and even your surgeon, be cautioned that volume does not equate to accuracy or responsibility.

Survivor Sites

You may stumble across or hear about a considerable number of Web sites run by cancer patients. In general, their medical advice is not highly rated by the professional oncology community. Fund-raising activities, items for sale, social activities, and things to write to Congress about are also posted on these sites.

If the experience of asking questions at one of these sites was disappointing—or disturbing—try the agencies and nonprofits listed in the Reference Center. The folks you reach are generally better prepared to serve your needs. The organizations they represent have met high standards. The survivor sites—which may also have met high standards—did not have to.

Commercial Sites

All drug companies and treatment centers have Web sites. So do many non-traditional treatment advocates, nutrition interests, manufacturers, and their professional associations. Those that deal across state lines must observe the laws governing interstate commerce, or at least appear to. You still have to be careful.

Garbage, Myths, and Cultural, Political, and Religious Bias

If a site is suitably accessorized with the blessings of the Better Business Bureau, *Consumer Reports,* Federal Drug Administration, American College of Surgeons, American Medical Association, or a similar generally recognized watchdog or authority, there is reason to accept its offerings. But there remains the possibility of misunderstanding or misinterpretation. If the Web site claims lesser authority, or none, you may not want to bet your health on its advice.

Government and Established Nonprofits

There are people in our nation's capital whom, as sportscaster Steve Young might put it, we hope to keep closer to the Gatorade than to the ball. Despite them, the National Institutes of Health, its National Cancer Institute, and other arms of federal government having to do with health matters are better today than they have ever been. And they are by far the best in the world. See the Reference Center for the Web addresses of these and other responsible voices.

Nutrition

Instructions for recovering at home from surgery other than operations that open the stomach or intestinal tract may not mention diet. That could be an oversight. Ask your doc if you should discuss your situation with the staff nutritionist (also see Chapter 28, "Nutrition and Fitness").

Thanks

There is a wonderful bumper sticker you may have seen: "If you can read this, thank a teacher." In the same spirit, consider the thanks due to the army of men and women whose treatment and nurturing skills are enriching and extending your life. A surprisingly small number of patients or their families write thank-you notes. Far fewer volunteer time or make a monetary donation to a related cause.

VI Related Issues

Topics You May Need to Know More About

42 Budgeting

You need to know this stuff.

To the person who is sick and worried, cost is beside the point. Find out what's wrong and fix it.

Shortly thereafter, still sick, now weary, with a bandage over a needle stick and a next-appointment slip in hand, you face a person who asks, "And what method of payment will you be using?" This medical team, like all the others, has an economic engine.

If not at this point, then very soon, the chorus of payment questions from people at desks, your health-insurance provider, and others gives you one more thing to be sick of. Even those served by HMOs are likely to have significant extra expenses. There will be complexities. Worst of all, there will be surprises.

Maybe your medical team or your insurer feels certain that your costs will be of little consequence. If not, you or one of those helping you through this ordeal may decide that a cost forecast is necessary. This chapter is here to help.

Avoiding This Subject

If you really don't care about costs, or if you just don't want to spoil a good mood, stop reading. The complexity and unfairness of this issue will at least confuse you and maybe dishearten you. You will learn that your insurer, your hospital, your medical team, your employer, and others you will be counting on for support can be callous. From this point forward, you may want a lawyer, an accountant, an insurance expert, and a junkyard dog in tow.

If you decide to read on, understand that the objective is to leave you stirred, not shaken. Try to be dispassionate. And please don't shoot the messenger.

Consultations

There are no pat answers when forecasting costs. People who work in the various areas of interest must give you carefully considered answers. Every case is different. You will want to consult with several different kinds of folks.

Medical Team

Somebody on staff should be able to analyze the elements of your situation and give you what the team considers a fair ballpark assessment of the drug and treatment costs facing you. Be aware that the costs quoted will cover only medical treatments and drugs administered by that team. While these are sometimes heady numbers, they may fall well short of your grand total.

Qualified Financial Planner

The American Cancer Society recommends that you hire a financial planner and offers a brochure on the subject. "How to Find a Financial Professional Sensitive to Cancer Issues" is free. To order, call the ACS at 800/224-2345, or visit www.cancer.org. You can also go to the Reference Center "Yellow Pages" to locate financial planners who may be qualified to help you.

A person with cancer brings a couple of special circumstances to a financial planner. Some of these folks may not be prepared to give you the level of help you had hoped for. Ask about experience with the particular problems of living with cancer. If you accept the ACS suggestion that you consult a financial planner, work with a veteran.

Health-Insurance Provider

People at health-insurance companies have statistical tables that tell them what your treatment and drug programs will probably cost. Once your case is understood and a nurse-advocate is assigned to it, you may be able to get data through that channel. Expect any numbers you get to be limited to direct medical costs—essentially, data on insurance-industry indemnities, though there could be more. If anything, cost indicators from one of these actuaries will be low. Multiyear databases are used at a time when the cost trends are up, up, up. New, more expensive procedures are constantly being introduced (also see Chapter 14, "Health Insurance").

Employee-Assistance Professional

If you work for a large organization, you may have access to an EAP or to someone who fills that role at work or in your community. This person has experience and may be able to help you. You may also come across an oncology social worker or a psychosocial nurse linked to a treatment center who can help you with medical cost data (more on this in Chapter 12, "The Patient's Workplace").

Second Opinions

We have discussed the advisability of second—even third—medical opinions in early chapters. While you're getting the opinions, get cost figures.

A Survivor of Your Kind of Cancer

Not everybody who has gone through the ordeal you face will know what things cost. Many—probably most—patients don't track it. If you can find a veteran who can discuss costs with you, it will be eye-opening. You don't need to find a twin, but things to match include the same type cancer, stage, part of the body, age, sex, lifestyle, hospital, medical team, type of insurance.

Finding a Survivor to Consult With

The charities and service organizations listed in the Reference Center, with counselors at toll-free phone numbers, are staffed by people with the background and training most apt to help you. You can also ask your oncology team to introduce you to another patient, a former patient, or the close companion of a patient. If you are fortunate, there will be a cancer-survivor support group of the Wellness Community nearby, or the hospital may sponsor a suitable support group. Support-group organizations and hospitals often have libraries of helpful data too.

If all else fails, sit down with friends and try to estimate what's ahead and its cost. But the exercise will be less effective because the experience factor is missing.

Sordid Nitty-Gritty

We are about to explore some of the nastiest, least-fair topics a recovering cancer patient faces. Please do not conclude that any of these costs are usual or even common. If they come along, some will be covered by insurance or paid for through some device such as a clinical trial. Some will be partly covered. Some may be forgiven if you holler loud enough.

This list is provided because these costs can appear, and you, as a person who is very serious about forecasting a budget for the time of your treatment, have demanded to know the possibilities:

- Insurance (includes HMO) goes up
- Insurance cap too low
- Time loss at work and its consequences, especially lost income and reduced health benefits
- Job loss due to the illness
- Transportation and living away from home for tests or treatment
- Prosthetic and cosmetic devices that insurance won't cover
- A prosthetic or cosmetic device superior to the one the insurance covers
- Elective cosmetic surgery
- Purchase of blood or blood products
- Search for a blood, stem-cell, tissue, marrow, or organ donor
- Things insurance doesn't cover that you must do to get on the list for a transplant or other highly specialized treatment
- Physical therapies that helped
- Family and personal professional counseling
- Home medical equipment and other needs related to treatment or recuperation
- Home-modifications, particularly structural accommodations
- Education and research, including this book
- Loans
- Legal matters
- Professional help to fight your health insurer, health provider, government agency ruling, or personal lawsuit

- Tax and accounting fees
- Wardrobe (smaller or bigger clothes, wigs, hats, scarves)
- New or special hearing aid or glasses
- Child care or elder care
- Ostomy supplies and maintenance
- Computer and other home-office needs
- Home phone, Internet, heating, and electricity add-ons
- Modifying or purchasing another motor vehicle
- Special arrangements for other family members in place of duties you performed

- Housekeeping, gardening, home maintenance
- Nontraditional, off-label, and "investigational" drugs, procedures, and devices that you need
- The difference between what is allowed for a drug or procedure and what you have to pay
- Some palliative drugs and procedures you may need, especially to relieve pain or nausea
- Some cosmetics and cosmetic procedures directly related to your cancer
- Others' expenses, because of your illness
- Other medical and dental needs required or recommended by your oncology team or radiologist
- The unplanned medical opinions that you needed during treatments
- Exclusions from medical insurance. (Transplants and off-label drugs are common. It is even more common to discover that, once treated, you can't go back for seconds of the same thing. For more, see Chapter 14, "Health Insurance.")
- Imaging using more sophisticated devices than are covered by insurance
- Imaging at facilities other than those covered
- Imaging and other services necessary before permission of the insurer or managing health agency could be obtained
- Special technical support, like digitizing patient image files for greater portability and avoidance of new Internet security measures

Notes on Planning

It may help the budgeting process to figure out when a cost is apt to come along. A successful battle with cancer may take years.

You may also benefit by not automatically assuming that you will have to pay the same for something as someone else did. The cost could be higher or lower, or you may discover that there is a new, improved alternative.

As you proceed with your cost investigation, you will meet people with specialized experience in various phases of treatment and recovery. Many are salespeople or counselors who represent eventualities you wonder about because you may need them: extended home care, special therapies, alternative prosthetics, visits to out-of-town centers of medical excellence, that sort of thing. Some of these people are very conversant with costs, benefits, and trade-offs.

Specialized Centers of Cancer Healing

There are treatment centers for cancer patients throughout the world that feature patent medicines and therapies. Highly technical terms are applied to their benefits: "holistic immunotherapy," "antineoplaston therapy." The price tags are often as impressive as the medical terminology. If you also meet "counselors" assigned to "help" you find the resources to pay for these, be reasonably certain that mainstream oncology is not being offered, and that you will be on your own when the bill comes.

Budget Software

By transferring budget items and costs to a computer-spreadsheet program, a patient or partner may find planning and cost forecasting much easier. The math sure is.

There are some wonderful software programs that help, starting in the range of fifty dollars. They can keep a cancer program on budget, point out discrepancies, transfer funds, write checks, address envelopes, forecast, prepare tax reports. Look at more than one software product before making a decision. Once you pick one and begin to use it, a change will be hard. Go online for convenient free demos. Go for more bells and whistles rather than fewer.

43 Care at Home

> Use the Wizard's instruction to Dorothy. Shut your eyes, click your heels, and keep repeating, "There's no place like home."

In-and-Out Cancer

M. D. Anderson, often ranked the top cancer hospital in the United States, treats about two thousand cancer patients per weekday with fewer than six hundred beds available. Even though Anderson attracts the sickest of the sick from around the world, almost everyone is treated and released the same day. It is the very model of a modern major hospital.

Even when the procedure is quite traumatic, your medical team will have you on your feet and headed for the exit long before you may think that's a good idea. Recuperation at home, even with tubes still attached, is now the norm.

Benefits of Home Care

In an environment of love and encouragement—with proper attention to hygiene—a home is often the best place a patient can go to recover. People who love and encourage—and include—the patient give healing powers and joy to a person in great need. This positive atmosphere requires work and attention to detail. When the love and close proximity are not maintained, when negative vibes enter the relationship, the patient's recovery suffers.

This is obvious stuff backed by good science. To review, make a quick trip back to Chapter 13, "Friends." Then consider getting an aquarium for the patient's room.

Family Stress and Costs

The power of family love goes a long way toward making the best of the major production that recovery at home can become. There is no denying, however, that taking care of someone who is very sick is at the least a distraction and an inconvenience. It brings extra expenses with it. The income of at least one of the family providers may also be reduced because of time away from the job. Careers can suffer. There are often odorous and onerous matters: shots, IVs, ostomy bags, bedpans, diapers, wound cleaning, bandage changes, bathing the patient, therapy. Someone has to attend to hospital equipment, a special bed, a wheelchair, and all that. Then you have to navigate around it all. Just walk into the house and you smell sickness instead of dinner. It can be awful.

Sick kids don't think about it. A sick spouse will. A sick grandparent may worry so much about being in the way that he or she may deplete critical financial resources to pay for a stay in a nursing home or other far less recuperative environment. It is up to the family of a person with cancer to provide—or to decide not to give—home care.

Family Nursing Skills

Wanting to give compassionate service gets you halfway toward being able to help the person recovering at home. The doctors, nurses, and therapists on the case can show you the other half. The Red Cross also offers excellent classes, as do many community colleges and some cities' agencies.

It may demand you learn new skills, such as how to give a shot. It might require you to get over some learned behavior or squeamishness. Just listen to your teachers and your heart. Take notes. Practice. Take pride. You can be absolutely, positively certain that your help is a healing gift.

A Support Team

If you live in or near a town of almost any size, there are people who can bring nursing and therapy skills to your home. There may also be visiting doctors. The oncology team knows the names and phone numbers of many of them (see the "Nursing at Home" listing in the "Yellow Pages" portion of the Reference Center for more).

Some of this help is provided without charge to those who cannot pay. Compassion is high on the list of motivations of people in the business of delivering home care. But expect these folks to ask you to provide any financial support you can and to attempt to find a third-party payer for the balance of the costs. Please cooperate with the effort. Volunteer programs have to be funded too.

The tensions of home care—especially the extra costs and disruption—can overshadow the mission of saving a critically ill person's life.

Special Discount on Electricity

You can get a special discount on electricity during the time a patient is recuperating in your home. The life-support and other special equipment installed for the patient qualifies you. Call your utility's customer-service people for details.

Cost

A Needs Evaluation

Professionals will want to formally assess the situation and its needs before beginning a home-care program. They may need an inventory of necessary equipment, a look at the patient's home environment, a visit with the patient's oncology team, nurses, or therapists. If these investigations take place during a phase of the process in which such teams are competing for your business, you are not apt to be charged for any of this. If this work follows your selection of a home-care crew, you have more chance of receiving a bill. If this work can be charged to a third party, such as a health-insurance company or Medicare, it's in everybody's best interests.

The Visiting Nurses Association estimates the rate for a typical home-health-care service evaluation at $50 to $150 per hour. If you are going to be paying for it, ask what the exact per-hour rate will be and get an estimate of the number of hours a study is apt to require. From those facts, some acceptable cost ceiling can be agreed to before the work begins.

Medicare

Medicare pays for home care under certain conditions. A doctor must prescribe it. You must require intermittent, not constant, professional care. You must be homebound, meaning that you're stuck in bed, though you might be able to drag yourself out the door ahead of a slow fire. Finally, the home health-care providers must be prequalified by Medicare.

If the patient meets the qualifications, Medicare will pay for:

- Skilled nursing, part-time
- A home-health aid who helps the patient with personal care such as bathing, toilet, and dressing
- Physical, speech, and occupational therapy ordered by a doctor
- Some help with social and emotional concerns. Don't assume that you can get the counseling you think you need or that the cost will be what you've heard. Carefully question your Medicare advisor
- Limited medical supplies directly related to the cancer treatment

---

Financial help with the purchase of prescription drugs for Medicare patients began in 2005 and continues to improve. But this is a transitional period. Assume nothing. Call 800-MEDICARE, 24-7, to learn more.

If Medicare does not provide the drug help you need, turn to the Reference Center "Yellow Pages." Look under "Financial Assistance" for organizations that provide free or very low cost drugs to cancer patients, and even assistance with co-pays. If you know the name of the manufacturer of the drug you need, look in the same place to see if it sponsors a nonprofit that will help you.

Medicare does not pay for around-the-clock care, meals delivered to your home, or homemaker services such as cleaning, laundry, and shopping. (Other service providers and volunteer agencies may; see the Reference Center.)

Medicaid

This joint federal-state program provides the same general services and terms as Medicare to the poorest of the poor and to cancer patients with specific types of disease.

Medicaid may have a different name in your state. To locate the state medical assistance office, call 877/267-2323, or visit Centers for Medicare and Medicaid, www.cms.hhs.gov.

Private Insurance

Home health care is a feature of many indemnity plans, PPOs, and HMOs. There is usually a co-pay, meaning that the patient pays a chunk. There are usually exclusions. There may be limits on the amount the insurance will pay for specific services you may need, and you may have a deductible to pay before cost sharing begins. Private insurers demand the same four qualifications discussed earlier for Medicare.

Recall from Chapter 14 that there is an employee at your health-insurance company called a nurse-advocate or case nurse who is charged with helping you get the most bang from your buck. Discuss the possibility of home health care with this person before the need is imminent. Some time for research and evaluation of circumstances may be necessary. If there are gray areas, you may need further time for negotiating and for insurance-company internal committees to staff questions. You may need time to get facts or a prescription from a doctor.

None of this will be a surprise if you had your health-insurance policy vetted by an expert who understood the demands your cancer would probably place on your policy (Chapter 14, "Health Insurance"). You took action and came to this place in your cancer ordeal prepared to get the most from coverage and other resources you have learned about.

Cash

It is amazing how deeply costs can sometimes be discounted when a simple cash payment at the time of services is proposed. When the government paperwork, insurance claims, processing correspondence, and cost of credit and accounting come out of the payment equation, half the burden on some services is eliminated. Folding money at the door—negotiated in advance—may work with doctors, in hospitals, just about anywhere. Cash is king, baby.

Assembling and Keeping a Support Team

Picking and Choosing

It is appropriate to interview candidates for at-home nursing care and for therapy. You want individuals who show an interest in your case and an enthusiasm for the contributions they can bring to the patient's condition. A candidate who has ideas for therapy or suggests novelties such as going on outings with the patient is going to be a better healer than a candidate with a boundless interest in daytime TV.

You probably won't be able to require it, so listen carefully during your interview for your candidate to suggest help with light cleaning and meal preparation. They all know that you're going to need it. Some of the best will pitch in.

Negotiation and Rewards

The rates of nurses and therapists are not mandated and will vary. Bargaining is a good idea. So are bonuses for patient-recuperation milestones and for good general service. Examples could include being reliably prompt for a month, or hanging around after hours when there was a need. You are going to discover that the home-care industry is not a well-paid place. What may look like a lot of money goes into many hands. A little palm grease is a wise investment. If there is no money, think of some small gift from your household resources, perhaps homemade candy or a something out of your garden.

Thank-yous

Always thank your home-care team for jobs well done. Good work deserves your appreciation. It is even more important to make it clear by your thanks that a job has been performed properly. This makes it possible to redirect a person more positively who is doing something you want stopped. These little corrections you need to make, like turning the volume of the TV down, are easy and effective when they are part of a generally upbeat, enthusiastic atmosphere.

In many cases, your home-care team is part of a larger organization with a supervisor in a business office somewhere. On occasions that deserve it, thank a supervisor for providing such an outstanding person for your home. This will be even more effective if you give the supervisor at least one specific reason for your praise, in a note.

Voluntary and Involuntary Replacements

Sometimes workers in the home-care industry leave a job before it is done. If one of your workers quits, it may be instructive to know why. It is often a personal issue. Your worker is bored or needs more time for some personal matter. If some part of the reason is your fault, you should know that. You may not want to repeat the mistake with the next person.

On occasion, a worker has to be asked to leave. If the person works for an organization, call the supervisor and request termination. Carefully consider the reasons you provide. This will have serious consequences for the worker.

If the worker is self-employed, give notice at the end of a shift. Try not to be overly negative or threatening. Just state that you will not require any further service. Thank the person if you can manage to. Give a full final payment. Make sure all personal possessions depart with the person. If gifts have been exchanged, be prepared to give them back. There may be a friendship with the patient to mitigate against this, but it is better if the person is asked not to come back. Have someone with you if companionship during this meeting is helpful.

The Nursing-Home Alternative

You should carefully evaluate nursing homes, recuperation wings of hospitals, and similar places before you allow them to become serious rest-and-recuperation options. Visit any facility you wish to consider seriously.

Be it ever so humble, there's no place like home.

John H. Payne, Clari, the Maid of Milan (1823)

Many of these places are little more than warehouses for people with nowhere else to go. The promise of twenty-four-hour doctoring and nursing care may be laughable. The food, the smell, and the environment could be awful. Serious new disease, on top of what the patient was admitted with, is distinctly possible.

Hospice Care

When cure of illness is no longer a possibility, hospice care can be requested through the oncology staff, Medicare, Medicaid, or directly from a hospice provider. Hospice care is usually home based. It is structured to provide for the physical needs of the patient during the last six months of life. All costs are paid through a consortium of Medicare and state and local agencies, with the cooperation of any private medical insurance that serves the patient.

The patient's physicians, nurses, physical therapists, and social workers cooperate under a hospice umbrella. All drugs and hospital equipment come to the home. Nursing visits and consultation with physicians are available 24-7, though around-the-clock nursing at the patient's bedside is not. Basic legal services related to wills and durable powers may be provided. If not, look for help in the "Yellow Pages" section of the Reference Center under "Legal Services."

Though hospice provides grief support to survivors for thirteen months following the demise of the patient, family counseling before the death of the patient may not be covered. If a professional counselor is brought in, hospice—not the patient or family—picks the person. If your place of worship provides counseling, this is the time to seek it.

Additional Resources

- The extensive Web site of the Visiting Nurses Association is at www.vnaa.org. It includes detailed discussions of issues. It offers checklists that organize and qualify home-care programs. It has a locator for available members throughout the United States by zip code.

- The free publication *How to Choose a Home Care Provider* is available from the National Association for Home Care. Call 202/547-7424, or go to www.nahc.org.
- The American Cancer Society has a free pamphlet titled *Caring for the Patient with Cancer at Home: A Guide for Parents and Families*. Call 800/ACS-2345, or order at www.cancer.org.
- The American College of Physicians offers a free publication, *Home Care Guide for Advanced Cancer Care*. Call 800/523-1546. Ask for Customer Services, extension 2600. (This organization's Web site is not very functional without a member's identification code.)

44 Clinical Trials

Well over 7,500 clinical trials are under way at any one time. About 2,000 of them are directly linked to the battle against cancer. Many will provide patients and their healing teams with cause for hope. Some will partly meet the goals their developers set for them. Some will take research teams to a wholly unexpected place. Some will simply fail.

Clinical Trials, Generally Speaking

You should favor the use of clinical trials. Nearly all the progress made in treating various kinds of cancer in the last forty years involved their use, according to the National Cancer Institute. The NCI and corporate developers heavily subsidize each one. Cost to the patient is rarely an issue, though cost to the health-insurance provider may be.

About 10 percent of cancer patients participate in one or more clinical trials. The most common reason the other 90 percent don't is that, for their illness, there is no reason to consider using an experimental drug or procedure. The illness has an effective, understood means of treatment. The case proceeds as the oncologist intended, meeting everyone's expectations.

Some patients decide not to participate in a clinical trial proposed to them. One of the common reasons is that travel makes it inconvenient. Another is the completely unfounded fear that you might end up in the group that gets the sugar pill instead of the real deal. Not only is travel inconvenient and difficult for ill patients to endure, but also it may be expensive. But the fear of finding out later that you didn't get the good stuff is unfounded. The managers of any clinical trial that includes a placebo-taking control group are duty bound to make certain that everyone in the test knows it.

Thanks largely to the findings of clinical trials, the five-year survival rate for all stages of breast cancer is nearing 84 percent, and rates for melanoma and cancers of the cervix, uterus, prostate, and bladder exceed 90 percent.

Jane E. Brody, "Personal Health" (New York Times, October 15, 2002)

Clinical trials are run by any of several sets of ground rules, none of which are kept secret from the patients. In one of the most common types of clinical trial, everyone gets the clinical trial medication. In another common format, patients receive either the investigational therapy or what medical science considers the best of the established therapies. In those cases, the best choice between the therapy being tested and the established route is hard to guess, going in. Sometimes the investigational therapy turns out to be best. Sometimes not. Sometimes parts of each test group enjoy the greater benefits. Sometimes everybody improves about the same.

Some people worry that some new drug might be harmful. Except in phase I trials, which are rarely open to the public, your chances of being harmed are low. Federal data indicate that only one in ten thousand patients in clinical trials has died of the effects of the drug being studied. "We're not doing enough to explain how medical research works, and the benefits and rewards of participation," says Mark Eisenach, chief executive of Acurian, a clinical trials company in Philadelphia.

Kinds of Clinical Trials

A clinical trial is a test of a new intervention to fight your disease. It could be a new drug. Many of the compounds used in chemotherapy are involved in clinical trials. Pain medications, vaccines, psychiatric compounds, wound-healing drugs, and many other sorts of FDA-controlled compounds may be offered as parts of trials.

All sorts of devices may also be parts of clinical trials. Some are implants, including pacemaker-type stimulators and artificial bones and joints. Some help make treatments more effective or improve the comfort of the patient. Some are diagnostic tools, notably ways to examine patient conditions non-invasively. There are devices related to surgical procedure recovery, including some used in supporting roles like ostomy. Trials test prosthetic devices. They test whole ranges of monitors and other things that assist the day-to-day life of a recovering cancer patient.

There are many laboratory analytical processes in a clinical trial. The detection of cancer cells remains an area of great challenge. Genetics are studied in hope of learning how to forecast cancer and to predict where it may travel from the place it originated. Another interesting field of study hopes to understand why some other diseases attack and sometimes obliterate cancers. Vaccine research also becomes more promising every day (see Chapter 31, "Vaccines").

Not all the drugs and procedures in clinical trials are new. Some have been used for other purposes for years, even centuries. Some cancer fighters are under consideration for new or different uses. Drugs that have been discarded may resurface in clinical trials. For example, thalidomide, a horror that caused birth defects in children in the 1960s, is now in clinical trials for the treatment of breast, prostate, brain cancer, and Kaposi's sarcoma, according to the FDA. Men and women of active reproductive age must be aware of its serious effect on the unborn. But it appears to be an excellent cancer fighter under at least some circumstances.

Preclinical Studies

The ideas that eventually trigger clinical trials usually come from laboratory-based research and discovery. The next steps in development try to strip away extraneous factors that may be making the discovery more or less effective. Once down to the nitty-gritty, laboratory experiments are common, followed by studies using animals. Ideas that pass these tests go next to clinical trial.

Animal studies are an irreplaceable step in learning as much as possible about medical science without subjecting a human being to unnecessarily dangerous experimentation. Researchers prefer other means of testing, where possible. But eventually, animals become necessary. This is a humane process, now defined and governed at every turn.

If you are uncomfortable knowing that animals are used in medical research, please don't let your distaste deter you from accepting treatment. This is not the time to decline help on principle. Just about every part of the fight against cancer that you have already benefited or will benefit from — surgical procedures, drugs, tests, and many teaching methods — required the support of live animals. This testing is also universal in the development of cosmetics, processed foods, and in many other parts of life you encounter daily.

Americans tend to be squeamish about animal research. Three-quarters of the world's pets live in the United States, according to the U.S. Census Bureau.

Stages of Clinical Trials

Clinical trials are experiments. To reduce the risk as far as possible, each trial goes through at least three phases. When invited to participate, a patient needs to know which phase a trial is in to make the most informed decision. In addition to learning the stage of a trial, evaluate, as best you can, the confidence level of those inviting you to be a part of the process. You may ask the person in charge of this clinical trial a simple question that takes the issue down to where the rubber meets the road: "If your child were in my situation, is this the next thing you would want for him or her?" If the reply to this question requires more than one word, there may be further complexities to be discovered and studied before you make your decision. You may also need to consult other experts.

Phase I

In clinical trials, phase I is the first step that studies effects on people. Something fewer than a hundred patients participate, typically patients who cannot be helped by other treatments. Safety is the first concern of researchers, even before efficacy. Researchers study how a drug is absorbed, metabolized and excreted during phase I trials. They measure side effects at varying dose levels. About 70 percent of new cancer drugs pass this test.

Phase II

A larger group of patients participate in phase II of development, which focuses on efficacy. Phase II testing may continue over months or years

until all test questions have been answered. Often, phase II tests involve
two groups. One receives the element being investigated, while the other
receives the standard accepted best treatment. Results are compared. When
possible, the researchers prefer not to let those in the study know which
group they are in. This eliminates several possible effects that might bias
the result. Only about one-third of experimental drugs pass both phase I and
phase II.

Phase III

Hundreds to thousands of patients are involved in a drug's phase III testing.
The FDA and the manufacturer amass statistically significant performance
results that can be applied to the nation as a whole. Randomly selected
patients receive either the test compound or the standard accepted best treatment. Testing may continue for several years. About 90 percent of drugs that
enter phase III pass. Once testing is completed to the FDA's satisfaction, the
manufacturer can request approval to market the drug. Permission may or
may not be given—or may be given provisionally.

"At the very least," reports Jane Brody, *New York Times* medical columnist, "you will receive the best established therapy. At most, you will be
among the first to receive a treatment that proves to be ... either more
effective or less hazardous. All participants in clinical trials also receive
high-quality care and are likely to be closely monitored and tested to assess
their progress."

Phase IV

The complexities of clinical studies are almost endless. Typically, questions
remain after phase III, or some side effect in a small number of patients
needs to be watched, or something else demands more work. This may be
called "late phase III" or phase IV. Studies in this phase may compare the
performance of the new drug to others already on the market.

One of the greatest causes of concern among clinical trial teams is the
almost predictable delay of final reports and studies. As of February 2002,
fewer than half of the phase IV studies the FDA was holding open, pending
final study reports from the manufacturer, were on schedule. In a report to
Congress, 882 of 2,400 commitments to the FDA's drug division had been
completed, and 44 of 301 had made it to its biologics division. This is no
scandal. As the FDA itself explained in its report, no one can accurately predict how long it will take to test unknowns.

Cost to the Patient

Clinical trials that involve experimental drugs and procedures are often
delivered to participants at little or no charge. Other trials that use established equipment, methods, or pharmaceuticals in new ways often come at
a cost to the patient. Some clinical trials have price tags that health insurers
balk at covering.

Mistaken Assumptions

"Taking Part in Clinical Trials," a free pamphlet published by the National Cancer Institute, points out: "New treatments under study are not always better than, or even as good as, standard care. They may have side effects that doctors do not expect or that are worse than standard treatment." New treatments can lead patients down unexpected paths that may cost more, exact greater physical discomfort, or take longer to provide the desired result.

A second point is commonly overlooked. Your body is not like anyone else's. Even though a new treatment does a better job on average during a clinical trial, that does not guarantee that you will benefit to any greater extent than the patient in the trial group who fared the worst. As you evaluate a treatment's potential, hope for the best but be prepared for lesser heights.

This is a good place to remember that medical insurance companies rather frequently take issue with "experimental" medicine. Both the providers that write checks to hospitals and the HMO types that decide what meds and procedures to offer you can be stiff-necked. There are several reasons for the static you may encounter, most having to do with cost. It is a good idea either to be certain that a new procedure is approved in advance or to come to the approval meeting prepared for a fight.

The Clinical Trial as a Cloaking Device

Cancer patients are slipped into free clinical trials every day so that they can receive effective treatment at a saving. Typically, the doc has every confidence in the positive effects of the treatment and the hospital owes the oncology group a favor. In other cases, the manufacturer donates its product to a worthy cause (you). When the insurance people share the savings, this is a dandy arrangement for all concerned.

The Sordid Past of the Clinical Trial

The clinical exploitation of the underprivileged was common until recently in the United States and continues in much of the rest of the world. Americans behind bars and children in orphanages were experimented on into the mid-1900s. During the early 1930s, four hundred black men were infected with syphilis without their knowledge by government researchers at Alabama's Tuskegee Institute. Treatment was then denied them for forty years to document the natural progression of the disease. As recently as the 1950s, the U.S. Army gave LSD to soldiers and marched others through the debris of fresh nuclear weapons tests.

As a result of this sordid history, 63 percent of black Americans and 38 percent of the white population believe that some doctors still experiment on patients without their knowledge or permission, according to a recent University of North Carolina study. The medical community and government watchdogs adamantly deny that irresponsible or involuntary drug experimentation happens anymore.

Evaluating a Proposed Clinical Trial

There are extensive lists of questions that experts suggest patients use to evaluate clinical trial proposals. Questions having to do with cost and duration of the experiment make sense. The manufacturer—at the insistence of the FDA—provides other information that is always interesting to patients or necessary to their well-being. You are supposed to be carefully briefed and then given this information in writing as part of the meeting in which a clinical trial is proposed to you.

If anything, this process overreaches. Some of the topics, while arguably important, bring up matters that cannot have full valid answers. One of the common questions is, "What risks are involved?" An honest answer would be, "We think this drug will do you more good than harm. But we don't know."

In the end, if you accept the offer of a clinical trial, it should be because you trust the doctor who recommended it. If you don't trust the doctor who recommends a clinical trial—or any other procedure—there is an unacceptable weakness in your team's cohesion that needs your immediate attention.

Searching for the Best Clinical Trial

More than eighty thousand sites in the United States are outlets for clinical trials of one kind or another, and many of these trials are critically undersubscribed. If they don't add more people to their rolls, they can't document enough case histories to make the test acceptable to the FDA. Without FDA acceptance, the medicine or device can't be sold. All the investment in R and D goes into the tank. You better believe they want your business.

That is why you may have seen brochures titled something like "A Patient's Guide to Cancer Clinical Trials." That is why you may have noticed magazine think pieces on how to decide which clinical trial to sign up for and clinical trial Web sites that promise "unique and powerful search engines for oncology professionals." These are all appeals for patients, just as are television commercials for drugs that can be obtained only with a prescription. It's a way of churning up the market in the expectation that excitement will generate sales.

Most people come to the realization that, for a patient with no medical training, the decision to "talk to your doctor about Doxorubicin" is silly. Your doctor will bring it up if it makes any sense.

The "Hail Mary" Clinical Trial

Abigail Burroughs, a twenty-one-year-old senior at the University of Virginia, died a few years ago of head and neck cancer. She had taken every medication her doctors could think of, according to a story about her struggle in the *Los Angeles Times*, "A Push for Wider Use of Experimental Drugs," by Judy Foreman, September 29, 2003. Her last chance, she believed, might be one of two new drugs. Her father, Frank, contacted the manufacturers. Both compounds were in clinical trials that target other forms of cancer. Not head and neck. On that basis, Abigail Burroughs was denied access to them.

Powerful forces believe that the decision not to give these experimental drugs to the thousands like Abigail Burroughs who attempt to gain access every year is proper. "We have a system in place to prove the safety and efficacy of therapies. We can't afford to undermine that system," the *Times* quotes Fran Visco, president of the National Breast Cancer Coalition. "The system is premised on (the idea that) drugs should not be available until they are proven safe and effective."

The history of sick people made sicker by untested or misunderstood drugs is a long one. The present FDA-adjudicated system of clinical trial is a direct result, which its adherents are determined to hang onto. Frank Burroughs, who founded the Abigail Alliance for Better Access to Developmental Drugs, is not among them. He has teamed up with the Washington Legal Foundation in an attempt to force the FDA to loosen its rules. He believes that once a drug completes phase I testing for safety (before the test of its efficacy has even begun), cancer patients should be allowed to use it under certain circumstances. Basically, a dying patient should be permitted a sort of "Hail Mary," last-chance pass into the endzone.

The Burroughs proposal "would rip the heart out of clinical research," Nancy Roach, a director of the Marti Nelson Cancer Foundation, is quoted as saying. "New drugs are far more likely to fail than to succeed, so the chances are that a patient will be hurt by a drug rather that helped," adds Dr. Marcia Angell, a former editor of the *New England Journal of Medicine*.

The other side of the coin has an obvious and persuasive argument: Once a patient's condition has failed to respond to all the known ways it might be improved, shouldn't a person have the right to try something experimental? If the scientists complain that some non sequitur would screw up their database, they are welcome to leave it out, aren't they? Equally, when someone is dying, isn't it a bit late to fret about the possible dangers of drug experimentation?

As an editorial writer for the *Wall Street Journal* suggested on April 2, 2003: "No one wants desperate patients placing their hope in elixirs or, worse, exposed to unnecessary risks. But with an increasing number of novel cancer drugs showing obvious safety and effectiveness—and yet far away from formal approval—ways need to be found to get them into the hands of more patients whose lives might be saved."

The only alternatives available to such patients right now come from a U.S. industry that does a multibillion-dollar-a-year business in nostrums that have never been submitted to the FDA for approval or that have failed the FDA trial process. It sells vitamins, herbs, "whole foods," and other "natural" substances through a variety of enterprises that offer "health" and "physical fitness." Surely the experimental development of a major pharmaceutical house is no worse a gamble.

A Useful Clinical Trial Checklist

Two nurses were talking about FDA and pharmaceutical house advisory literature on drugs with a group of patients in the Chemo Room at the Angeles

Clinic and Research Institute in Santa Monica, California. These are some of the points they thought were most important:

How many people are signed up? For a number of reasons, you don't want to be one of the first ten.

What side effects have you seen? If the person recommending the drug claims that there are no side effects, you are probably not speaking to an informed individual.

Will this clinical trial take away other options I may want? If yes, name them and tell me why.

How long will I have to wait to begin the trial? The answer should be "in no more than a few days," or "you start immediately following brief qualification tests." You ask this question because sometimes the wait is longer, which is unwise if your cancer is behaving aggressively.

Have some or all of the elements of this clinical trial been through this process before? If the answer is yes or maybe, learn more. If this is round two for a drug that failed the first time, your chance of benefiting may be significantly better or worse.

What's new about this test? Listen carefully and critically. Make certain you understand the technical terms. Statistical data are sometimes misleading, too.

How long has this clinical trial been going on? If less than one year, it is particularly important that you receive a written risk assessment.

What phase is the trial in? Less is known about drugs in phases I and II than those in phase III or IV. Data on both effectiveness and side effects are far more complete after a drug has been in phase III trial for a year or two.

What do responsible medical reports on the Internet say about it? Look for reports prepared for medical journals and meetings (sometimes called "symposia") by people with affiliations to major healing centers and schools. These are indications that the drug is probably of general professional interest. Then carefully read at least the introductory summaries (often called "abstracts") to see if the author gives the subject a thumb's up or down.

Are there Web sites or Internet chat rooms devoted to this drug or procedure? If so, are they manned by enthusiastic cheerleaders or by grim survivors trying to guide others to safety?

Can your doc give this to you, or do you have to travel? If you have to travel, how far? How often? Is it a nice place? Who picks up the expense tab?

Will I get a placebo? You're sure you won't. Ask anyway.

45 Personal Health Disclosure Guidelines

> Two psychiatrists pass in the street. "Hi! How are you?" the first
> one says. "I'm fine, how are you?" the second replies. As they go on
> their ways, each thinks, "Now what did she mean by that?"

When someone asks, "How are you?" you've got to think about what to say
back. Does this person know you're a cancer patient? Does the person care?
How much detail should your reply have? Do you even want to engage this
person in conversation? If not, what's the best way to politely dismiss the
question?

Times aren't normal. You're of special interest. Prominence demands
social grace. You probably need to give a minute or two to deciding on a strategy for replying to people you know, which is about as long as this chapter
will take to skim.

You also need to know that there are commercial interests that trade in
health data. Some of them will hurt you to make a buck.

A Practiced Short Answer

By now you have learned a good deal about your illness and about the interests of the audiences around you in the everyday world. You have probably
tried explaining your disease by simply saying "cancer." You have seen what
a violent and frightening word it is to many folks. You may have also tried out
more specific answers, such as "Hodgkin's disease." If your cancer began in
the breast and you say "breast cancer," you cannot avoid noticing how peoples' eyes fly to your chest appraisingly. If your cancer began in a sex organ,
you may feel awkward saying so.

The result of this experimentation with various forms of explanation
should produce your elevator speech. This is a pat statement you are comfortable with—something that is minimally disturbing, makes sense, and
avoids any need for follow-up questions. To be successful, it must also be
deliverable in a few seconds, about the time it takes an elevator to move from
one floor to the next.

Once you've got it down, teach it to your partner, your family, your team
at work, your friends at church, so that everybody you are close to has the
same pitch to give to the rest of the world. The great value of this consis-
tent message is that it stops rumors and misunderstandings. Once everyone
has learned the description that works best for you—for example, "It's a
small tumor in the left lung"—you are free of all manner of less attractive
speculations.

Your Partner and Closest Family Members

You can uncover any of our nation's most closely held military secrets by having lunch in the U.S. House of Representatives. Before the first bowl of Congressional Soup has made it to your table, someone will have spilled the beans. The details of your condition will travel at the same rate of speed among your closest family members. Do your best to keep these people current. If the talk remains free of speculation and innuendo, be content.

If you can keep the inner circle repeating the mantra "a little tumor in the left lung" to the rest of the world, you are as close to public relations nirvana as this world permits.

Kids and Elderly Relatives

Your small children and certain aging relatives—you know the ones—have no way of dealing with the facts of your disease, much less its implications. The least harmful alternative for you is to give them your elevator speech— face-to-face, sooner rather than later. Get your inner circle to help you monitor the unfolding evolution of what follows. There may be some consequences, but the mess will be less.

You should not consider trying to keep your condition a secret from the kids and elderly. First of all, you're sick, which is all too self-evident. Second, these people rub elbows in an inner circle that can't help leaking some version of the situation. Much better it comes from you first. If your aging relatives find out from scuttlebutt at the kitchen table, they will know exactly what you did, understand why, and be hurt.

Your Medical Team

In the beginning, tell your family medical professionals and oncology teams everything that might have a bearing on your condition. After a while, you will learn how to shorten the narrative to pertinent facts. General rule: If uncertain, tell.

If, by the way, you're stuck for just the right words for your elevator speech, discuss it with your oncology-team leader.

Health-Providing Organizations

The rule of thumb is to tell your health-insurance company and other health-providing organizations the absolute minimum. You can always add information later, but data can never be taken back. These are meticulous record keepers that are not very good at protecting confidential information.

Your health insurance company's case nurse is usually an exception to this recommendation. He or she should be duty-bound to confidentiality, if you request it.

Some databases managed for the benefit of life-insurance companies and others want your name and as much information as possible about your condition. They will use against you whatever data they gather, both to determine your insurability and to set your rate. (If you learn that a database manager has a file on you, ask to review it for accuracy. A garbled message can make a bad situation worse.)

Your employer may use the same information against you for career decisions. A boss can probably get away with this for the first five years after you have completed treatment. After that, you may have a case—if you can prove that management's using your health history to deny advancement.

If you change jobs and your former employer gives your medical history to your new one, that's a major indiscretion. It shouldn't happen. If it does, consider discussing your options with an attorney.

Questioners' Varied Motives

There will be occasions during your sickness when you will not want to discuss how you feel. To the general question, "How are you?" you shrug and say, "I'm fine." Then smile and change the subject.

On other occasions, it will be evident that the question was simply a courtesy. "How are you? I was calling about the bicycle you have for sale." Forget the wellness issue. Go right to the bicycle question.

You probably have friends and relatives with some knowledge of medicine. If you see scholarly curiosity in a friend's eyes, a dispassionate recitation of the diagnosis and the treatments may be the best course. Provide it selectively, keeping in mind that some version of what you say is apt to be repeated.

46 Project Management Suggestions for Partners

By organizing for the journey ahead, more of the things that need to be accomplished will be accomplished. But planning can be overdone or adhered to with unnecessary rigidity.

Perspective for Partners

Do you remember the pencil box you were so sure you'd need for third grade? Or maybe it was a Mickey Mouse thermos or a fancy notebook. You were shopping for the things you'd need before the first day of school. You told your mom you just had to have it. She smiled and bought it for you, knowing full well that you'd never really need it. But that was okay.

Some of those who want to help cancer patients also overdo it. The suggestions in Chapter 11, "The Patient's Personal Organization," could well be more than you will need to concern yourself with. If you thought you might need something else and wasted a few bucks to have it on hand, that's okay, too, isn't it?

The main thing is that you are—rightfully—worried about your special patient. This is a serious situation. You'd like to know all you can about how to prepare for and anticipate what may come along later. Just be cautioned that overpreparation, though better than surprise, is also a wasteful and taxing condition.

Learning What You Can from the Experts

If the patient has any of the more common kinds of cancer, the medical team can use its experience to show you the probable path from now through the next few months to years. The health-insurance company—especially if it is of the HMO variety—will probably have a similar treatment profile in its files. The American Cancer Society and the National Cancer Institute also have treatment profiles and related details available for you to look up on their Web sites. For more information, find survivors and other counselors in the Reference Center to talk to. While you should consider what you learn to be rough and general, you and the patient will have at least an inkling of the near-term picture.

Savoring the Good Things of Normal Life

Both you and the patient will still face many of the demands of normal life. Cancer just changed the priorities and complexities. As you look at the mess this disease has caused, try not to let it take any more of the joy and goodness from your life or the patient's than is absolutely necessary. To do otherwise would be like helping a thief steal your stuff.

Things That Cancer Can Screw Up

The needs of family, employers, and schools, along with social obligations, are apt to take second place during this process of making room for cancer. Government programs to help you deal with treatment needs can also take time away from normal life. Both you, as the primary caregiver, and the patient have to safeguard the important things in your lives. Those who love you two may be neglected. You could also lose your job or your school course credits.

If you don't know the details of any of these broad subjects, you will find discussions in chapters that focus on them. The point here is that planning may be necessary, and it could become complex. You need to be watchful and ready.

Talking to the Patient about What-Ifs

There are apt to be times during this fight against cancer when the patient will not want to face questions. Think through the dilemmas that have some chance of surfacing. Get others in the patient's close family circle to give you lists, too. If appropriate, ask the patient for a list. Put all this gloom and doom on a piece of paper. If possible, come to some sort of agreement as to what you should do in each case. Where no agreement is obtained, see if someone can at least be nominated to take responsibility.

Sometimes written declarations and even legal documents are needed for these contingencies. You, the partner, need to be the coordinator for these things and probably the keeper of the contingencies. The patient may want some actual what-if to be attended to by someone else, but you may still play a role. If so, know what it is.

The Course-Correction What-If

Even the sorts of cancer treatment that are well understood can produce nasty surprises for your patient and the medical team. We tend to discount the good things that happen. But we bitterly resent the bad turns in the road, which are also parts of living with cancer.

If the patient takes a serious turn for the worse, the medical team will quickly respond with changes to the treatment plan. You and the patient need to be prepared to do the same thing—to set your emotions aside as best you can and go through a practical revaluation process.

It is a whole lot easier to write these words than it will be for you to force aside the sudden fear and get your job done properly.

47 Stuff Happens

> A cancer patient recently announced to a Chemo Room of sympathetic listeners: "I have been told that God doesn't give us more than we can handle. Yes he does."

Piling on is a long-established, predictable human condition. Do you remember at work saying, "Please stop giving me extra things to do. I can't get my job done"? Cancer, which began as an additional "thing" for you, will attract its own coterie of hangers-on.

Focus, Focus

There are people who cannot allow the telephone to ring unanswered. There are people who must pluck a loose thread from someone's sweater, turn off an unnecessary light. Compunctions like those will invite cancer to create additional distractions for you. For the sake of the twenty-four-hour limitation on the day and your own sanity, you must learn to let unimportant things go.

- Your prime directive is this: Focus on the things that matter.
- If there is someone available to take care of something, let them. If it hasn't been done to your satisfaction, it is still probably good enough.
- Try to understand the difference between a demand of your disease and one of its whims. Demands come with penalties. You respond to them or else. Whims are all the other things that cancer waves in your face: the people you aren't fond of who want to talk to you, superfluous errands, pointless correspondence, the unwashed car, the

unpulled weeds—things that can wait. Respond immediately to the demands of your disease. It's job one.

- Seek protection. Help your family and your employer understand that you're no good to them if cancer wins. Ask them for shelter from distractions until cancer has been effectively dealt with.
- Understand that anger and frustration are the normal emotions of those bumped from first positions in your life by cancer. Anticipate these emotions from people who are used to having you do things for them—children, spouse, employer, social groups. Sometimes pettiness results. Sometimes—not often enough—reason prevails.

And on Top of That . . .

Being severely frightened, inconvenienced, subjected to all manner of medical mumbo-jumbo, faced with huge bills—all while enduring discomfort and illness—is not enough. More will be put on your plate.

You face other serious health conditions on top of cancer.

- It is likely that you will receive surgery. Afterward, recovery and physical therapy will demand top billing.
- Chemo may have physical side effects. It can also change your appearance for a while. This deeply upsets some patients. If it happens to you, try not to dwell on it. This is another way that cancer messes with you if you let it.
- Drugs used in chemo and pain relief can cloud a person's mind and reduce thinking ability. Your faculties come back after the drugs have left your system, though not always right away.
- Additional diseases may come along. It doesn't help that the average cancer patient is diagnosed at age fifty-one, the beginning of prime time for things that happen to "old" people. Examples: Some cancer patients experience heart attack or stroke. Diabetes is a possibility. Lymphoma is known to encourage meningitis. Chemo causes anemia. Radiation can bring on lymphedema. Trauma and exhaustion encourage cachexia, a serious opportunistic disease.
- Treatments that degrade parts of the patient's immune system invite serious infections. The places that patients go for treatments and the other people a patient meets there provide additional opportunities for infections.

Your marriage collapses. The complexities and frustrations of the human condition are made worse when life-threatening illness comes along. Unknowns and new demands are hard to deal with. The money problems make it worse. Some spouses and life partners leave.

A yoke mate responsible for being your cancer-fighting partner is less apt to grow apart from you than is a spouse you have sidelined. But the fear either of losing you or of your permanent disability also promotes desertion.

Consider making family counseling a core element of your cancer-fighting program.

A natural disaster occurs. As the crescendo of the battle against cancer rises, a sewer pipe is going to fail under the kitchen floor. There will be a small fire in the garage. The hexserver in your car is going to spifflecate. Locusts will eat your lawn. Zeus has not singled you out for punishment. It happens to everybody. These are just things. Let them go. When you get well, you can make it all better.

The patient or the partner—or both—get fired. Chapter 12, "The Patient's Workplace," was included because problems with employment are such a common part of being indisposed for any period of time.

The IRS announces an audit. At least our government has a policy regarding very sick people. If you are called for jury duty, are selected for tax audit, get called up by your army-reserve unit, or have some other business with state or federal government, you will be excused from it until you have recovered.

Your adult child divorces and moves home—with two dogs, a baby, and a friend. Some young adults whose wings are still in the developmental stage seem to have an affinity for thoughtless, inappropriate behavior—which they are the last to recognize for what it is. The good news is that the kid knew where home was. Treasure that.

You can count on having serious billing and service disputes. The health-insurance carrier, the hospital, the professional corporation of one of your medical team, or all of them will create administrative and financial headaches for you. Make a point of reviewing Chapter 11, "The Patient's Personal Organization," recalling the emotion of the nasty moment when some simpering idiot brought this crisis to your bedside.

The point of reviewing all this potential horror is to impress upon you the importance of focusing on the game. Don't let distractions take you too far away from this new center of your life. Tip: You will be more successful at this with the support and cooperation of your partner and family. At times during your illness, you may be physically and mentally dependent on them.

Dealing with Crises

First, understand that all this is temporary. Do not allow anything, most certainly not a cancer-whim sort of problem, to take over ownership of your life. After all, where will this issue be a year from now? Keep your priorities in order. Then find somebody to hand the shovel to. Candidates include:

The person who handed it to you
Your partner
The medical team
The medical team's administrator
Your case nurse at the insurance company
A social worker or hospital volunteer
The EAP (see Chapter 12)
Your boss at work

Your parents
Your children
Your pastor
Your family counselor

Or take the issue to a support-group meeting. See what sorts of solutions others suggest.

48 Travel For Medical Purposes

Patients from outside the local area, some from other countries, visit all the major cancer-treatment centers in the United States. You too may need to travel.

All oncology departments have exceptional people on staff. But no oncology department can serve the needs of all cancer patients. The family of cancer diseases and the consequences of cancers are far too varied. So cancer medicine has developed a sort of UN spirit, with docs exchanging whatever is needed across organizational boundaries for the ecumenical good.

Physical distance is the least of oncology's concerns. Scientists across the country routinely discuss challenges and triumphs. A highly specialized department in one city can evolve for the benefit of patients everywhere. On one level, this is a competitive process: Every center wants to be first with the newest innovation. But economic imperatives also force cooperation and sharing.

- A new cancer-transplant facility may cost hundreds of millions of dollars. You can't put one on every corner. If the one you need isn't nearby, you will have to travel—and stay—where it is.
- Many clinical trials require patients to live near a certain medical team or research hospital. You travel if you want the juice.
- Many forms of cancer are considered rare. The specialists who know the most about each one will be concentrated in a single treatment center, or at most in a few. The small number of specialists and the few patients with the rare condition must be brought together for both practical and economic reasons.
- The collateral damage done by successful cancer treatment at one center may require the help of a specialist located somewhere else. Common reasons for travel include transplants, amputations, artificial organs, cosmetic surgery, and repair work in places to which only a few can go, such as into the brain.
- There are testing facilities that produce strange and wonderful insights. The research, development, and capital costs are obscene. Do you need this special sort of imaging? This genetic evaluation? You go there.

The Cancer-Patient Travel Industry

If you are advised that you should leave a perfectly wonderful center of medical excellence and go to some other clinic, particularly if you have never been on an airplane, you may find the idea bizarre. Travel for treatment may also be unnerving—most certainly time-consuming, expensive, uncomfortable, and exhausting.

Do not be disheartened. An industry has sprung up to accommodate the tens of thousands of cancer patients like you who travel for treatment every year. It understands your problems and special needs.

Your Traveling Companion

You are expected to travel with a spouse, nurse, or some other partner. Airplane accommodations routinely make allowance for this. Places you will stay, with the exception of the isolated, antiseptic ones, will be configured for at least two. Some of the nonprofit organizations that provide financial help may have money for only one traveler, but that's a consequence of underfunding, not of a belief that you should travel alone.

Help with Arrangements

The first step is to make the examination and treatment appointments. Your medical team or its administrator will take care of that.

Once the reason for the travel is established, your destination hospital will help you. It probably provides full travel-agency services and a concierge to take care of you. Age eight or eighty, with or without special travel needs, you should receive every conceivable assistance.

There are also low-cost and free services specifically configured for cancer patients and their parties. Lists of those waiting to serve you can be found in the Reference Center. You'll find help with food, lodging, local transportation, and flights. The quality of the offers varies, as you should expect.

Free air transportation is not what you may imagine. The aircraft are seldom if ever like the ones the airlines have. Some are private prop-type craft. Some are corporate jets. Many times, they use smaller airports with none of the parking, help with luggage, or food amenities—or security inconveniences—of the majors. These aren't bad things, only different.

More significant, these flight services are not managed the way commercial airlines are. You fly "space available." You must either have commercial airline tickets as backup or not care when you depart or arrive. Your destination isn't guaranteed either. The flight you thought was landing at JFK may be diverted to Albany. You've got to be prepared with the cash for a bus ticket to the Big Apple.

All that said, the volunteers who offer free air travel are well intentioned and do their absolute best for those they serve. If you are well enough and the air travel begins and ends at good places for you, it should be a memorable adventure.

NEWS FLASH!
Suicide Bomber, Posing as Cancer Patient, Nabbed at O'Hare

If you receive a radioactive compound as part of chemo or an imaging procedure, you could set off a radiation detector at a security checkpoint. You will need to carry a doctor's note of explanation for the half-life of the drug.

Detectors of this sort are now in use at all commercial airports in the United States. They are also more and more commonly found at entrances to courthouses and other key public buildings.

As examples, fluorine-188, used in PET scans, is active for up to twenty-four hours. Technetium-99, a radioactive tracer used in kidney, liver, thyroid, and bone scans, stays hot for three days. Thallium, used in cardiac exams, can produce excitement at checkpoints for up to thirty days. Iodine, used in thyroid treatments, may get you spread-eagled up to three months later.

"Irrevocable" Airline Tickets and Getting Your Money Back

The need to have a commercial airline ticket as backup for a free trip can present a refund problem. The ticket you were forced to buy may have strict terms: Use it or lose it; no refund or flight change allowed.

You may have bought such a ticket with every intention of using it. Then plans changed because of sickness or because the doctor you were traveling to see had to reschedule.

For whatever reason you came to be stuck with a no-refund ticket, the airlines make an exception in your case. You must submit a note from your doctor explaining that you were unable to use the ticket due to your critical illness. If you need help with the wording, the airline will tell you what the note should say.

Credit-Card Deals

Chances are that if you have to make one trip for medical purposes, others will follow. Some credit cards accrue travel miles. Perhaps making use of one now could pay for a leg of a trip later or for nights in a hotel. If such a card makes sense and you don't have one, a few useful notes follow.

A bank, airline, credit union, or somebody else will make you a terrific credit-card offer. You'll be urged to use the card for all your expenses. In addition to free miles and gifts, you may receive a monthly or quarterly itemized statement. That's going to help your tax preparer. Discounts on hotel rooms and car rentals and who knows what else can also be parts of the deal.

Be wise. There are many competing offers. Look at several. If you are not sure which is best for you, any frequent traveler can probably help you decide.

If you do not plan to fully pay the invoice every month, the card's credit terms are its most important feature. Look for low, fixed rates. Watch out for very high and variable interest. Some of these offers could do you more financial damage than your cancer.

Free Financial Arbitrator

A credit card can help you in arguments with people over purchases. If you want to return something or if you were charged the wrong amount, reason with the merchant. If that fails, call the toll-free number on the back of the card. Ask for help. The bank behind the card wants you to be happy and has quite a bit of clout with merchants who accept its credit services.

Should you travel outside the country, your credit card will guarantee you the most favorable exchange rate for local currency. Put the charge on your card. The bank does the rest.

The Tax Man's Stingy Stipend

For those who have always wondered how to qualify for the IRS medical expense allowance, this is a grand day. Those who haven't and don't care still need to know a little bit about this subject.

To begin with, deductions permitted by the federal and state authorities are not generous. A very sizeable deductible reduces this expense before you qualify the first penny of a claim. You certainly won't get anything close to your expenses back. Maybe less than ten cents on the dollar.

You will need the help of a tax preparer. The rules governing tax reports have gotten completely out of hand. Go see this person before you begin making trips to doctors. There are worksheets and simple guidance that will help.

Double-Duty Receipts

The Leukemia and Lymphoma Society, and perhaps other nonprofits, will help with rebates on actual expenses of travel to treatments. These cover long-distance as well as local travel. To apply for help, you must submit a form with copies of receipts attached as soon after the expenses were incurred as possible.

Do not apply to the leukemia and lymphoma people for help with costs unrelated to leukemia and lymphoma. Don't count on money until the check comes in. This opportunity may change at any time.

Perhaps a more important general suggestion is to review the listings in the Reference Center that apply to your circumstance. See what help may be there. Remember too that many of the nonprofits you come across provide volunteers, transportation, hot meals, treatments, subsidized or free prescription medicines, and many more valuable services in lieu of cash.

Car Rentals

The car-rental industry is competitive and volatile. You can't count on much of anything about renting a car to be exactly the same from one transaction to the next. As much as you might like to rely on Avis because it always tries harder or on Hertz because it is number one, you can't. Rates and the quality of service may differ even between branches of the same rental company located just a few miles apart.

To illustrate, the office at the airport may offer a full-size Ford for sixty-five dollars a day. The car they give you is hosed down, not really washed, and it reeks of air freshener to disguise the recent presence of a cigar smoker. Five miles away, another branch may offer the same car for thirty-eight dollars per day. You get a clean, fresh-smelling vehicle and an additional 20 percent off with your AAA or AARP card.

More Car-Rental Tips

Check out the eight or nine Internet travel sites that compete for this business. These Web sites can make great offers when the rental companies give them excess inventory at fire-sale prices. Just don't count on it. The twenty-dollar-a-day car you found at Logan last time probably won't be there again.

Incredible low rates most often appear in the five-to-ten-day advance window. Rental companies are most apt to cut rate offers to the bone about two weeks before the rental date. Rock-bottom rates are not necessary earlier. The people who plan travel that far ahead want to have their car rentals confirmed at the same time, and they don't quibble.

The real deals vanish about five days before the rental date. That's prime time for business-traveler sales. A low rate is far less important to the business traveler than the guarantee that the right car will be waiting.

Special equipment is probably available. Many car-rental companies can provide autos and vans that are configured for the handicapped. Call the company's home office, not the branch where you expect to pick up the vehicle. Explain exactly what special modifications your rental will need. There may be an extra charge.

Accommodations

Marriott and other hotel chains manage specially equipped lodgings near major treatment centers throughout the country. The Rotary House, with an elevated passageway directly into the bowels of the M. D. Anderson Cancer Center in Houston, is a fine example. The price is fair. The quality of the rooms and service is top-drawer. Just about anything that patients and their parties could need is available. To find out about hotels serving the clinic you will be visiting, ask the hospital's travel agency or concierge.

The Reference Center also lists independent housing services for patients. The rates are often based on the patient's ability to pay. Free services, including transport back and forth to the hospital and airport, and meals may be included.

More Tips

1. This book has eleven chapters in Part IV, "Supporting Resources," devoted to help. There's more in the Reference Center.
2. If you will be gone for more than a month, ask your utility and telephone companies for reduced rates. You will probably need to tell

them that you will be receiving cancer treatments. You may need to show proof.

3. You should be able to stop subscriptions to newspapers and cable-television programming without penalties.

4. The best deal on long-term care of your pets may be at a friend's house.

5. Consider the benefits of paying someone to take care of your place and pick up the mail.

6. If your house or apartment will be empty during your absence, tell the police that you will be gone, and why. Leave a phone number where you can be reached.

VII Relationships

*Critical Elements
of Patient-Partner
Relationships*

49 Basic Patient-Partner Relationships

Truths and consequences of this very special sort of kinship deserve discussion.

In Chapter 3, we explored the idea of partnering from the patient's point of view and outlined its benefits. Chapter 9 covered the things a partner needs to do. This chapter begins a section of the book on the appropriateness and end results of various sorts of partnering.

In late winter and early spring, as the snow is melting on the slopes, ski lodges begin tacking up notices to warn skiers that they may suddenly come across bare spots and exposed rocks. That's the kind of thing we're going to cover here— the places in partnering that may or may not cause problems. Please carefully consider your coping skills.

Teaming Up

A cancer patient needs comfort from a physically and mentally tough partner. All cancer cases are scary. All cancer cases cause stress. All cancer treatments have trade-offs that demand sober, levelheaded reflection and that usually challenge financial resources. Cancer treatments also leave the patient exhausted or too doped up to drive or do much else for a while. And those are just the easy ones.

For these and many other reasons, every patient should have one or more partners to go through this thing with. This person or persons must understand that "partner" is not an honorary position. It requires maturity, energy, time, caring, and thoughtfulness. And willingness to get your hands dirty.

Affectionate Attentiveness

The first quality of a partner should be loving, attentive care—only when necessary—making sure the patient does not lose control or dignity. Please be certain that you, as a partner, can provide this kind of affectionate attentiveness to this particular cancer patient and not overdo it.

Should care be necessary, it's the partner's job to see just what is called for and to provide it. This help is mental as well as physical. Notably, the partner is responsible for hearing the whole story during meetings with the medical team and prompting or asking the right questions if the patient needs this help. Partners also take good notes and find out answers to questions.

Forty thousand times every year in the United States, a motorist climbs into an automobile and is later scraped out of what remains of it. Not one of them thought there was any chance their life would end that day, but it did.

Unlike a car, cancer has already made its threat public. You'd think that a cancer patient and partner would have more respect for the unexpected than those motorists have. But some don't. Please take this situation seriously. Even though the test or treatment is routine, be alert. A test may turn up something unexpected. A chance remark may lead to consideration of a new treatment or a way to save big bucks or time, or the reading you did last night may prompt a question that inspires the medical team.

Possibilities

The Harlequin Factor

Of the wrong reasons to become a partner, one of the most dangerous is the idea that a romantic attachment could result. Both patients and partners can be guilty of holding this expectation. In fact, romance will flower without much encouragement. The elements of a classic romance novel are all there. If either the patient or partner has a third party in their life, further complications are obvious. Please be sure you know what you're getting into.

Unhappy Endings

Some patients do not recover from their disease. Others are physically, mentally, or psychologically changed. For the good of the patient, a partner needs to stay the course. Patients consciously need to think this matter over too. Is the person you are considering as a partner strong enough and stable enough and thoughtful enough to fill this slot on your team? It is not good for a partner to bail out, nor is it good for the patient to have to seek a replacement.

Mistakes and Amends

During this stressful, dangerous period in the patient's life, social mistakes are predictable. There may be angry words or deeds. What then?

If you, the potential partner, are harboring a grudge against someone close to the patient, or if there is anyone in the patient's circle of family or friends who harbors ill feelings toward you, it is going to cause trouble for the patient. Consider making amends right now. Negative vibes are a special, very dangerous circumstance.

Falling Outs

Patients and partners have falling outs. If it happens to you, try to fix it, of course. Failing that, see if a third party can help patch things up. Once past that point, a graceful exit from the relationship is a wise course. Try very, very hard to keep the parting amicable.

Partner Recognition

Should you, as a partner, receive less credit or thanks for the job than you deserve, don't mention it to a soul. If everyone else is receiving rewards of cash or goods and you have been forgotten, say nothing. Continue to serve with all your heart and ability. Your reward may come to you—perhaps when you least expect it. Then again, it may not. Remember that this isn't about you. Be content with the gift you've given.

50 Parent-Child Partnerships

This may be parenting at its most challenging.

If you have turned to this chapter, it is likely that your child has cancer. That is excruciating and terrible news. You need time to deal with the shock and to grieve. You must also realize that you are inside a burning house. You must control as much of this situation as you can—now—before it gets worse.

There is no formula for success here, except to note the obvious: So long as shock and fear control the situation, you will be a less effective helpmate to your sick child.

The Precognitive Parent

As a parent, you are aware of the mountains of books available on the general subject of child rearing. You also know that the authors often disagree with one another. Perhaps a writer you know of would violently disagree with comments made here. You can modify the suggestions to suit your circumstance. But please do not reject the subjects as inconsequential. The points made reflect the experiences of parents who walked this road ahead of you. You may have a better solution, but you will be crossing the same bridges with the same trolls beneath them.

The Cumulative Nature of Observations in This Chapter

Most of what generally applies to early-age cancer is also relevant to cancer in middle-age children and teenagers. A comment that applies to all levels of childhood development is noted only where it first pertains. It is not repeated in section after section, to avoid tedium. If information in one section seems to pertain to the next, expect that it does.

The Handicaps of Being a Single Parent

Being the single parent of a sick child is a long and lonely road. It is far easier to have another parent to share the anguish and indecision with. If you are a single parent, you are going to be further tortured by finding references throughout this chapter to married couples and to the advantages that a team brings to the fight against a child's illness. From your point of view, this is tasteless and maybe hurtful. With sincere apologies, it is nevertheless true.

On the positive side, an experienced single parent has already developed compensating skills that will minimize the handicap. Other members of the family—grandparents, brothers and sisters, and maybe an ex-spouse—can also help.

The Precognitive Child

For our purposes here, we can think of children as passing through three general stages of development. From birth to about age four or five, a huge sluice is open through which pour languages and libraries of information at a rate far greater than happens later in life. But the child has no experience or judgment to speak of. During this period, parents *tell* children. They do it lovingly, but neither enthusiasm nor agreement is needed before moving on.

The Team: Parents and Child Only

This should be a time with tender, personal moments that embody the best strengths of the special union between child and parent. If you are fortunate enough to be part of an active marriage, the two of you join in fighting for the survival of your precious loved one.

Single parent or couple, this is a time of focused sharing with your child. You may allow some input to your management decisions by your doctor, your spiritual advisor, or some other person. But you and your spouse own this experience, all its costs, all its consequences. This is a responsibility that cannot be delegated. Even if you run and hide, it is still all happening on your watch. And you, the parent, will always know it in your heart, no matter who excuses you or what they say.

Parents as the Decision Makers

Although doctors and other experts may offer valuable advice, you must decide. Relatives, perhaps including your own parents, may have views. You will find in the Reference Center parents to call who have gone through much of your experience. But none of them can lift the heavy weight of responsibility from your shoulders.

This point will be unimportant if things go well during the treatment and recovery of your child. If they do not, this issue is central. No matter what the circumstance, no matter what some lawyer tells you about whom you can blame and how good your case is, you were and are responsible. Stay on your toes. Do the best you can.

Key Parent-Child Differences

You cannot expect your child to understand the anguish you may face over a treatment decision. It is probably not helpful to share it. Remember, too, that your young child may seem to have some reasoning ability, but it is probably too immature and too fragile to be put to great use just yet.

Advance Agreement on Key Issues

Some of the worst dilemmas parents may face involve the reconciling of their differing religious or cultural backgrounds. These problems are worse when they clash with strong recommendations of a medical team. Certain tests, the sharing of blood and blood products, transplant procedures, amputation or organ removal, and other matters may bring you smack up against a mile-high wall with your spouse or family on the other side. Dear friends, if you do not resolve the matter on behalf of the life of your child, you will live with an open wound for the rest of your life.

Note Making

You will never forget the grave illness of your child, but you'll forget some of the details. The astigmatic optic of memory, further conditioned by what happens later in life, will also come into play. Make notes and take pictures. They will help you with family history. They may also be priceless to some future parent in desperate need of hope and good information.

Death

If your child dies:

Point 1: This wasn't your fault. It was cancer's.
Point 2: We are not emotionally equipped to bury our children. We expect them to bury us. We count on it. You're going to have to get over this shock.
Point 3: People will say things to you in their attempts to console that will strike you as outrageous or cruel. They don't mean to be hurtful. Don't hold them accountable. Among them may be someone who has lost a child. You're surprised. You don't understand. Let it go. This is tragedy without redemption. People don't have any idea what to say.
Point 4: Spend time with a counselor with specific past experience helping parents recover from the loss of children. Do it immediately. Four out of five marriages that lose a child break up because of it.

The Child of Cognitive Age

Parents know when children begin linking complex factors together to arrive at sophisticated conclusions. If your child has figured out some of the key implications of being a cancer patient, you don't have to guess: You have a cognitive child.

Notes on Briefing Your Patient

A child who can understand that cancer is not normal and that serious consequences may follow needs to have parents add some specific information to the equation. Repeating for emphasis: *parents*. Your child looks to you. Keep it that way. Your child needs to be as close to your loving assurances as possible throughout this difficult time.

The information your child needs will include some details of what this cancer is and where it is in the body. Logically, how tests and treatments may help should be the next thing to teach and discuss. Your child must also have lots of verbal and physical assurances (holding, hugs, kisses, pats) that the family is and will remain protective and loving. The child must also be certain that nothing about this situation is the result of anything the child is responsible for. Most assuredly, cancer is not punishment.

Cancer and treatment information needs to be conveyed positively, without flinching. It must be at the child's intellectual and emotional level. It needs to be passed on to the patient in bite-sized pieces without delay. Any explanation that goes on for more than 120 seconds contains too much information for the average child of this age to assimilate. Also be careful to define new words as you use them.

Another reminder: Your child learns both verbal and nonverbal lessons from you. When you cry, your child learns. When you have hysterics, it leaves an impression. When you are confused and don't know what to do, your child feels the same way. This does not mean you should hide your emotions from your child. It is meant to suggest that you be certain that your emotions are always genuine, and that you explain them so that your child always understands you fully.

Other points to specifically cover with your patient: Cancer is a natural disease that other children get too. Cancer is not good. We are all sorry that this has happened. Mommy, Daddy, and the doctors are all working very hard to fix it.

No Lying

Never play bluff poker with a six-year-old. Never, never, never try it with *your* six-year-old. They always know.

Lying is another very bad idea. If you've been talked into a corner and your choices seem to be either making up something or opening a can of worms, try changing the subject or simply refusing to say anything further. Don't compound a mistake already made. Understand, too, that you will eventually have to confess a major indiscretion and apologize for it.

No Outside Experts

Grandparents and older siblings can feel especially driven to comment to your child. There are things they just have to say about cancer or about some related experience of theirs. Or someone in the extended family has instructions on how to act or what to expect or do. Make it as clear as you can that this information is welcome—so long as it comes to you or your spouse privately. Questions about the condition of the patient, the efficacy of treatments, the competence of the doctor, the progress of the disease, exciting new cancer drugs, and so forth are also welcome in private—not around the patient. Explain that the circumstances are far too complicated and serious for more than one hand to be on the wheel at any one time, and that the only hands permitted on the wheel are yours or your spouse's.

You don't want to gag these people. They have to talk, so some outlet is only wise. Allow times of sharing with the patient. Encourage the child to lead a general discussion of how things are going. Let the group learn about the treatments or the hospital from the patient's viewpoint. Let the patient talk about being sick. Emphasize listening and interest. Cut off the people with advice to interject.

Medical Meetings

Include your child in meetings with doctors and other health providers. Even though young for the experience, the patient is still the patient and deserves to be there. There may be exceptions. You will know what they are, both as a parent and through earlier experiences. At some point, your child may also give you pointers as to which meetings should include him or her, and which may not.

If you are forced into a difficult and heart-wrenching experience in which the topic is the worst imaginable, remember that most children take these disclosures better than adults do. Also ask yourself, Is there ever going to be a better time or place to discuss this? There may be. Probably not.

Medical Meetings II

Your doctor is leading the fight against your child's cancer along with cases in all those other meeting rooms in the clinic. This condition will—sooner or later—force your doc to leave before all your questions have been answered. Since all those other cases are waiting, you'll need to schedule another meeting. Do it immediately. If possible, tell someone the general areas to be covered so there'll be at least a partial agenda and the doc can prepare as necessary.

If some of the missing information has to do with an urgent need, be sure to tell someone on the medical staff. Provide a means for the doctor to reply to you without delay, such as a telephone number.

Medical Meetings III

Help your child feel like a peer in meetings about the disease. It will improve retention. Also help your patient/partner to ask questions. "Do you remember what we were talking about at breakfast, honey? Wouldn't you like to ask the doctor that question?" When you believe it helps, ask questions for your child. Try not to sound childlike in the process. You don't want your kid to laugh at you.

Medical Meetings IV

You'll probably think of very important questions sometime between right after the door has banged you in the behind and the middle of the next night.

You have other resources for answers to some general types of treatment and disease questions. But the patient-pertinent stuff needs an answer by your patient's expert. Before ending the next meeting with the doc or chemo nurse or radiologist, ask, "How will I be able to get back to you with the questions I forget to ask you now?" Most of these people have personal cell phones, general office numbers, e-mail addresses, or an assistant you can contact. If someone tells you that none of those things are available, ask why not. Get the phone number you'll need.

The Pubescent Youth

Transitions from child to adult are gradual, with only approximate beginnings and completions visible. But somewhere in the development of the flower, a seedpod forms and new life complications are only too evident.

Communication

Forthrightness may be more difficult for a teenager than for a preteen. The process of withdrawal from Mom and Dad, along with the hormone-driven need for private turf, confuses everybody. There are people in the oncology community who can provide cohesiveness to these patients and their parents. If you are lucky, you will have one on your team. If you are not, you may be able to bring order to this situation yourself. If you can't, get outside help. Solve it somehow.

Without putting too fine a point on it, trust and candor in communications are harder. Severe depression and absolutely wacky progressions of illogic by your teen are almost predictable. At a minimum, discuss the matter with a family counselor.

Respect

Critical illness may swing the maturation process either toward adulthood or back toward juvenility during these transitional years—perhaps as often as several times a day. Pay less attention to the foibles of the moment than you do to the trend toward maturity over time. Reward progress by releasing parts of the treatment process to your young person's control. Respect the adult who is trying to get out. It will encourage a process that is generally constructive.

Treaty Negotiations

Your young adult's need for "space" may lead to conflicts you didn't know you created. Negotiate treaties to help stabilize the organizing for treatment. For example, give the patient responsibility for taking medication or testing samples. Reward with respect and trust. Try not to punish at all. Also be alert for the effects of illness and drugs. Explain them to the patient as best you can.

Data Overload

If a cognitive child may assimilate up to 120 seconds of carefully organized medical information, a teenager will have some greater capacity. It will vary based on many factors such as happiness, wellness, and security. You may find on one day that the patient has seeming limitless capacity or has gone on the Internet and studied ahead of both you and the doc. On another day, the brain is mush.

Encourage questions. Get feedback. Watch for anger, lost attention, and other indications that the discussion period is over. Be patient. Don't force. Don't despair.

Spurious Transmissions

Your child may have a considerable amount of false and misconstrued information that needs to be separated from cancer's core issues. Be unruffled. Reply to situations at whatever level is most effective. When the going gets too scientific, find an expert to toss the ball to. Don't delay or put off your sincere questioner.

You will also hear the dissident voices of relatives, friends, and neighbors coming back to you through the patient. You are going to have to provide good, solid explanations as to why Aunt Jean opposes blood transfusions and why John from church says you're better off dead than going to *that* hospital, which he says is run by heretics. Further, be prepared to add to the moral teachings of your young adult. As an example, suppose you hear: "If there comes a point when the sickness gets too bad, the best thing is to take an extra bottle of pills and escape it all." Even though this sounds like a conviction, it is a question, and you had better have a thoughtful reply.

Treatment Options

There are always treatment options. They run the gamut from the latest scientific discovery to things that call themselves "alternative medicine" but probably aren't. All these options are always in play, despite what you may believe. You will be required to take a pruner to the tree if you want to reduce the number of limbs. Consider the strategy of studying treatment options with your partner-patient, so that you share a common ground for deciding among the choices the medical team presents. This may also eliminate much of the credibility that might otherwise be given to baseless poppycock.

51 When the Patient Is Your Spouse

Share this chapter with the love of your life in full resolve to keep the bonds of your union strong in sickness as in health. We who have gone before you make this promise: Successful trial by the fire of cancer will produce a great love story.

A Wake-Up Call

Many times, cancer visits a marriage that has been running on less than all cylinders, perhaps harmoniously, for a long time. Quite suddenly, its weaknesses are probed. Marriage partners are forced to see each other through reopened eyes. Priorities and values take on new implications. Some unions fail. In others, one partner is unable to deal with the pain or the physical manifestations of the disease. Those unions often crumble too.

If you are coming to the realization that one of these issues or some other part of your life is threatening the holding power of your relationship, the problems are obvious though the remedies may not be. The path you are sworn to take by the nature of your relationship is clear. Even so, your situation may not be so simple that you can decide how you will cope unless you get qualified help. Perhaps you should speak to a spiritual counselor. Perhaps a respected friend or relative. The oncology center you are becoming familiar with probably has both chaplains and psychosocial nursing professionals trained to help you with this problem.

The one thing you must not do is to ignore the issue. Cancer is an ultimate test. You must strip off any encumbrance that could get in the way of the challenge of a lifetime.

To an Ex-Spouse Back in the Picture

The wisest man or woman alive may not be able to see much farther down this road than the immediate needs of a threatened person whom you still value. The decision to help, while generous, may become more complex than anyone could have predicted. Open the closest, most caring and honest communication link possible with your partner in this venture. Share your feelings and dilemmas as best you can. Think about other resources that may support you. There is no way to predict how this noble decision to return and help will turn out. Be aware that both blessings and curses came with it.

New Demands

Expect the unexpected. Things began with a diagnosis that surprised and shocked both of you. Tests, searching, bewilderment, and decisions have followed. The raw emotions that you and your spouse have experienced to this point will continue. Each of you is being changed in little ways that may catch you off guard. Something will come up, and you will wonder, "How could he (she) say such a thing?" "I never, ever felt that way. What in the world did she (he) mean?" Keep in mind that you are both having unpleasant new experiences. Once in a while, each of you needs to remind the other to take a break. Lighten up. Smell a rose. Smile. Remind yourself of the love you share.

Third-Person Helpers

Many marriages require the intimate help of third persons during cancer recovery. The spouse is physically or mentally incapable of lifting, bathing, wound dressing, giving shots, or dealing with ostomy or problems of incontinence. Many spouses must continue to earn the family livelihood and perhaps be away from home on business.

When more partner caregivers are needed, the most satisfactory choices are usually blood relatives of the patient. This minimizes the modesty and emotional issues. The other good choice is a professional home nurse. This alternative is apt to be expensive, though insurance or a government program may help. Discuss recourse possibilities with your medical team or pick a listing to telephone in the Reference Center "Yellow Pages" under "Nursing at Home." By the way, home-nursing candidates are apt to be well versed in your payment and claim options.

There are agencies and charities that provide people, too. The professionals and volunteers who come into your home from these sources can also be excellent solutions to the problem. Neighbors or friends may also be good choices, but they can cause problems. A minuscule number will be dishonest. A larger number will prove unreliable. The greatest problem could be emotional. Someone in the house who is not a relative and is intimate with the patient over a period of time is potentially divisive to family unity.

Make Decisions Together

Parents and others may be more than eager to help you and your spouse make key decisions. The medical team may also try to help you weigh treatment choices and other decisions. They may all be right. But you will miss an important component of recovery if you allow any of them to take control of your decision making. Don't you or your spouse make important decisions on your lonesome either. Emotions can leave you off balance. The political pandering in the news media about "it" being "your body" is way too pat and shallow to influence an important decision that may affect the remainder of your days. Take the advice of whomever you value, certainly. But go into private session with your life partner to settle things.

Marriage Encounter, Promise Keepers, and Similar Seminars

Most couples who take healthy, stable relationships into these marriage seminars enjoy a strengthening result. But a marriage already struggling with issues can be further weakened. If you and your spouse are considering the use of one of these programs to help with a dilemma caused by cancer, you may find it helpful or disastrous—pretty much one extreme or the other. Counsel with someone you can trust with the future of your marriage who knows the program. If, at the end of the day, you remain in doubt about participating, the likelihood is that you shouldn't go there, at least not right now.

A Special Set of Tools

Marriage teams often manage critical cancer decisions with all the aplomb of a hog on ice. You know what the situation is and where you want to go. You just lack the traction. Here's a toolkit that may help.

Lists

Dr. June McCarroll, who got tired of having her car run off the road in 1917, came up with the idea of painting a line down the middle of streets. Simple organization can make a huge contribution to success. Start with a pad and pencil. Make lists. Define things. Put them in order. Think about what has been written. Revise. Your objective is to end up with a master document that diffuses the madness of these uncertain times. As a subset to your master organizer, make lists of things that are required to make complex projects and treatments successful.

Roles

The role of one of you is to be sick, and of the other to be helpful. Are there other roles? Who is going to keep track of medications? Who will monitor the billing and payment processes? Who gets to argue with the hospital when the bills are wrong? Are there kids or parents who need to be included? Do you have trips to plan for? Who takes charge of medical research? Look at the lives you lead together as a team, and list all the roles that apply. You will probably find that you disagree on a few points. This is a dandy time to sort it all out.

Responsibilities

Roles come with responsibilities. There are also backups. Much of this is obvious until you begin looking at the detail and seeking agreement. As a partnership, you will often share responsibility, with one of you grinding the organ and the other passing a cup around. It's really smart to hash this out, and as your lives fill with even more new things, continue the practice of looking to see whose role and whose responsibility falls where.

Ownership

Sickness usually comes and goes. When it is less, a patient may crave normal activities. Though this is an extreme example, a beautiful lady named Karen insisted on painting the garage door of the family home during the final stage of succumbing to her disease. She died two weeks after she finished. A partner needs to be understanding and flexible, caring when care is needed and supporting in better times.

Love

A spouse's first commandment is to provide unconditional love, un-conditionally.

Physical Strength

The illness and its treatments take physical strength from even the most powerful of us. Sometimes the ability to do something is taken away suddenly. A spouse needs to be vigilant. And the patient must remember to ask for help. It is even good for a patient, on occasion, to ask for help that isn't needed. Let a spouse, son, daughter, or friend give a gift.

Sleep

Cancer patients have trouble sleeping. Pain and the aftereffects of many treatments cause insomnia. Sleeping pills and booze may be okay with the doc, but the patient may tire of how they make one feel later or worry about addiction. Consider getting up with your sufferer, turning on the TV, and making some popcorn. Or get out the playing cards. Make a silk purse out of that sow's ear. You'll do fine, even if you miss a whole night's rest.

Personal Care

People who spend too much time doing nothing get "bed head" and bad breath, fingernails that need clipping and painting, divots, and dings. You need to help. If you have never shaved a man, if you have never given a pedicure, it is time you learned. If you have never given a massage, find out how (though you may also need to discuss this with the doc.)

Some care needs are very personal. Should you discover that your patient cannot "wipe," for instance, you must find a way to help that preserves the lovers' relationship between you.

Professional Obligations

In addition to continuing your life as best you can, you may need to help with your spouse's professional obligations. Answering mail, reading journals, taking messages, writing notes, and maybe even attending meetings or taking over other duties in your spouse's name may be required. Be open to learning and doing.

Nursing Skills

Nobody stays in a hospital long. Outpatient care is the name of the game. Patients are sent home with all sorts of tubes and bags attached, with shots to be given, tests to be taken. You, a home-care nurse, or both draw the duty. It cuts no ice that you are too squeamish to stick in a needle. The nurse at the treatment center is going to show you how, and then it's up to you. If urine and stool samples have to be checked, you'll get the test kit. If wounds have to be dressed, if bags have to be changed, if diapers are needed—you'll learn all about it.

Take on these challenges gladly. Your spouse is blessed to receive loving care from you. Even if you are clumsy or inexpert. Even if you screw up. Unless you visit one of those nursing homes where people without partners receive "assisted-living care" from the "staff," you will have no idea how great a gift you give.

Blood and Body Parts

You are the wreck in the junkyard that they will come to first when your spouse needs spare parts. Your children should be next in line, followed by parents and other blood relatives.

If the search must widen, you should take charge of it. Finding a donor could be a major expense that insurance frequently does not cover. Depending on what's needed, you may find an association in the Reference Center "Yellow Pages" that helps. Your hospital also has resources, which are automatically put in play in most cases.

All the Money, All the Assets, All the Credit, All the Time

Marriage isn't a fifty-fifty deal. It's 100 percent, pedal to the metal. Use every speck of common sense and every available help that's out there. But in the end, if the choice is between a cost of treatment and keeping the house or sending the kids to college, you spend the money. You do this because when all this is behind you, you will need to look back and know that every nail was pounded in all the way. You did not shortchange your sweetheart.

Management of Patient Rights

Both the patient and the spouse will have moments of hysteria over this thing that's messing with life. In hopes it helps, here are some notes on ownership that you may want to ponder.

The cancer patient has final say on matters having to do with cancer. So long as the patient is of sound mind, the doc is going to bring decisions to the patient, and the patient is expected to make choices. A spouse can express an opinion, as can anyone else. But after due deliberation, the patient decides. The first duty of the spouse after a decision has been rendered is to support and to shelter the patient from criticism. (The second duty of a spouse with a dissenting opinion is to keep I-told-you-so's out of later conversations. The third duty of the spouse is to point out, and apologize for, being wrong.)

The partnership stays fifty-fifty on family matters. No fair claiming more than half the votes on family matters just because you're sick. Patients may be able to rant and get away with it when arguing with third parties, but respect the circumstances and wisdom of a spouse.

Partners must represent the patient viewpoint when the patient needs it. When the patient is too sick to stand up for issues, the partner must do so, even when the matter is disagreeable. Nor is the partner permitted to apologize for it. The patient has decided the case. The spouse is the enforcer.

It would be naughty to reorganize his shop or sell her golf clubs.

Topics That May Need to Be Discussed

It is difficult to face some issues squarely. The only reason to get these out for discussion now is that it may be far more difficult to do later.

Household Business

Recovery from cancer is a time when household chores must be redistributed. Some men have particular trouble with household chores. Some women find heavy yard work and home maintenance unappealing. But this stuff has to be discussed and settled.

Children

All the school, sports, church, and other stuff that involves your children needs regular discussion and coordination. This has to be more organized than it was in the past because there is less time for it. The children's relationship with the sick parent is a new core issue. Through all of this, everyone has to have free access to everyone else. The recovery process must come to seem as open and normal a part of family life as possible. In thinking about this, it may be helpful to remember the famous photo of John John playing under President Kennedy's desk while he worked in the Oval Office. Be as natural a parent as that, if you can.

Family Business

Money and all the things that compete for it will continue to demand parental attention. This becomes a big problem for most cancer patients.

Critical Care Decisions

Even though you may see none at the moment, expect treatment and care decisions to come along. Expect that discussions with spouse, medical team, insurance company, your employer, and others may be necessary.

Last Will, Living Will, Final Dispositions, Advance Directives

If both parents have not gone through the process of formalizing contingency decisions, this is the time to do it. This is also the time to make certain that your medical team is instructed as to "heroic measures" should you be concerned by the dignity, or lack of it, that may accompany your passing. If you have children, consider how they may be loved and sheltered until maturity should both parents die. Talk to the person or family who would take them in. Come to a formal understanding, complete with financial arrangements.

Disposal of a Business

If you own controlling interest in an organization that others count on for their living, please decide what you want to happen to it. For a few suggestions and thoughts, see the final section of Chapter 12, "The Patient's Workplace."

Funeral Arrangements

Make your own funeral arrangements, now. Buy the plot if you want your body buried. Pay for the funeral ceremony. You can even buy a casket in advance. Sometimes flowers too. It's all cheaper. You take a huge load from the shoulders of those who love you. Besides, you get it your way.

52 When the Patient Is a Parent

This is an open letter to the son, daughter, or other young relative of a senior patient.

If your parent has come to you for help, you obviously have their admiration and respect. You also qualify because you have the energy and resources, and because you can be trusted with intimate feelings and estate protection. But this whole thing of becoming a caregiver to one who brought you life is probably unsettling, just as it is for your sick parent. It involves an exploration of new territory, a place where two generations learn new things about each other, about strength and wisdom.

Any Elderly Relative

As time passes, the membership of every generation shrinks. Seniors sometimes find that the closest blood relative with the necessary qualifications to help them is a niece, nephew, or cousin. If there is a friendly, familial relationship with this person, he or she is apt to be far preferable to any alternative. In what follows, substitute aunt, uncle, grandfather—whoever the senior relative is—for parent if it applies in your case. The guiding principles are the same.

The Qualifications of Younger Caregivers

You may be an adult so far as your generation is concerned and a big deal at work, but the cancer patient you are helping changed your diapers. Your business or professional skills are almost beside the point so far as your partner-parent is concerned. Their expectations that you will be attentive to needs and that you will be respectful are your most essential qualifications. If you also know something about the health-care system or estate management, that's a bonus.

The Spouse and Siblings of Your Patient

A present or former spouse may be the proper partner instead of you. Now, be careful. Don't miss the true point here. Your patient has chosen you. You are essential. But there may be an emotional, legal, or family reason for at least a ceremonial copilot. Discuss this with the mom or dad you're helping. You two may come to realize that the spouse is capable of discharging most, if not all, of the cancer-patient duties. Or that it doesn't matter.

There are numerous reasons for concluding that you should step back from the partnership title and vest it in the spouse. You remain the load-bearing timber supporting them.

But you have probably been brought into this situation because neither the cancer patient's spouse nor a closer blood relative from that generation has the necessary energy and resources. Please spend a moment to contemplate this situation. Perhaps they're infirm, but if a spouse or siblings are still around and if there remains the possibility of a familial tie, it may be wise to involve them in this situation. Ask your partner-patient about it. Can you create places of honor within the caregiving circle for these folks?

An aging spouse, most particularly, needs to feel included in what is going on. Respect the love. Reinforce the sense of belonging. Give dignity to this person, and value.

- Can you name them to an auxiliary-care team, to take turns sitting with the patient after surgery?
- Can you put them on a telephone tree to pass along treatment news?
- Can they start a prayer chain?
- Can they help with physical therapy?
- Can you organize periodic luncheons for everybody?

None of these suggestions may suit your situation. The purpose of listing them is to germinate a creative process so that you will come up with the right way to involve your patient's generation and the rest of the family in a positive way.

Recruiting a Support Team of Experts

You may not know nearly as much about your parents as you think you do. Or you may need to know more about some aspect of your parents' lives to be prepared for subjects you may be forced to bring up later. As a place to start, make a list of the key people in your partner-parent's life: spiritual advisor, friends at work or at the service club, tax preparer, lawyer, people in your parents' social circles. If your ill parent sits on a board or has some other advisory capacity, you may need to meet people from that group. Get your parent's permission to chat with these folks. Learn what you can and begin making the contacts that you may need in the future.

The Power of "We"

Any person with an emotional tie to the cancer patient should be offered the opportunity to help out. Visits, food, cards, flowers, bed care, games—there are plenty of ways. Briefing friends on the situation and organizing support activities help broaden the circle of warmth and friendship around your sick parent.

Pigheadedness

It is common for the patient to refuse to do something important at some point during treatment. The consequence is abominable. You, the partner, are convinced that you've got to change the patient's mind.

A good first step may be to consider the possibilities. More than one may apply.

1. You may have been pushing too hard or be just too bossy in general. Your parent wants a partner, not a keeper.
2. Fatigue, pain, loss, confusion, sorrow, or fear has made the road harder to travel. The patient wants to stop or at least slow down.
3. Your parent has objections to a doctor, a treatment, a cost, the travel, or something else. Find out what it is. Approach solutions from the same side of the issue as your parent, as a friend should. Do not allow yourself to become a defender of the problem. It puts you on the wrong side of the issue, and gives your parent a convenient target (you).
4. The subject is embarrassing, perhaps the object of ridicule.
5. Your parent begins to deny that a problem exists or that the solution in question will help. Resolving denial takes love, ingenuity, and patience.
6. Your parent associates going on with the prospect of death or physical loss. If this is the root, and if you cannot move the parent beyond this objection, this powerful, permanent factor will color every additional decision that comes along.
7. The patient has had enough, or you have, or you both lack the will to continue the fight. We've got at least three possible issues here, maybe intertwined. Sometimes one issue is blamed because another is too emotionally painful to acknowledge.

For more on all this, see Chapter 2, "Personal Decisions," and Chapter 26, "Nine Easy Ways to Shoot Yourself in the Foot." Discuss the issue with your doc, a counselor, or a qualified person you find through the Reference Center.

Side Issues to Know About

Is there a business liability you may have to deal with? Is the IRS after your parent or after a family holding? Is a complaint about to be filed? Can any other civil or criminal matter jump out of the bushes and bite?

This all seems to be a bit removed from the care of a person with cancer. It isn't. Any major concern that demands emotional energy, time, and money takes recuperative power away from the patient. If something is coming up, you can minimize it through planning. If nothing's there, you've covered the bases.

The Spouse as Healer

The healing powers of a spouse may be considerable. Even though this person proves incapable of assuming the role of strength giver and project manager, your parent-partner needs other gifts that the spouse can give in abundance.

Joyousness, Humor

Partners share happy moments effortlessly, just by being together. Nothing heals better than the comfort this association brings.

Memories

The older you get, the greater the store of memories, and the more valuable they become. Even after short-term memory starts to go, most people have fond recollections of other times. A spouse is an instinctive source of memories.

Tradition

Just imagine Tevye (Zero Mostel), in *Fiddler on the Roof,* bellowing "Tradition!" and breaking into song. Tradition is a taproot to life's sustaining juices. Husbands and wives have applied its teachings to family decisions since their life together began. They will apply it now to the decisions before them.

Sex

You're never too old.

Friendship

With age, there seem to be greater opportunities for friendship. Just sitting in the same room, each with a book, with not a word exchanged can be a satisfying act of friendship between senior people.

Reality Check

The spouse of your patient-parent may intuitively sense more about the sickness and recovery picture than you or the doctor will. You need the spouse like a fort needs a lookout.

Marriage Chores

A spouse knows what to do for a partner to keep the atmosphere comfy. A spouse can stop hurtful things from happening. In these and other roles, the spouse is irreplaceable. Nobody else could imagine them. For example, some couples take sustenance from occasional bickering.

Toxic Spouses

Some relationships go bad because of infidelity. Sometimes accident or illness damages one of the partners. A tendency to be scatterbrained has gained ground. Love has turned to hate, possibly from addiction or mental illness. This is a judgment call, but in some of these cases, bringing an estranged spouse back into close proximity with your patient-partner will make matters worse.

Pass the Soap, Partner

Have you ever bathed your father? Diapered your mother? This may be your chance. We observe conventions of modesty for good reasons, but cultural norms must sometimes be set aside. You may find yourself in the room when a physician examines the private parts of your parent. You will also need to be a caregiver at home. Make nothing of a catheter up the penis or an ostomy bag. These things require good care, which has become your job. Deal with them soberly. You may be surprised to hear the patient compliment you on your work in front of others. It is still wise to make no contribution to the conversation beyond a modest smile.

Planning Together

A Positive Recovery Plan

A written recovery plan has the distinct advantage of presenting a list one can use as a reminder, item by item. Its other benefit is that you and your parent have a method in front of you for listing everything either of you thinks needs to be included to be sure all the bases are covered.

Go back through the pertinent parts of this book to derive the areas to plan for. Call cancer survivors in the Reference Center to be sure you have things in a generally workable order.

A Budget

With a recovery plan made, base a budget on it. Don't forget to add a contingency-cost factor for the incidentals that come out of pocket. Parking, snacks, meals, gas, flowers, a movie after the treatment, and all the rest can reach an astonishing total.

Decide whom you will show this plan to and agree on why including each of these people is a good idea. You will need outside input from informed sources and family, but this plan will not be an appropriate piece of paper to pass around the dining-room table. If you do a good job of preparing it, the list will be graphic—and perhaps unsettling. There are circumstances in which it should reserve money for a wig, a prosthetic device, a transplant, or funeral arrangements.

Make no joke of personal matters at the time you are giving care, and never, ever discuss them with anyone except medical professionals who require the information.

Cash Flow

One of the most sensitive parts of your relationship with your parent is the question of who spends money for what, when, and how much. It's safer to be as specific and conservative as possible. Once the costs are listed, choreograph income and spending.

Never, never charge your parent for anything you provide or ask for a consideration later, such as in the will. It is apt to poison the relationship.

If you are offered a gift, make sure it comes from love of you (or your spouse or children), not as a form of compensation. If the gift is out of balance with portions of the estate given to others, somebody else in the family may become a problem for you later.

More on Money

Here's a secret map of the enemy harbor that shows where many, but not all, of the mines are tethered. You must sail in. Good luck.

Handling the Issue

Bring up money issues for discussion before there is any pressure to commit. Consider having your parent control the checkbook unless money management is confusing.

Provide regular, written statements of cash flow. This will help you both. Often Mom or Dad has a sense that the dollars are flying by in a blur. This recap will provide a clearer view of the situation.

We have already made reference to possible criticism you may face from other members of the family over money matters. Written statements will also help calm the dissidents. Keep all the potential scenarios in mind as you design the layout of these statements.

Recording All the Assets

Your parent has asked for your help. You need to know exactly what tools the parent has available for the job. Wealthy parents and some others may bridle at a financial disclosure, or they may be cagey. You have to decide if limited information is enough for you to work with. If not, politely but firmly resign your partnership position. You can't fly with one wing. Don't try. If you mess up the financials, the same person who held out on you is going to lay the blame for failure on your shoulders.

Presuming that the parent's assets can be known, at least between the two of you, make a list of everything that can help pay the bills. Include all sources of regular income, health insurance, life insurance, cash on hand, negotiable securities, real estate, anything significant that can be sold for a fair price, plus collectable debt. Sources of credit should also be noted, to the extent that the partner has a reasonable means of paying off the amount one might borrow. Mortgaging or refinancing real estate is one likely source of cash. Commercial lines of credit, particularly those of businesses your parent has an interest in, can also be good producers.

Credit-card debt is a bad idea. The interest rate and payment terms can be crippling. Moreover, reports of credit-card debt fly immediately into the records of those scoring your parent's overall credit worthiness. This little worm will grow big teeth the instant you attempt to obtain a real-estate loan or apply for an expensive hospital stay.

Millionaires and Debtors

When net worth exceeds $1 million or the estate is deeply in debt, involve an attorney. You will need an expert's management plan that protects the two of you from slings and arrows from all sides. This may be a significant expense unless you can get help from one of the legal resources listed in the Reference Center. Go forward. Do not allow cost to deter you. Hope that the attorney, your biggest cost, will show you ways through the problems ahead.

Certified Power of Attorney

Discuss frankly the possibility that a day may come when your parent will be indisposed. Write down the reasons why you may have to act without the parent's consent. To facilitate this written plan, get an unrestricted power of attorney. It must be unrestricted, because nobody thinks of everything. Have this agreement witnessed and certified.

Probable Sharks in the Water

There is always some family interest in the selection of treatments and hospitals. You may be criticized for choices that you and your parent-partner make. But money matters bring out the biggest guns. Any hint of impropriety with Uncle Mort's egg money is going to land you in unbelievably hot water. Relatives, usually led by people who believe they have a vested interest in the estate, may attack you.

You may also be attacked by third parties, such as the Medicare case supervisor or the county's welfare representative. They will come at you suddenly and forcefully from the lofty perch of "client interest." They hit the door with court orders in hand. You will be at least stuck with the time and cost of defending yourself, plus a fine or jail if you get nailed. You will be dealing with sanctimony personified. Guilty until proven innocent. Beheading before trial. Even your parent-partner may have limited success beating these monsters back into their caves.

Estate Pilfering

The possessions of the patient and spouse become susceptible to pilferage as soon as illness destabilizes normal life. "I mean, holy cow! She's never going to drive it again anyway. Why can't I take her car back to school next semester?" The interesting and creative ways that loved ones go through the pockets of the wounded will amaze you.

Your parent can add further complexity to this situation by deciding to give things to people who have asked for them. You may need to prepare a little lecture with a chorus that goes something like this: "Have you considered the possibility that you may need (fill in the blank) for a few more years? Your heirs can wait. Let them."

Estate pilfering is a hot rock that may be handed to you at any time. Unless you enjoy being the villain to multiple sides, explain this liability to your parent and come up with a policy that keeps you out of hot water. A suggestion: Nobody gets anything until Mom or Dad has fully recovered.

Managing Your Parent's Business

You may be forced into management of your parent's business. As the cancer patient's confidant and primary caregiver, you will begin getting the business-related phone calls when the boss is indisposed. You dutifully pass along the notes. Your parent, who is too sick to do more, waves a limp wrist and mumbles, "Just handle it." Don't panic. Toss the problem back to the company. Tell the senior person to do the best that he or she can. There's a good chance that you've made a stellar move, with little risk that the ship will falter.

A Supervising Committee

Someone is apt to get the bright idea that a committee should be formed to deal with the complexities of "Pop's condition." You respond by pointing out that your father has made you responsible for his care and estate management. This riposte passes neatly over the head of the person with the bright-eyed suggestion, who continues, "So when shall we get together to talk about this?" Stand your ground. Do not permit this plot to be homesteaded.

A committee is usually a terrible idea. It makes tough decisions concerning health care even more difficult. And it is a breeding ground for needless arguments about money and other estate matters.

For purposes of this discussion, a committee has been formed to supervise the cancer patient's caregiving and estate despite your best efforts. Some thoughts are offered for your safety should you choose to go near this disaster on wheels.

If you accept the chair position, be prepared to lose a lot of time you thought you would be able to give to other matters, and to pay for a string of surprising and often unnecessary costs out of your pocket.

Somebody has to hold durable power of attorney, for the protection of the patient. If that person is not on the committee, you've got a royal mess on your hands. If that person is on the committee or in the employ of the committee, the situation is no better.

When problems become complex, the committee is going to need legal counsel and the services of a CPA, in all likelihood. The sick parent whom this is supposed to be helping is not responsible for this bureaucratic bungling. Committee resources, not those of the patient, should pay the ensuing bills.

Patient Dementia

Pain and some cancer-treatment drugs are hard on reasoning abilities and judgment. You never know when a patient may lose sharpness, or for how long. As a senior, other deficiencies of old age can make this condition worse. As a part of dying, patients may also slip into unworldly places with or without the assistance of drugs.

If dementia has taken hold of your parent, you may hear from your doctor or a psychiatric oncologist that mental recovery is possible, and they will instruct you as to next steps. If the professionals have no expectancy of recovery, they will help you understand how to treat dementia as part of a terminal condition.

Sometimes dementia occupies a frustrating middle ground. As time passes, the patient may or may not return to a more lucid state. Meanwhile, you inherit a foul-mouthed juvenile who knows exactly how to find the hot buttons of the medical staff and maybe yours too. Your patient may refuse to take medicine. The doctors will lose interest in treatment. Attendants will begin using psychotropic medications and restraints. The patient will be isolated. Violence can follow.

Managing a Business-Leadership Transition

If your parent loses to cancer, causing a family-owned business to teeter, you may find yourself in the middle of it. If you have business experience and the confidence of the family behind you, emulate Howard Hughes or Katharine Graham, who took command of small ventures and did right well for themselves. Otherwise, hire a consultant to sell the enterprise on behalf of the estate. If it is a viable company, one of its competitors may make an attractive offer. Lots of times, a good company can be sold at an excellent price to a group of its employees, though the estate will probably have to agree to time payments. Don't try the initial public-stock-offering solution without an expert at the helm—way, way too many perils. As a last gasp to salvage something, there are vultures in the investment banking community who will offer about a tenth of real worth (and then try to cheat you out of that).

53 When the Patient Is Not a Relation

While there are hospital volunteers and paid companions available to help, a patient with a personal partner or partnering team is much better off.

Being alone is mentally tough on a cancer patient, as well as a dangerously slipshod way to treat a serious condition. So it is good that you have turned to this chapter, which is written to both the patient and to the person or persons contemplating a helper's role.

The Stranded Patient

Some patients have outlived everyone they know. Some have spouses who must work, perhaps even live, elsewhere. Many adult children think that they cannot spare the time, or won't. A surprising number of family members fear medical things. They'd sooner walk into a lion's den than a cancer clinic.

Dear stranded patient: You may feel hurt that no one is helping you. You may not accept the excuses of those you had hoped would be there for you. But, as you may have already observed, cancer-clinic waiting rooms are full of patients in need of partners. It is probably more practical to come up with a new strategy for getting help than to hope to change the mind of someone who has left you in the lurch.

Solutions for Stranding

As a patient without a partner, your solution may be as simple as asking for help. Tell a potential helpmate about the values discussed in Chapters 3 and 9. People don't realize that partnering has such great importance.

If there isn't someone to ask directly, look around:

- Tell the next person who asks, "How are you?" that you need help.
- Ask your parent, adult child, or another close relative to help you with this search. You never know when just admitting that there is a situation can return major benefits. The busiest person you know may find a way to change priorities after learning about your search.
- Your doctor, one of the senior nurses, someone on the psychosocial care team, or a hospital chaplain may have a solution.
- The American Cancer Society has a companionship program in many cities, as do other groups such as the Leukemia and Lymphoma Society. You will find toll-free phone numbers for these and other help organizations in the Reference Center.
- The YWCA in some cities has an active support program for women. The Salvation Army and Catholic Charities USA help both men and women. (These aren't the hopelessly old-fashioned organizations that some imagine. You'll enjoy the people you meet. Also, you don't have to profess any faith to be served by either of them.)
- Ask a leader in your church.
- Ask the president of a club you belong to.
- Paid companions are available, of course. Health insurance, Medicare and Medicaid, and some hospitals provide transportation and companionship to those who qualify. Generally, the emphasis is on transportation, often group transport. You need more than that. You need eyes and ears and friendship in the treatment room. But if you're starting with nothing, one of these services is an improvement.

Just don't keep your need for a partner a secret. Tell everybody. You've heard that old adage about how the squeaky wheel gets the grease. Be pleasantly persistent.

Partnership Options

No logical partner? Your situation can be solved in other ways. One of them is to let yourself become a group project. Let several people take turns helping you. This is a difficult challenge if you have a small circle of acquaintances, particularly if your friends have the limited resources of many seniors, but it can be done. Think creatively.

The concept of becoming a group project is important. Anybody may help you a time or two each and then go on to other things. But a support group is likely to be more effective and longer lasting if you help each person feel that he or she is part of a group, Project *(your name goes here)*; make up a calendar of times and places when you need help; and coordinate related needs such as runs to the drugstore or the market or helping you with physical therapy or medications at home.

To the Prospective Companion

Don't let perfect be the enemy of good. Just do your best. You don't need to be a nurse. Your love is the essential gift.

If you've been invited to consider helping someone through the experience of cancer treatment and have your nose in this chapter to find out more about it, most of what remains in this chapter is for you.

First of all, cancer is a lengthy affair, not six weeks and the cast comes off. By deciding to help, you provide a strong shoulder for the patient to lean on, which the patient will count on for a long time, perhaps years. The treatment and healing process demands that you and others helping the patient keep up the sheltering and caring program. Please don't desert your post without provision for a replacement.

The other core value is the loving concern you give. This attention to needs, both the ones you see and the ones the medical staff shows you, fills a critical gap that no one else takes care of. The recovery and positive mental attitude of the patient benefit enormously.

You will be drawn into the life of this person you are caring for. You will share, and you will care. You will grow in maturity and knowledge, and you will never forget this experience.

Dividing Things Up

The role of partner can be divided up. And it's good to pass out pieces of the job, at least on occasion, so that nobody hefts too large a load. You may want to consider five general areas of help to contribute to the needs of a cancer patient.

1. Friends with cars who can take a person to tests and treatments, take notes if necessary, and maybe find something to share a smile over will be important.
2. People who can help keep a household together—the kids, the meals, the cleaning, and all that—will be needed on the team. Help informing and coordinating with the rest of the patient's family seems to be part of this function, too. If it turns out that another person is needed to take care of answering questions and passing along news, a sixth category may be in order. This can be particularly important if communication is better in more than one language.

3. People with the ability to manage business matters may be needed.
4. A researcher with access to the Internet who will call listings in the Reference Center and talk to associates and medical staff is always valuable. On the Web, there are also things to find, travel arrangements to make, or shopping for a better deal.
5. Most people have only the vaguest idea of what a cancer patient's medical team is talking about most of the time. Someone who can help with a basic understanding of what's really going on helps a lot. This same person will also think of good questions to ask. (Don't doctors and nurses help with this? Yes. Fortunate patients have medical teams that keep them fully informed. The rest can expect a willing and sincere effort to be helpful anytime within the fifteen-second window during which you have the attention of one of them.)

Government Intervention

Patients who are minors without the support of a functional family unit, and senior people receiving welfare, Medicare, VA, or certain other government programs, may become wards of the state. Some may not realize that there is an agency that considers itself to be a responsible party. If you learn that your cancer patient is part of one of these programs, have a meeting with the patient and all interested groups. The people from the government agency are usually focused on good results, just as you are, and will be pleased by the team approach. Things can work out quite well.

Legal Matters

Patients own things. You will want to help protect them. Patients have friends and relatives who may not live nearby. You will want to help protect their rights and possible future property. You may also find that there are people watching you from the sidelines in questioning ways. For many reasons, discuss the details of the help you are providing with one of the free legal counseling services listed in the Reference Center and be guided by the recommendations you receive.

Age Difference between Patient and Partner

If there is an age difference of more than twenty years between patient and partner, it may be helpful to read about general relationships with the other generation; see Chapter 50, "Parent/Child Partnerships," or Chapter 52, "When the Patient Is a Parent."

One More Thing . . .

You Have a Golden Opportunity

Please consider how fortunate you are to be where you are. Your cancer took aim but you haven't gone down. You have a great team supporting you. You have resources. You are experienced. You don't stare into the future blindly.

Yes, you continue to struggle with a nasty, expensive, scary, disgusting, disruptive thing that has done major damage. It is also true—as hard as optimism may be for you—that progress has been made on at least some fronts.

Sixty years ago, standing in London's smoldering ruins, Winston Churchill proclaimed an "end to the beginning" of the war against Nazi Germany. In the same way—though the conflict is far from over—it's time for you to strike back, time to bomb Bremerhaven.

As sick and as preoccupied and as broke as you may be, you can retaliate. Perhaps a way has already come to mind, or:

- Let your medical team know that you are available to talk to new patients.
- Ask how you can return the service to a group that has helped you.
- Adopt a patient. And be available for phone calls from partner and family.
- Adopt a counselor, someone who needs your insight to help others.
- Ask your doc if there is a promising clinical trial that needs your case.
- Start a support group at your hospital, place of worship, workplace or service club.

Don't try to make a grand gesture. Do something easy. But do something. You are, right now, what someone dreams of being. Help that dream.

Reference Center

A Note on the Reference Center

The Reference Center is intended to be a reasonably good first tour around the cancer-support neighborhood. Like all such lists, it is imperfect.

The "White Pages" list organizations alphabetically. The "Yellow Pages" is an alphabetical listing of organizations by topic: acupuncture, financial help, lung, pancreas, support groups, and so on.

Important organizations have doubtless been omitted by mistake. Others have been created or have passed out of existence since this listing was compiled. Sometimes organizations merge, though in the crowded and complex world of cancer treatment and recovery, probably not often enough. Names and phone numbers change. The objective is to lead the reader in the right direction, hoping that this imperfect service is sufficient and not too frustrating.

All the listed organizations claim national scope of service. (Many more local groups await your discovery.) These groups often have extensive Web sites and bookstores, which will be helpful to those with access to the Internet. Some also publish public-interest newsletters, guides, catalogs, and magazines.

A reminder: Most public libraries provide Internet access at no charge. Libraries also subscribe to magazines and get books their patrons ask for.

If your search of these listings does not produce an obvious group to contact, the American Cancer Society and the National Cancer Institute, both listed, are good places to start. If you know the name of the organization you need to reach, an Internet search engine, such as Lycos or Google, will likely be of service.

White Pages

This section characterizes most listings into one of the four listed types; the symbol that denotes the organization's category follows its name.

G   Government site: Thoroughly chewed information offered in conservative, nonsectarian terms. Often public service at its best.

N   Nonprofit private organization, often with a charitable mission: Services range from very broad to extremely narrow. Some are huge. Others are quite small in terms of both people power and budget. Some also teach. Some fund research. Some engage in advocacy.

P   Professional association: The high standards of a profession, as determined by its leadership, dictate the information offered. Words and attitudes common to the group are used, which may take some getting used to.

S   Sponsor products or services: Offered in a helpful way from a commercial point of view. Valuable insights into areas of patient need are often found.

Note: This information was last reviewed in August 2005. Please go to aboutmycancer.com for the latest version of this directory.

Organization	Contact Information	Description
Accelerate Brain Cancer Cure *N*	650/685-2200 abc2.org	Funds research on brain treatment techniques; screens drugs.
Abledata *N*	800/227-0216 abledata.com	Database lists 25,000 of the most demanded products for the special needs of cancer patients. Call an operator or go online. Free service of the National Institute on Disability and Rehabilitation Research.
AboutFace *N*	800/225-3223 800/665-3223 (Canada) interlog.com/~abtface	Support and info network for people with face and neck disfiguration—birth defects, injuries, and surgeries. 25 U.S. chapters. Publishes *AboutFace* newsletter.
About Herbs, Botanicals & Other Products	mskcc.org/html/11570.cfm	Pharmacist specializing in oncology provides info about herbs and

(continued)

Organization	Contact Information	Description
N		botanicals, with clinical summary for each. Lists potential benefits, side effects, interactions, other problems.
Adenoid Cystic Carcinoma Resource Center *N*	home.paonline.com/ knippd/acc/	Helps those with Adenoid Cystic Carcinoma find sources of info and support. Extensive links (some to wrong sites).
Adrenocortical Carcinoma *S*	pages.zdnet.com/ beverlin/ adrenocortical carcinoma/	Extensive links and contacts from Richard Beverlin. Invites patients and caregivers to join a closed support group.
AirLifeLine *N*	877/247-5433 877/727-7728 airlifeline.org	National network of private aircraft provides free trips to treatments for patients and family members. Demonstrate financial need. Must be medically stable and ambulatory.
Alliance for Lung Cancer Advocacy, Support, and Education *N*	800/298-2436 360/696-2436 alcase.org	Publishes *The Lung Cancer Resource Guide* for patients. Offers custom searches of medical databases. Sponsors *Phone Buddies* for peer counseling. *Spirit and Breath* newsletter.
American Academy of Dermatology	847/330-0230 aad.org	Info about melanoma; resources for patients.
American Academy of Medical Acupuncture *P*	800/521-2262 medicalacupuncture.org	Acupuncture locator; medical topics, continuing education, newsletter, journals.
American Academy of Pain Medicine *P*	708/966-9510 painmed.org	Provides education, training, advocacy, access to research. Site serves physicians. Not patient-friendly.
American Alliance of Cancer Pain Initiatives *N*	608/265-4013 aacpi.org	Provides leadership and advocacy for state and regional pain initiatives.
American Amputee Foundation *N*	501/666-2523 americanamputee.org	120 support groups in 36 states. Helps with insurance disputes, locating financial aid for artificial limbs and home modifications. Publishes *Life Care Planning* newsletter and a national resource directory.
American Association for Cancer Research *N*	215/440-9300 aacr.org	Devoted to basic, clinical, and translational cancer research. Promotes communication among professionals.
American Association for Respiratory Care	972/243-2272 aarc.org	Has locator for respiratory therapists; info on lung care,

G = Government, *N* = Nonprofit, *P* = Professional, *S* = Sponsor

Organization	Contact Information	Description
N		home therapies, continuous positive airway pressure (CPAP).
American Association of Naturopathic Physicians (AANP) P	206/298-0126 naturopathic.org	Patient info, ND locator, publications, explanation of naturopathic medicine.
American Association of Oriental Medicine P	866/455-7999 aaom.org	Member site; promotes highest ethical and academic standards for Chinese herbal medicine and acupuncture. Site links, referral service, educational info.
American Brain Tumor Association N	800/886-2282 847/827-9910 abta.org	Free publications about brain tumors; support-group lists, referral information, pen-pal program. *Message Line* newsletter.
American Cancer Society N	800/ACS-2345 cancer.org	Dedicated to eliminating cancer as a health problem. Provides educational materials, including custom booklets, in direct response to individual needs.
American College of Physicians P	800/523-1546 aponline.org	Primarily serves physician and med-student members. Customer Service: ext. 2600.
American College of Surgeons: Cancer Programs P	312/202-5085 facs.org/cancer/ index.html	Verifies that your surgeon is certified in the surgical specialty you need, other cancer-specific surgical information.
American College of Gastroenterology P	703/820-7400 acg.gi.org	Educational materials, including glossary of GI terms and digestive-system health tips.
American Foundation for Urologic Disease N	800/822-5277 410/468-1800 afud.org	Info for the public, patients, and health-care professionals on prostate cancer treatments, bladder health, sexual function.
American Gastroenterological Association P	301/654-2055 gastro.org	Info and referrals for colorectal cancer.
American Hospice Foundation N	202/223-0204 americanhospice.org	Helps locate hospice organizations nearby.
American Institute for Cancer Research N	800/843-8114 (Nutrition hotline) 202/328-7744 airc.org	Research and public education in areas of diet, nutrition, and cancer; pen pals; free publications.

(*continued*)

Organization	Contact Information	Description
American Lung Association N	800/LUNG-U.S.A 212/315-8700 lungusa.org	Dedicated to conquering lung disease and promoting lung health.
American Pain Foundation P	888/615-7246 painfoundation.org	*Pain Action Guide,* information, support, advocacy.
American Pain Society P	847/375-4715 ampainsoc.org	References to nearby centers and clinics from a database and of 3,200 professionals.
American Psychosocial Oncology Society N	434/971-4788 apos-society.org	Association of health professionals that strives to make psychosocial services available to cancer patients.
American Society for Blood and Marrow Transplantation P	847/427-0224 asbmt.org	Promotes advancement of the field of blood and bone-marrow transplantation. Members in clinical practice, research.
American Society for Gastrointestinal Endoscopy P	978/526-8330 asge.org	Info about gastrointestinal endoscopy techniques, patient experiences.
American Society for Therapeutic Radiology and Oncology P	800/962-7876 astro.org	Locator for radiation oncologists; brochures and videos for patients and friends; research data.
American Society of Anesthesiologists P	847/825-5586 asahq.org	Referrals to society members specializing in pain management.
American Society of Clinical Oncology P	703/299-0150 peoplelivingwith cancer.org asco.org plwc.org	Info on more than 50 forms of cancer. Discusses treatments, clinical trials, coping, side effects. Oncologist locator. Chat with counselors "live" by e-mail. Drug database; links to patient-support organizations.
American Society of Colon and Rectal Surgeons P	847/290-9184 fascrs.org	Patient info on GI conditions, colon and rectal surgery.
American Thyroid Association N	718/920-4321 thyroid.org	Scientists and physicians dedicated to better understanding and treatment of all thyroid diseases. Patient support info.
Amgen Safety Net S	800/272-9376 *amgen.com/patient/ assistance.html*	Pharmaceutical manufacturer; offers its cancer-fighters at low or no cost to those without financial resources.

G = Government, N = Nonprofit, P = Professional, S = Sponsor

Organization	Contact Information	Description
American Thoracic Society P	212/315-8700 thoracic.org	Locator for thoracic (chest) surgeons.
Amputee Coalition of America N	888/267-5669 amputee-coalition.org	Educates people with limb loss about resources, opportunities, options. *First Step: A Guide to Adapting to Limb Loss,* highly recommended.
Amschwand Sarcoma Cancer Foundation N	713/838-1615 sarcomacancer.org	Suggestions for the newly diagnosed. Lists most significant treatment facilities in U.S., with private homes nearby that host patients.
Anderson Network N	800/345-6324 mdanderson.org/ andersonnetwork	Patient-matching program; support for caregivers; educational forum. Quarterly newsletter.
Angel Flight America N	800/446-1231 angelflightamerica.org	Network of 5,000 pilots transports cancer patients and their families.
Area Agencies on Aging (AAA) G	800/677-1116	660 in the U.S., federally mandated by the Older American's Act. Services such as transportation, home health care, homemaker help, and legal assistance to those age 60 and over.
Association for Applied Psychophysiology and Biofeedback P	aapb.org	Lists nearest biofeedback therapists.
Association of Community Cancer Centers N	301/984-9496 *accc-cancer.org*	Looks after the economic and regulatory well-being of its 650 member oncology centers.
Association of Cancer Online Resources P	212/226-5525 acor.org	Discussion groups; links to cancer-specific sites; info on most kinds of cancer. Locator service for patients looking for others with same cancer.
Association of Oncology Social Work P	215/599-6093 aosw.org	Dedicated to the enhancement of psychosocial services to cancer patients and their families.
Association of Pediatric Oncology Nurses P	847/375-4724 apon.org	Leading professional organization for registered nurses caring for children and adolescents with cancer and their families
AstraZeneca Foundation Patient Assistance Program S	800/424-3727 astrazeneca-us.com	Pharmaceutical manufacturer; offers its cancer-fighters at low or no cost to those without financial resources.

(continued)

Organization	Contact Information	Description
Autologous Blood and Marrow Transplant Registry P	414/456-8325 ibmtr.org	Does *not* aid in searches for transplant donors. Info on about 50% of autotransplants done in North and South America since 1989.
Aventis Oncology S	800/996-6626 aventisoncology.com/ reimbursement.htm	Helps patients with reimbursements, financial assistance; may help reduce obstacles to third-party payment when health-care providers use certain of its products (same org. as PACT Plus).
AVONCares Program for Medically Underserved Women N	800/813-4673 cancercare.org	Pays for supportive services such as child care, transportation, and home care for breast and cervical cancer patients of very limited means. (Program managed by Cancer Care, Inc., also listed.)
Beyond the Cure N	314/446-5215 beyondthecure.org	Info from the National Children's Cancer Society pertaining to all areas of a survivor's life.
Billy Foundation N	510/264-9078 bfmelanoma.com	Raises funds to find cures for late-stage melanoma, to educate the public regarding cause and prevention. Free literature and educational programs.
Biological Therapy Institute Foundation N	615/790-7535	Leading resource for physician and patient info regarding the use of biopharmaceuticals in cancer therapy.
Bloch Cancer Foundation N	800/433-0464 816/932-8453 blochcancer.org	General info, peer counseling, help obtaining medical second opinions. Cancer-patient support group. Free books on how to fight cancer for patient and caregiver.
Blood & Marrow Transplant Information Network N	888/597-7674 bmtnews.org	Practical help for stem-cell, bone-marrow and cord-blood transplant patients. Counsel by survivors of the procedures. Links to financial and technical aid. Info on 200 U.S. transplant centers.
Bone Marrow Foundation N	800/365-1336 212/838-3029 bonemarrow.org	Provides financial aid, education, and emotional support to bone-marrow transplant recipients.
Bone Marrow Transplant Newsletter N	888/597-7674 847/433-3313 bmtinfonet.org	Matters of interest to patients, bimonthly. Also sells a book. Attorney referrals for those having difficulty obtaining reimbursement for treatments.

G = Government, N = Nonprofit, P = Professional, S = Sponsor

Organization	Contact Information	Description
Brain Tumor Foundation *N*	212/265-2401 braintumor foundation.org	Counseling and peer-matching services.
Brain Tumor Society *P*	800/770-8287 617/924-9997 tbts.org	Research and education organization. Hot line, support groups, free literature. *Heads Up* newsletter.
Breast Cancer Action *N*	877/278-6722 bcaction.org	Provides info and organizes people to demand effective treatment and true prevention.
Breast Cancer Advisory Center *N*	301/984-1020	Information clearinghouse.
Breastcancer.org *N*	breastcancer.org	Aims to provide the most complete and reliable info available.
Burger King Cancer Caring Center, Pittsburgh, PA *N*	412/622-1212 (Also a hotline)	Info for people diagnosed with cancer. Helps patients, friends, and family cope with emotional impact.
Caitlin Raymond International Registry *N*	800/726-2824 508/792-8969 crir.org	Worldwide database of 2.2 million volunteer marrow donors. Umbilical-cord blood banks. Counseling and financial aid.
CAN ACT (Cancer Patients Action Alliance) *N*	718/522-4607	Advocacy and public policy. Does not offer services to individuals.
Cancer411.org *N*	877/226-2741 cancer411.org	Searchable list of all current clinical trials; news articles; other patient resources.
Cancer Aid and Research Foundation *N*	623/561-5893 canceraidresearch.org	Awards scientific research grants. Provides supplies and equipment to alternative therapy programs.
Cancer Care, Inc. *N*	800/813-4673 212/712-8080 cancercare.org	Emotional support, information, referral, and practical assistance for people with cancer and their loved ones. Toll-free counseling line, educational teleconferences, online chat rooms. Ask for its excellent resource brochure: *Helping Hand Newsletter: Cancer Care News.*
Cancer.com *N*	800/325-7504 cancer.com	Info about forms of cancer, current therapies, advances, prevention, detection. Current news, treatments, side effects. Physician locator.

(*continued*)

Organization	Contact Information	Description
Cancer Conquerors Foundation N	800/238-6479 717/533-6124	Cancer-survival training programs and self-study materials with specific emphasis on body/mind/spirit integration.
Cancer Control PLANET N	cancercontrolplanet .cancer.gov	Tools for cancer control planning, implementation, evaluation. Joint project of the National Cancer Institute and the American Cancer Society.
Cancer Genetics Network N	epi.grants.cancer.gov/ CGN	Links to a national network of centers specializing in inherited predisposition to cancers.
Cancer Hope Network N	877/467-3638 908/879-4039 cancerhopenetwork.org	Free one-on-one support to cancer patients in treatment and their families. Counselors are trained volunteers who have survived similar treatments.
Cancer Info Net N	cancerinfonet.org	Info about diagnosis and treatment; prevention, research, and resource links.
Cancer Information and Counseling Line N	800/525-3777 amc.org	Current information, emotional support, and short-term counseling to callers.
Cancer Legal Resource Center N	213/736-1455 lls.edu (or) wlcdr.org	Info on cancer-related legal issues for people with cancer and those who support them.
CancerQuest N	cancerquest.org	Emory University site teaches the biology of cancer.
Cancer Research Institute N	800/99-CANCER 212/688-7515 cancerresearch.org	Supports research to develop new methods for diagnosing, treating, and preventing cancer.
Cancer Research and Prevention Foundation N	800/227-2732 preventcancer.org	Manages projects for the prevention and early detection of cancer through scientific research and education.
CancerSource N	cancersource.com	Education, news, support. Detailed info on complementary and integrative therapies.
Cancer Support Network N	412/361-8600	Emotional and psychological support through peer support groups, educational programs, community workshops, advocacy, social gatherings.
Cancer Survivors Coalition N	888/650-9127 cansearch.org	Supports cancer survivors, families. Washington, D.C.–based advocate of patient rights.
Cancer Survivors Gathering Place N	geocities.com/ cancer_survivors	Bulletin board, chat rooms, links, and inspirational materials for cancer survivors.

G = Government, N = Nonprofit, P = Professional, S = Sponsor

Organization	Contact Information	Description
Cancer Survivors Network N	877/333-HOPE acscsn.org	Phone and Web counseling and info services for patients, families, caregivers, friends. Sponsored and maintained by the American Cancer Society.
CancerTrialsHelp.org N	cancertrialshelp.org	See Coalition of National Cancer Cooperative Groups
Cancer Trials Support Unit G	888/823-5923 ctsu.org	Helps physicians participate in National Cancer Institute–sponsored phase III cancer-treatment trials.
Cancervive N	800/486-2873 310/203-9232 cancervive.org	Support groups; educational materials; insurance information, assistance, and advocacy. Cancervive newsletter.
Cancer Warriors N	cancerwarriors.org	Encourages and supports children, siblings, and caregivers during treatment for childhood cancers.
Candlelighters Childhood Cancer Foundation N	800/366-2223 301/9623520 candlelighters.org	Info, support, and advocacy for families of children with cancer, survivors of childhood cancers, and the professionals who care for them. Lists financial resources and eligibility criterion.
CaP Cure N	800/757-2873 capcure.org/	Supports research, mostly at eight affiliated U.S. treatment centers (also known as the Prostate Cancer Foundation).
Carcinoid Cancer Foundation N	888/722-3132 carcinoid.org	Education, support groups, transcripts of lectures, nutritional information.
Catholic Charities U.S.A N	703/549-1390	Provides free or low-cost transportation, family counseling, home health care, respite care, etc., regardless of religious affiliation.
Center for Clinical Trials and Evidence-Based Healthcare N	trialscentral.org	Links to summaries of clinical trials and reviews. From Brown Univ., affiliated with Cochrane Collaboration, U.K.
Center for Information and Study on Clinical Research Participation N	ciscrp.org	Facts, figures, and info about participating in clinical trials.
Center for Mind-Body Medicine N	202/966-7338 cmbm.org	Addresses the mental, emotional, social, physical and spiritual sides of health and fitness. Combines modern science with ancient healing practices.

(continued)

Organization	Contact Information	Description
Center for Patient Advocacy N	800/846-7444 703/748-0400 patientadvocacy.org	Phone counselors; helps patients with treatment problems navigate the managed-health-care morass. Washington, D.C., lobbyist on health-care issues.
Center to Advance Palliative Care N	212/201-2670 capcmssm.org	Tools and training for health-care professionals to start and sustain palliative- care programs.
Centerwatch N	617/856-5900 centerwatch.com	Lists 41,000 government- and industry-funded clinical trials that are actively recruiting patients. Most oncology trials included. Patient-notification services available.
ChemoCare N	800/55-CHEMO 908/233-1103	One-on-one emotional support from trained and certified volunteer survivors for those undergoing chemotherapy and radiation.
Chemotherapy Foundation N	212/213-9292	Supports laboratory and clinical research to develop more effective methods of diagnosis and therapy. Conducts professional and public-education programs.
Children's Brain Tumor Foundation N	866/228-4673 212/448-9494 cbtf.org	Free resource guide; Parent-2-Parent Network; Family Outreach Project; newsletter; school issues; summer camps; annual teleconference.
Children's Cause N	301/562-2765 childrenscause.org	National catalyst to stimulate drug discovery and development for childhood cancers, expand resources for research and treatment, and address the needs and concerns of survivors.
Children's Hospice International N	800/242-4453	Services for gravely ill children.
Children's Oncology Camps of America N	803/434-3533	Provides normal life experiences for children, siblings, and their families.
Civilian Health and Medical Program, Dept. of Veterans Affairs (CHAMPUS) G		*See* Tricare.
Coalition of National Cancer Cooperative Groups N	877/520-4457 cancertrialshelp.org	Info about clinical trials offered by seven cooperative groups; links to patient advocates.

G = Government, *N* = Nonprofit, *P* = Professional, *S* = Sponsor

Organization	Contact Information	Description
Colon Cancer Alliance N	877/422-2030 212/627-7451 ccalliance.org	Patient-support services and info. Supports public education, research; sponsors events.
Colon Cancer Support Group N	415/885-7546	Peer counseling.
Colorectal Cancer Network N	301/879-1500 colorectal-cancer.net	Survivors and caregivers provide access to colorectal-cancer support groups.
Coming Home Network N	800/664-5110 740/450-1175 chnetwork.org	Someone is waiting to pray with you, M–F, 9 A.M.–5 P.M., Zanesville, Ohio, time. All Catholic and Protestant denominations.
CONVERSATIONS! N	806/355-2565 ovarian-news.org	Free monthly ovarian cancer patient newsletter: general info., treatment options, coping skills, humor, connections with survivors.
Coping with Cancer Magazine S	615/790-2400 copingmag.com	Bimonthly for people whose lives have been touched by cancer.
Corporate Angel Network N	866/328-1313 914/328-1313 corpangelnetwork.org	Searches for free "space available" on corporate aircraft for cancer patients traveling for treatment, bone-marrow donors, and their parties.
Crohn's and Colitis Foundation of America N	914/328-1313 ccfa.org	Sponsors research; educational programs and support services for patients with Crohn's disease and colitis.
Cure for Lymphoma Foundation N	800/CFL-6848 212/213-9595 cfl.org	Supports an integrated, nationwide research strategy to increase cure rates. Develops programs for patients, caregivers, and professionals.
CURE Magazine S	800/210-CURE curetoday.com	Quarterly for patients, survivors, and caregivers. Contact for free subscription.
Cutaneous Lymphoma Network N	513/584-6805	University of Cincinnati Hospital research program.
Dave Dravecky's Outreach of Hope N	719/481-3528 outreachofhope.org	Special experience with amputation. Prayer, comfort, outreach and hope for cancer patients.
Department of Social Services G	(See your phone book's white pages)	State, local, and city departments coordinate Medicaid and Temporary Assistance for Needy Families ("welfare"), food stamps, state-funded financial aid.

(continued)

Organization	Contact Information	Description
Doctor Evidence S	310/650-8657 doctorevidence.com	Reports on products, procedures, outcomes, and other matters of concern to a patient. Fee charged.
Eli Lilly's Patient Assistance Programs S	800/545-6962 elilly.com/products/access/ direct_patient.html	Pharmaceutical manufacturer; offers its cancer-fighters at low or no cost to those without financial resources. Also provides reimbursement info to patients and health-care providers.
Encore Plus N	800/953-7587 ywca.org	Post-op peer-support and exercise programs for women (YWCA).
Esophageal Cancer Awareness Association N	866/730-3222 ECaware.org	Promotes understanding and support for esophageal cancer patients and their caregivers.
Exceptional Cancer Patients N	814/337-8192 ecap-online.org	Emotional support and education for patients.
Eye Cancer Network S	212/832-8170 eyecancer.com	Paul Finger, MD, discusses the diagnosis and treatment of eye-tumor patients. Eye-tumor info links; locator for eye-tumor specialists.
Facing Our Risk of Cancer Empowered (FORCE) N	866/824-7475 954/255-8732 facingourrisk.org	Support, info, and resources for women with breast or ovarian cancer.
Families Against Cancer (FACT) N	315/446-5326	Federal lobby for greater spending on early diagnosis and intervention.
Federation of Chiropractic Licensing Boards P	970/356-3500 fclb.org	Promotes excellence in chiropractic regulation. Consumer info; member locator.
Fertile Hope N	888/994-4673 fertilehope.org	Information, support, and hope regarding cancer and fertility through programs of awareness, education, financial assistance, research.
FindCancerExperts N	findcancerexperts.com	Referral service for those needing a second opinion on a biopsy.
Foundation for Digestive Health and Nutrition P	301/654-2635 fdhn.org	Public-education initiatives related to digestive diseases. Also disburses grants. Sponsored by the American Gastroenterological Association.
Foundation for Hospice and Home Care N	202/547-7424 nahc.org	Helps locate accredited home-care aid.

G = Government, N = Nonprofit, P = Professional, S = Sponsor

Organization	Contact Information	Description
Friends Network N	805/565-7031	Publishes *The Funletter,* a national newsletter about cancer activities. Proceeds benefit children with cancer.
Gilda Radner Familial Ovarian Cancer Registry N	800/OVARIAN ovariancancer.com	Registry tracks families with a history of ovarian cancer; help line, education, info, and peer support.
Gilda's Club N	888/445-3248 917/305-1200 gildasclub.org	Social and emotional support for people with cancer and their families. 16 locations.
GIST Support International N	gistsupport.org	Supports patients, families, and friends and ongoing research to treat and cure gastrointestinal stromal tumors. Clinical trial information.
GlaxoSmithKline's Commitment to Access S	866/265-6491 *commitmenttoaccess .gsk.com*	Pharmaceutical manufacturer; offers its cancer-fighters at low or no cost to those without financial resources.
Good Health for Life N	530/647-9047 ghfl.org	Knowledge and direction for cancer patients seeking jobs.
Gynecologic Cancer Foundation N	800/444-4441 312/578-1439 wcn.org	Promotes gynecologic cancer prevention, early diagnosis, proper treatment. Supports research and training. Women's Cancer Network at the Web site helps women assess their own risk for developing gynecologic and breast cancers, plus info on screening, detection, treatment, clinical trials. Forum for gynecologic cancer survivors. (The foundation arm of the Society of Gynecologic Oncologists.)
Heal Magazine S	214/820-7152 healtoday.com	Focuses on life after recovery from cancer. $20/year.
Health Resource Inc. S	800/949-0090 thehealthresource.com	Reports on products, procedures, outcomes, and other matters of concern to a patient. Fee charged.
Helping Patients.org N	800/762-4636 helpingpatients.org	Helps patients get free and low-cost medicines. Site sponsor, the Partnership for Prescription Assistance, offers a single point of access to more than 275 public and private patient-assistance programs, including more than 150 programs offered by pharmaceutical companies.

(continued)

Organization	Contact Information	Description
HER2 Support Group Organization *N*	760/602-9178 *her2support.org*	Christine and Joe Druther's Web site; shares achievements and offers help and encouragement to cancer patients.
Hill-Burton Program *G*	800/638-0742	Directs callers to hospitals and other health providers with free or very low-cost services. 1,800 U.S. hospitals participate.
Hereditary Colon Cancer Association *N*	608/263-1017 *hereditarycc.org*	Promotes awareness of hereditary colon cancer and the need to find better treatments for those who are at risk or have been positively diagnosed.
Hole in the Wall Camps *N*	holeinthewallcamps.org	Network of summer camps for critically ill children. Organized by Paul Newman.
Hirshberg Foundation for Pancreatic Cancer Research *N*	310/472-6310 pancreatic.org	Dedicated to advancing pancreatic-cancer research and providing information, resources, and support to pancreatic-cancer patients and their families.
Hope Street Kids *N*	800/227-2732 hopestreetkids.org	Kid-oriented education and advocacy.
Hospice Foundation of America *N*	800/854-3402 hospicefoundation.org	Supports organizations and efforts that assist the terminally ill and their families.
Hospice Education Institute *N*	800/331-1620 hospiceworld.org	Referrals from a list of 3,000+ local hospice providers; free info and counseling.
Impotence Institute of America *N*	800/669-1603 301/262-2400 impotenceworld.org	Lists physicians specializing in treatment of impotence resulting from prostate cancer therapies. Support groups. *Impotence Worldwide* newsletter.
Inflammatory Breast Cancer Research Foundation *N*	877/786-7422 ibcresearch.org	Links to clinical trial info. Education and background info. Active in research.
Institute for Myeloma and Bone Cancer Research *N*	310/623-1210 myelomasource.org	Focuses on new approaches to lengthen the lives and relieve the symptoms of myeloma and bone-cancer patients. Free consultation, news, events, links.
Intercultural Cancer Council *N*	713/798-4617 icc.bcm.tmc.edu	Promotes policies, programs, partnerships, and research to eliminate "an unequal burden of

G = Government, *N* = Nonprofit, *P* = Professional, *S* = Sponsor

Organization	Contact Information	Description
		cancer among racial and ethnic minorities and medically underserved populations in the United States and its associated territories."
Intergroup Rhabdomyosarcoma Study *N*	804/786-9602	Special study of young children with this sarcoma.
International Association of Laryngectomees *N*	800/227-2345 209/472-0516 cancer.org larynxlink.com	Sponsors 300 U.S. "lost chord" or "new voice" IAL clubs. Speech instructor referrals; peer counseling; *IAL News* newsletter. (Part of the American Cancer Society.)
International Bone Marrow Transplant Registry *N*	414/456-8325 ibmtr.org	Does *not* aid in searches for transplant donors. Info on about 40% of all allogeneic transplants done since 1970.
International Cancer Alliance *N*	800/422-7361 icare.org	Free cancer-therapy review: description, detection and staging, treatment, diagnostic tests, and clinical trials for a specific cancer. *Cancer Breakthroughs* quarterly.
International Myeloma Foundation *N*	800/452-2873 myeloma.org	Myeloma education for physicians and patients. Research, clinical and scientific conferences, quarterly *Myeloma Today* newsletter.
International Psycho-Oncology Society *N*	434/971-4788 ipos-society.org	Focuses on the clinical, educational, and research issues of psychosocial care for cancer patients.
International Waldenstrom's Macroglobulinemia Foundation *N*	941/927-4963 iwmf.com	Information, resources, a communications network, and experience on how to live with WM.
Its Time to Focus on Lung Cancer *N*	877/646-5864 lungcancer.org	Offers education, resources, clinical-trial info, support groups, teleconferences, quarterly e-newsletter, news. (Newly renamed the Lung Cancer Awareness Campaign.)
Kidney Cancer Association *N*	800/850-9132 847/332-1051 kidneycancerassociation.org	Research, materials on diagnosis and treatment, support groups, physician referral service, *Kidney Cancer News* newsletter.
Kids Cope *N*	404/892-1437 kidscope.org	Helps children understand the effects of cancer or chemotherapy on a loved one. Comic book and video.

(*continued*)

Organization	Contact Information	Description
Kids Konnected N	800/899-2866 949/582-5443 kidsconnected.org	Friendship, education, and support for kids who have a parent with cancer.
Lance Armstrong Foundation N	512/236-8820 laf.org livestrong.org	Dedicated to enhancing the quality of life for people living with, through, and beyond cancer. Survivorship programs, national advocacy initiatives, scientific and clinical research grants.
Let's Face It N	360/676-7325 faceit.org	Resource locator, educational info, and support groups for people with facial disfigurements.
Leukemia and Lymphoma Society N	800/955-4572 212/573-8484 leukemia-lymphoma.org	Research, patient financial and educational aid, public and professional education. Support groups for patients, family, and friends.
Leukemia Research Foundation N	847/424-0600 leukemia-research.org	Research grants.
Liddy Shriver Sarcoma Initiative N	liddyshriversarcoma initiative.org	Support and info for sarcoma patients; e-newsletter.
Life Raft Group N	liferaftgroup.org	Support and info about clinical trials for gastrointestinal stomach tumor (GIST).
Light of Life Foundation N	732/972-0461 lightoflifefoundation.org	Aims to improve the quality of life for thyroid cancer patients, educate public and professionals, promote research.
Liver Cancer Network, Allegheny General Hospital N	412/359-6738 livercancer.com	Regional program; part of national network for the few hospital programs focused on liver cancer.
LiverTumor.org S	877/306-3114 livertumor.org	Guidance for colorectal- and liver-cancer patients explains treatment options and specialized terms. Specialist locator.
Living Beyond Breast Cancer N	800/753-5222 610/645-4567 lbbcresearch.org	Educational materials, calendar of events, quarterly newsletter, Young Survivors Network, phone counseling.
Living with It N	livingwithit.org	Support program for women with breast cancer; education, diet, exercise, financial advice, personal stories.
Look Good . . . Feel Better	800/395-5665 lookgoodfeelbetter.org	Techniques that help people undergoing cancer treatment improve

G = Government, N = Nonprofit, P = Professional, S = Sponsor

Organization	Contact Information	Description
N		their appearance. Sponsored by the Cosmetic, Toiletry, and Fragrance Association Foundation.
Lumetra N	415/677-2000 lumetra.com	Dedicated to measurably improving the quality, safety, and integrity of health care.
Lung Cancer Awareness Campaign N	877/646-5864 *lungcancer.org*	Education, resources, clinical-trial info, support groups, teleconferences, quarterly e-newsletter, news. (New name for It's Time to Focus on Lung Cancer org.)
Lustgarten Foundation N	866/789-1000 516/803-2304 lustgartenfoundation.org	Advances sciences related to diagnosis, treatment, cure, and prevention of pancreatic cancers. Guidance, support services, info on clinical trials, locations of comprehensive treatment facilities.
Lymphoma Information Network S	lymphomainfo.net	Lists Internet lymphoma-info resources.
Lymphoma Research Foundation N	800/500-9976 310/204-7040 lymphoma.org	Patient-to-patient hot line for the newly diagnosed; *Lymphoma Update* newsletter; referrals to other resources, specialized oncologists, clinical trials, support groups.
Make-a-Wish Foundation of America N	800/722-9474 602/279-9474 wish.org	Works with gravely ill children.
Make Today Count N	800/432-2273	Support group for persons with life-threatening illness; *The Messenger* newsletter.
Malecare N	212/844-8369 malecare.org	Info on prostate, testicular, and male breast cancers. Support groups, links to specialized sites, glossaries, news.
Mautner Project for Lesbians With Cancer N	202/332-5536 mautnerproject.org	Provides transportation to treatments; legal help, support groups, bereavement counseling, education, smoking-cessation program.
Medicaid G	877/267-2323 cms.hhs.gov	*Also see* Centers for Medicare and Medicaid, a joint DHHS site.
Medicare G	877/267-2323 cms.hhs.gov	*Also see* Centers for Medicare and Medicaid, a joint DHHS site.
Melanoma Center N	melanomacenter.org	Info and resources to deal with melanoma and its prevention. Topics: early detection and diagnosis, staging and treatment, symptom

(continued)

Organization	Contact Information	Description
		management, where to turn for support. Link to a pediatric melanoma site.
Melanoma Patients' Information Page N	mpip.org	Community bulletin board with research links and news.
Men Against Breast Cancer N	866/547-6222 menagainstbreastcancer.org	Mobilizes men in fight against breast cancer. Support for men caregivers of women with breast cancers.
Merck Patient Assistance Program S	800/994-2111 800/727-5400 *merckpap.com*	Pharmaceutical manufacturer; offers its cancer-fighters at low or no cost to those without financial resources.
Mercy Medical Airlift N	888/675-1405 800/296-1217 mercymedical.org patienttravel.org	Multiple charitable medical air-transport networks serve financially strapped patients and their parties.
Mesothelima Applied Research Foundation N	805/560-8942 marf.org	Funds research. Patient-awareness campaign; free literature.
Mothers Supporting Daughters with Breast Cancer N	410/778-1982 mothersdaughters.org	One-on-one support by volunteer mothers. Hand book; companion brochure for daughters.
Moving Forward Foundation N	713/669-0908	Lymphoma recovery group.
Multiple Myeloma Research Foundation N	203/972-1250 multiplemyeloma.org	Research grants, symposia. Referrals and info packets for patients.
Mycosis Fungoides Foundation N	248/644-9014 mffoundation.org	For patients with all forms of cutaneous T-cell lymphoma: locate physician specialists, clinical trials, latest treatment modalities, live Webcasts.
National Adrenal Disease Foundation N	516/487-4992 medhelp.org/www/nadf.htm	Primarily for people with Addison's disease, not cancer. Of benefit to cancer patients needing to know about life after adrenal-gland-removal surgery. Support groups in many states.
National Alliance of Breast Cancer Organizations N	888/806-2226 212/719-4154 nabco.org	Advocates for legislative and regulatory concerns of the breast-cancer community. Current clinical trails list, free literature, *NABCO* newsletter.

G = Government, N = Nonprofit, P = Professional, S = Sponsor

Organization	Contact Information	Description
National Asian Women's Health Organization N	415/989-9747 nawho.org	Supports needs of Asian women patients and their families.
National Association for Continence N	800/252-3337 nafc.org	Lists urologists specializing in treating incontinence caused by cancer treatment. Resource guide, audio and videotapes, *Quality Care* newsletter.
National Association for Home Care N	202/547-7424 nahc.org	Will provide a list of state-licensed home-care agencies nearby from database of 28,000 home-care and hospice agencies, info also on its Web site.
National Association of Hospital Hospitality Houses N	800/542-9730 nahhh.org	Finds low-cost accommodations for patients and their families away from home for treatment. Typical rate per person: $5–$15/day.
National Bone Marrow Transplant Link N	800/546-5268 248/358-1889 nbmtlink.org	Info 24-7 for those affected by bone-marrow transplantation. Promotes public understanding and peer support.
National Brain Tumor Foundation N	800/934-2873 510/839-9777 braintumor.org	Support and education for brain-tumor patients; research. Tracks clinical trials and medical center procedures; free consultations with neuroscience nurse; *Search* newsletter.
National Breast Cancer Coalition N	800/622-2838 202/296-7477 stopbreastcancer.org	300 member organizations, plus individuals, dedicated to eradication through action, policy, and advocacy.
National Breast Cancer Foundation N	nationalbreastcancer.org	Raises breast-cancer awareness.
National Cancer Institute G	800/422-6237 cancer.gov	Info related to specific cancers, treatments, and coping strategies; highly useful print materials free; news and announcements. CANCER-FAX: treatment guidelines, with current data on prognosis, relevant staging and histologic classifications. Free Protocol Data Query surveys the U.S. to match cancers with treatments. Currently conducts or sponsors 1,700 clinical trials.
National Cancer Survivors Day Foundation N	615/794-3006 ncsdf.org	NCSD observed on the first Sunday in June; free celebration-observance kits.

(continued)

Organization	Contact Information	Description
National Carcinoid Support Group N	members.aol.com/ thencg	Steers queries to nearest specialist; sponsors monthly conference calls for patients. *Rays of Hope* newsletter.
National Center for Complementary and Alternative Medicine G	888/644-6226 nccam.nih.gov	National Institutes of Health site; news, research, events, and clinical trials in complementary medicine.
National Center for Homeopathy N	703/548-7790 homeopathic.org	Explains homeopathy. Homeopathic locator; extensive bookstore; *Homeopathy Today* magazine.
National Center for Jewish Healing N	212/399-2320 jhhrn.org	Practical and spiritual healing resources for cancer patients.
National Certification Board for Therapeutic Massage and Bodywork P	800/296-0664 703/610-9015 ncbtmb.com	News; member locator; background and explanation of arts; member services.
National Certification Commission for Acupuncture and Oriental Medicine P	703/548-9004 nccaom.org	Professional association for practitioners. Locator for closest member; links; educational services; general info.
National Cervical Cancer Coalition N	800/685-5531 818/909-3849 nccc-online.org/	Cooperative site for general info. Materials available.
National Childhood Cancer Foundation N	800/458-6223 nccf.org	Supports research and treatment programs for the cancers of children and young adults.
National Children's Cancer Society N	800/532-6459 children-cancer.com	Improves the quality of life for children through financial and in-kind assistance, advocacy, support services, and education.
National Coalition for Cancer Research N	202/663-9125 cancercoalition.org	Lobbies on behalf of the National Cancer Act.
National Coalition for Cancer Survivorship N	877/622-7937 301/650-8868 canceradvocacy.org	Run by and for cancer survivors. Info and links to sites by cancer type; clearinghouse for job-discrimination and health-insurance issues; *Networker* newsletter.
National Colorectal Cancer Research Alliance N	800/872-3000 eif.nccra.org	Funds research and raises awareness; emphasizes the importance of screening. Sponsored by the Entertainment Industry Foundation.

G = Government, N = Nonprofit, P = Professional, S = Sponsor

Organization	Contact Information	Description
National Comprehensive Cancer Network *N*	888/909-6226 nccn.org	Alliance of 19 of the world's leading cancer centers develops, updates, and disseminates a complete library of clinical practice guidelines.
National Council for Reliable Health Information *N*	909/824-4690 ncrhi.org	Watchdog group.
National Council on Aging *N*	benefitscheckup.org	Finds programs that help pay costs of prescriptions and medical services for those over age 55.
National Council on Skin Cancer Prevention *N*	skincancerprevention .org	Shares the resources and research of its member organizations to maximize the impact of skin-cancer prevention programs and funding.
National Family Caregivers Association *N*	800/896-3650 nfcacares.org	Association of professional family caregivers.
National Familial Lung Cancer Registry *N*	410/614-1910 path.jhu.edu/nfltr .html	Seeks families with two or more people diagnosed with lung cancer for advanced research.
National Foundation for Facial Reconstruction *N*	212/263-6656 nffr.org	Reconstructive plastic surgery for children (and some adults) at New York University Medical Center, regardless of ability to pay.
National Foundation for Transplants *N*	800/489-3863 901/684-1697 transplants.org	Assists in funding and searches for bone-marrow and organ transplants; small grants for immunosuppressive drugs. Helps transplant candidates with insurance and hospital-waiting-list negotiations.
National Hospice and Palliative Care Organization *N*	800/658-8898 nhpco.org	Helps hospice professionals, volunteers, and the general public understand and best serve the terminally ill and their loved ones.
National Infertility Association *N*	617/623-1156 resolve.org	Advocacy, education, local chapters, support groups, help line, physician referral, magazine, and fact sheets.
National Institute for Jewish Hospice *N*	800/446-4448 nijh.org	Hot-line counseling, national database for Jewish resources, publications on core subjects.
National Institute of Neurological Disorders and Stroke *N*	800/352-9424 ninds.nih.gov	Sponsors clinical trials. General research into disorders of the brain and nervous system, including cancer.

(continued)

Organization	Contact Information	Description
National Library of Medicine G	medlineplus.gov	Consumer site; bibliographic database cites clinical trial abstracts from 4,500 journals; glossary and drug directory.
National Lymphedema Network N	800/541-3259 510/208-3200 lymphnet.org	Info on the prevention and management of primary and secondary lymphedema for the general public and health-care professionals; *NLN Newsletter*.
National Marrow Donor Program N	888/999-6743 800/627-7692 612/627-5800 marrow.org	Single point of access for all three types of blood cells used in transplantation: marrow, peripheral, and umbilical cord. Registry of five million potential donors, including 30,000 cord-blood units; some consulting services for transplant candidates.
National Meals on Wheels Foundation N	616/531-9909	Free and low-cost meals for patient and caregivers delivered to your door.
National Organization for Rare Disorders N	800/999-6673 203/744-0100 nord-rdb.com rarediseases.org	Federation of 140 health organizations serving people with rare disorders of all sorts. Manages a used medical equipment exchange; *Orphan Disease Update* newsletter.
National Ovarian Cancer Association N	416/971-9800 x.1320 ovariancanada.org	Raises awareness of ovarian cancer. Points to Canadian financial and educational resources for prevention and treatment.
National Ovarian Cancer Coalition N	877/682-6622 561/393-0005 ovarian.org	National U.S. membership organization. Promotes awareness, education, early detection and research through state chapters; referrals to gynecologic oncologists; extensive Web site databases; peer counseling; *NOCC Newsletter*.
National Pancreas Foundation N	866/726-2737 617/578-0382 pancreasfoundation.org	Supports research and provides info and services to people suffering from diseases of the pancreas; cancers are a major focus.
National Patient Travel Helpline N	800/296-1217 patienttravel.org	Locates best available travel options 24-7 for patients and their parties.
National Prostate Cancer Coalition N	888/245-9455 202/463-9455 4npcc.org	Advocates seek research and detection funding.
National Transplant Assistance Fund	800/642-8399 610/527-5056	Locates nearest center, helps calculate costs, locates funds sources. Makes

G = Government, N = Nonprofit, P = Professional, S = Sponsor

Organization	Contact Information	Description
N	transplantfund.org	modest grants direct to patient for relocations, medicines, home care, and transportation. *New Start News* newsletter.
Native American Cancer Research N	303/838-9359 natamcancer.org	Community-based nonprofit resource; seeks to reduce incidence of cancer in Native Americans.
NeedyMeds N	215/625-9609 needymeds.com	Finds programs that help pay for treatments and related costs.
Norman Endocrine Surgery Clinic S	813/991-6922 parathyroid.com	Private Tampa, Florida, clinic specializing in minimally invasive parathyroid cancer surgery; consult personally with James Norman, MD.
Neuroblastoma Children's Cancer Society N	800/532-5162 neuroblastomacancer.org	Volunteers run the site, help the sufferers, serve as a support group for families, and *raise money* for operations and research.
Nueva Vida N	202/223-9100 *nueva-vida.org*	Informar, apoyar y educar a las mujeres Latinas cuyas vidas han sido afectadas por el cáncer; facilitar y abogar por el acceso a servicios médicos de alta calidad para la oportuna detección, diagnostico y tratamiento del cáncer. (Informs, supports, and empowers Latinas whose lives are affected by cancer; advocates and facilitates timely access to state-of-the-art cancer care, including screening, diagnosis, treatment and care for all Latinas.)
Oley Foundation N	800/776-OLEY 518/262-5079 oley.org	For home intravenous and tube-fed patients and their families. Newsletter, conferences, and other support activities.
ONCOLINE Roche Reimbursement/Patient Assistance Program S	800/443-6676 xeloda.com	Pharmaceutical manufacturer; offers its cancer-fighters at low or no cost to those without financial resources.
OncoLink N	215/349-8895 oncolink.upenn.edu	Info about specific types of cancer, treatments, and news.
Oncology Nursing Society N	412/859-6100 ons.org	Organization of 32,000 registered nurses and other health-care providers, promotes excellence in oncology nursing.

(continued)

Organization	Contact Information	Description
Oral Cancer Foundation *N*	949/646-8000 oralcancerfoundation.org	Education, research, prevention, advocacy, and support for oral-cancer patients. Forum, chat room, message board.
Ortho Biotech Procrit Line *S*	800/553-3851 procritline.com	Pharmaceutical manufacturer; offers its cancer-fighters at low or no cost to those without financial resources.
Ovarian Cancer National Alliance *N*	202/331-1332 ovariancancer.org	Increases public and professional awareness of ovarian cancer and advocates more effective diagnostics, treatments, and cure.
Ovarian Cancer Research Fund, Inc. *N*	800/873-9569 ocrf.org	Early diagnostic treatment programs and research; educational research materials.
Ovarian Plus International *N*	703/715-6075 monitor.net/ovarian	*Gynecological Cancer Prevention Quarterly* newsletter carries recent info on research, diagnosis, and treatment for ovarian and other gynecologic cancers; targets risk-reduction, screening, early-detection, psychosocial, and policy issues.
Ovarian Problems Discussion List *N*	acor.org	E-mail support group.
PACT Plus *S*	800/996-6626 aventisoncology.com/reimbursement.htm	Helps patients with reimbursements, financial assistance; may help reduce obstacles to third-party payment when health-care providers use certain of its products (same org. as Aventis Oncology).
Pancreatic Cancer Action Network *N*	877/272-6226 pancan.org	Advocacy, awareness, and education for patients and professionals. Info about support groups, clinical trials, reimbursement programs.
Partners Against Pain *N*	partnersagainstpain.com	Pain-control guides, news, support groups, and tech info for professionals.
Partnership for Caring: America's Voice for the Dying *N*	800/989-9455 202/296-8071 partnershipforcaring.org	Crisis hot line; free living wills and medical powers of attorney for all states. Advocates for improved health care near the end of life. (Formerly known as Choice in Dying.)
Partnership for Prescription Assistance *N*	888/477-2669 pparx.org	Single point of access to 275+ public and private prescription-assistance programs for patients.

G = Government, *N* = Nonprofit, *P* = Professional, *S* = Sponsor

Organization	Contact Information	Description
Patient Advocate Foundation N	800/532-5274 757/873-6668 patientadvocate.org	Legal advice or representation for patients; liaison between patient and insurer, managed-care provider, employer, and creditors.
Patient Advocate Foundation's Co-Pay Relief Patient Assistance Program N	866/512-3861 copays.org	Helps with prescription co-pays for those in need.
Patient Advocates for Advanced Cancer Treatments (PAACT) N	616/453-1477 paactusa.org	Association for diagnostic and therapeutic treatments of prostate cancer. Serves patients and physicians.
People Living With Cancer N	703/797-1914 plwc.org	Oncologist-approved info to help people make informed decisions about their health care; links to all American Society of Clinical Oncology info.
Pfizer's Patient Assistance Programs S	800/707-8990 800/984-1500 877/744-5675 pfizerhelpfulanswers.com	Pharmaceutical manufacturer; offers its cancer-fighters at low or no cost to those without financial resources.
Pharmaceutical Research and Manufacturers of America S	202/835-3400 phrma.org	Directory of patient-assistance programs offered by pharmaceutical companies. (Tip: Have your oncologist's office make the request on your behalf.)
Phoenix5 N	phoenix5.org	Prostate-cancer education, treatment options, resources, side effects, and sexuality issues.
Physician Data Query (PDQ) G	800/4-CANCER cancer.gov	Lists the most recent info on cancer treatments, research studies, clinical trials, new treatments, organizations and physicians involved in various care programs. A National Cancer Institute program.
Planet Cancer N	planetcancer.org	Info-sharing Web site for young adults with cancer.
Prostate Cancer Education Council N	303/316-4685 pcaw.com	Encourages nationwide screenings for men; funds research. Education programs; extensive link network; Webcasts.
Prostate Cancer Foundation N	800/757-2873 prostatecancer foundation.org	*See* CaP CURE.

(continued)

Organization	Contact Information	Description
Prostate Net N	888/477-6763 prostate-online.com	Info on treatment options, side effects, research, news, and advocacy. Helps you understand the issues to cover with your doctor. Brochures and CDs.
Pulmonary Hypertension Association N	800/748-7274 phassociation.org	Info for lung-cancer survivors with PH. Encourages research into the disorder.
Quackwatch N	610/437-1795 quackwatch.com	Consumer-protection service
Rare Cancer Alliance N	206/600-5327 rare-cancer.org	Locates the closest support group for Sarcoma patients.
Research Advocacy Network N	877/276-2187 researchadvocacy.org	Advocates for medical research, often through clinical trials; encourages education, support, collaborations.
Ronald McDonald House N	630/623-7048 rmhc.org	Provides "refuge" from the hospital, a home away from home.
RxAssist and Rx Outreach Patient Assistance Programs N	800/332-2056 rxassist.org	Assists patients without drug coverage who meet income requirements.
Sarcoma Alliance N	415/381-7236 sarcomaalliance.com	Education and support for people with sarcomas and their families; info on treatment options. Locates specialists.
Sarcoma Foundation of America N	301/520-7648 curesarcoma.org	Sarcoma research. Patient-to-patient network, info on clinical trials, resource links.
Schering-Plough Pharmaceuticals Commitment to Care Program S	800/521-7157 schering-plough.com	Pharmaceutical manufacturer; offers its cancer-fighters at low or no cost to those without financial resources.
Schine On-line Services N	800/346-3287 findcure.com	Reports on products, procedures, outcomes, and other matters of patient concern. Fee charged.
SHARE: Self-Help for Women with Breast or Ovarian Cancer N	866/891-2392 sharecancersupport.org	Hot line for women with breast or ovarian cancer (English and Spanish). Peer-led support groups, wellness, education, and advocacy programs.
Sharsheret N	866/474-2774 sharsheret.org	Helps young Jewish women recently diagnosed with breast cancer.
Simon Foundation for Continence N	800/237-4666 simonfoundation.org	Local chapters of the foundation's National Continence Cooperative make bulk purchases of absorbent

G = Government, N = Nonprofit, P = Professional, S = Sponsor

Organization	Contact Information	Description
		paper products to reduce patient cost. Sponsors online discussion groups; *The Informer* newsletter.
Sisters Network N	866/781-1808 sistersnetworking.org	African-American women's breast-cancer survivorship organization. Peer counseling.
Skin Cancer Foundation N	800/754-6490 212/725-5176 skincancer.org	Public and professional education programs. Supports medical training and research; helps reduce incidence, morbidity, and mortality of skin cancers.
Society of Gynecologic Nurse Oncologists P	312/434-8639 sgno.org	Nurses' organization dedicated to patient care, education, and research.
Society of Gynecological Oncologists P	312/644-6610 sco.org	Physicians' organization dedicated to improving the care of women with ovarian and other gynecological cancers. Physician-referral list.
Society of Surgical Oncology P	847/427-1400 surgonc.org	Locator for board-certified thoracic (chest) surgeons specializing in lung cancer.
South-Eastern Organ Procurement Foundation N	800/543-6399 804/323-9890 seopf.org	63 transplant centers, organ procurement organizations, histocompatibility laboratories and tissue banks in 19 states. Offers life, medical, and disability insurance to donors.
State Children's Health Insurance Program G	877/543-7669 cms.hhs.gov	Free or low-cost health Insurance for those under age 19.
STARBRIGHT Foundation N	800/315-2580 310/479-1212 starbright.org	Helps children and adolescent patients cope with psychological and medical problems. Free materials and counseling.
Starlight Foundation N	323/634-0080 starlight.org	Transforms the lives of seriously ill children and their families through imaginative programs that educate, uplift their spirits, foster a sense of community, and help alleviate the pain and fear of prolonged illness.
Steve Dunn's Kidney Cancer Guide N	cancerguide.org	Helps patients weigh clinical trial options. By a kidney-cancer survivor and clinical trial participant.
St. Jude Children's Research Hospital N	866/278-5833 www.stjude.org	Completely free medical treatment and associated costs. Also consults. Focus is on specific cancers and

(*continued*)

Organization	Contact Information	Description
		hematologic, immunologic, or genetic diseases. Patients must be under age 20. Psysician referrals only.
Support for People with Oral and Head and Neck Cancer N	800/377-0928 516/759-5333 spohnc.org	Educational support, survivor-to-survivor network, list of clinical trials, newsletter.
Sunshine Foundation N	800/767-1976	Children's services.
SunWise School Program G	epa.gov/sunwise	Teaches protection from overexposure to the sun; classroom-, school-, and community-based components.
SuperSibs! N	866/444-7427 supersibs.org	Support services that help children redefine the "cancer sibling" experience.
Susan G. Komen Breast Cancer Foundation N	800/462-9273 komen.org	Advances research, education, screening, and treatment of breast cancer. Survivors counsel callers.
Team Survivor N	teamsurvivor.org	Free exercise and health-education programs for women with past or present cancer diagnosis.
Teens Living With Cancer N	585/334-0858 teenslivingwithcancer.org	Info about cancer and its treatments specially prepared for a teen audience.
Testicular Cancer Resource Center N	tcrc.acor.org	Info and support; patient- friendly comprehensive Web site. Contacts cancer survivors by e-mail for electronic or phone conversations.
ThyCa: Thyroid Cancer Survivors' Association N	877/588-7904 thyca.org	Support, education, and communications for thyroid-cancer survivors, their families, and friends.
Thyroid Foundation of America N	800/832-8321 617/726-8500 tsh.org	Professional services, patient info, *The Bridge* newsletter.
Together Rx Access N	800/444-4106 togetherrxaccess. com	Assists patients without drug coverage who meet income requirements.
Tricare G	800/538-9552 (Eligibility line) tricare.osd.mil	Comprehensive health-insurance program for retired military and military dependents.
Ulman Cancer Fund for Young Adults N	888/393-FUND 410/964-0202 ulmanfund.org	Free support programs, education, and resources for young adult patients, families, and friends.

G = Government, N = Nonprofit, P = Professional, S = Sponsor

Organization	Contact Information	Description
United Ostomy Association *N*	800/826-0826 uoa.org	International association of 450 ostomy chapters dedicated to the complete rehabilitation of all ostomates (those with intestinal or urinary tract diversions). International. Volunteers visit new patients; *Ostomy Quarterly* magazine.
Us Too! International *N*	800/808-7866 630/795-1002 ustoo.org	Educational and emotional support for prostate-cancer survivors and their families. Chapters internationally.
VHL Family Alliance *N*	800/767-4845 617/277-5667 vhl.org	Comprehensive info site for those interested in Von Hippel-Lindau (VHL).
Visiting Nurse Associations of America *P*	888/866-8773 vnaa.org	400 Visiting Nurse Associations provide health care, social work and counseling, hospice care.
Vital Options International *N*	800/477-7666 818/508-5657 vitaloptions.org	Weekly radio call-in cancer talk show, *The Group Room,* links callers with other patients, survivors, family members, physicians, researchers, and therapists. Sundays, 4–6 P.M., EST. Live Web simulcast.
Waldenstrom's Macroglobulinemia Foundation *N*	941/927-4963 iwmf.com	Info, resources, multiple communications networks, links, and contacts.
Wellness Community *N*	888/793-9355 thewellness community.org	Free emotional support, education, and hope for people with cancer and their loved ones. In 21 locations nationwide.
Women's Cancer Network *N*	wcn.org	News, risk-assessment tool, "doctor finder," and info on cancers affecting women.
Y-ME National Breast Cancer Organization *N*	800/221-2141 800/986-9505 (Español) 312/986-8228 y-me.org	Counseling, educational, and self-help programs for breast-cancer patients, 24-7; *Y-ME Hotline* newsletter. *Men:* Male counselors available.
Young Survival Coalition *N*	212/916-7667 youngsurvival.org	Network for women under age 40 with breast cancer.
YWCA *N*	202/467-0801 ywca.org	Helps underserved women in need of early detection, education, breast- and cervical-cancer screening; support services.

Yellow Pages

This section lists organizations by topic.

   Note: This information was last reviewed in August 2005. Please go to aboutmycancer.com for the latest version of this directory.

Acupuncture

American Academy of Medical Acupuncture	800/521-2262
National Certification Commission for Acupuncture and Oriental Medicine	703/548-9004

Also see Pain, Nausea, Anxiety Relief

Adrenal Gland

American Cancer Society	800/ACS-2345
American Society of Clinical Oncology	703/797-1914
Anderson Network	800/345-6324
Association of Cancer Online Resources	acor.org
Bloch Cancer Foundation	800/433-0464
Cancer Control PLANET	cancercontrolplanet.cancer.gov
Centerwatch	centerwatch.com
Coalition of National Cancer Cooperative Groups	877/520-4457
National Adrenal Disease Foundation	516/487-4992
National Cancer Institute	800/4-CANCER
National Coalition for Cancer Survivorship	877/622-7937
National Organization for Rare Disorders	800/999-6673
OncoLink	oncolink.upenn.edu

Amputee

American Amputee Foundation	501/666-2523
Amputee Coalition of America	888/267-5669
American Cancer Society	800/ACS-2345
Dave Dravecky's Outreach of Hope	719/481-3528
National Cancer Institute	800/4-CANCER

Anus

American Cancer Society	800/ACS-2345
American Society of Clinical Oncology	703/797-1914
American Society of Colon and Rectal Surgeons	847/290-9184

Association of Cancer Online Resources — acor.org
Bloch Cancer Foundation — 800/433-0464
Cancer Control PLANET — cancercontrolplanet.cancer.gov

Centerwatch — centerwatch.com
Coalition of National Cancer Cooperative Groups — 877/520-4457
Colorectal Cancer Network — 301/879-1500
National Cancer Institute — 800/4-CANCER
National Coalition for Cancer Survivorship — 877/622-7937
National Colorectal Cancer Research Alliance — 800/872-3000
OncoLink — oncolink.upenn.edu

Bile Duct
American Cancer Society — 800/ACS-2345
American Society of Clinical Oncology — 703/797-1914
Anderson Network — 800/345-6324
Association of Cancer Online Resources — acor.org
Bloch Cancer Foundation — 800/433-0464
Cancer Control PLANET — cancercontrolplanet.cancer.gov

Centerwatch — centerwatch.com
Coalition of National Cancer Cooperative Groups — 877/520-4457
National Cancer Institute — 800/4-CANCER
National Coalition for Cancer Survivorship — 877/622-7937
National Organization for Rare Disorders — 800/999-6673
OncoLink — oncolink.upenn.edu

Biofeedback
See Pain, Nausea, Anxiety Relief

Bladder
American Cancer Society — 800/ACS-2345
American Foundation for Urologic Disease — 800/242-2383
American Society of Clinical Oncology — 703/797-1914
Anderson Network — 800/345-6324
Association of Cancer Online Resources — acor.org
Bladder Cancer Webcafé — blcwebcafe.org
Bloch Cancer Foundation — 800/433-0464
Cancer Control PLANET — cancercontrolplanet.cancer.gov

Centerwatch — centerwatch.com
Coalition of National Cancer Cooperative Groups — 877/520-4457
National Cancer Institute — 800/4-CANCER
National Coalition for Cancer Survivorship — 877/622-7937
OncoLink — oncolink.upenn.edu

Blood (leukemia, lymphoma multiple myeloma, others)

American Cancer Society	800/ACS-2345
American Society of Clinical Oncology	703/797-1914
Anderson Network	800/345-6324
Association of Cancer Online Resources	acor.org
Bloch Cancer Foundation	800/433-0464
Cancer Control PLANET	cancercontrolplanet.cancer.gov
Centerwatch	centerwatch.com
Coalition of National Cancer Cooperative Groups	877/520-4457
Cure for Lymphoma Foundation	800/CFL-6848
Cutaneous Lymphoma Network	513/584-6805
Institute for Myeloma and Bone Cancer Research	310/623-1210
International Myeloma Foundation	800/452-2873
Leukemia and Lymphoma Society	800/955-4572
Lymphoma Research Foundation	800/500-9976
Moving Forward Foundation	713/669-0908
Multiple Myeloma Research Foundation	203/972-1250
Mycosis Fungoides Foundation	248/644-9014
National Cancer Institute	800/4-CANCER
National Coalition for Cancer Survivorship	877/622-7937
OncoLink	oncolink.upenn.edu
Waldenstrom's Macroglobulinemia Foundation	941/927-4963

Bone

Institute for Myeloma and Bone Cancer Research	310/623-1210

Also see Sarcoma

Bone Marrow

American Cancer Society	800/ACS-2345
American Society of Clinical Oncology	703/797-1914
Anderson Network	800/345-6324
Association of Cancer Online Resources	acor.org
Bone Marrow Foundation	800/365-1336
Bone Marrow Transplant Family Support Network	800/826-9376
Bone Marrow Transplant Newsletter	888/597-7674
Caitlin Raymond International Registry	800/726-2824
Centerwatch	centerwatch.com
Coalition of National Cancer Cooperative Groups	877/520-4457
National Bone Marrow Transplant Link	800/546-5268
National Cancer Institute	800/4-CANCER
National Coalition for Cancer Survivorship	877/622-7937
National Marrow Donor Program	888/999-6743
OncoLink	oncolink.upenn.edu

Brain

Accelerate Brain Cancer Cure	650/685-2200
American Brain Tumor Association	800/886-2282
American Cancer Society	800/ACS-2345
American Society of Clinical Oncology	703/797-1914
Anderson Network	800/345-6324
Association of Cancer Online Resources	acor.org
Bloch Cancer Foundation	800/433-0464
Brain Tumor Society	800/770-8287
Cancer Control PLANET	cancercontrolplanet.cancer.gov
Centerwatch	centerwatch.com
Children's Brain Tumor Foundation	866/228-4673
Coalition of National Cancer Cooperative Groups	877/520-4457
National Brain Tumor Foundation	800/934-2873
National Cancer Institute	800/4-CANCER
National Coalition for Cancer Survivorship	877/622-7937
National Institute of Neurological Disorders and Stroke	800/352-9424
OncoLink	oncolink.upenn.edu

Breast

American Cancer Society	800/ACS-2345
American Society of Clinical Oncology	703/797-1914
Anderson Network	800/345-6324
Association of Cancer Online Resources	acor.org
Bloch Cancer Foundation (and hot line)	800/433-0464
Breast Cancer Action	877/278-6722
Breast Cancer Advisory Center	301/984-1020
Breastcancer.org	breastcancer.org
Cancer Control PLANET	cancercontrolplanet.cancer.gov
Centerwatch	centerwatch.com
Coalition of National Cancer Cooperative Groups	877/520-4457
Encore Plus	202/628-3636
Facing Our Risk of Cancer Empowered (FORCE)	866/824-7475
Inflammatory Breast Cancer Research Foundation	877/786-7422
Living Beyond Breast Cancer	610/645-4567
Living with It	livingwithit.org
Malecare (men's breast cancer)	212/844-8369
Men Against Breast Cancer	866/547-6222
Mothers Supporting Daughters with Breast Cancer	410/778-1982
National Alliance of Breast Cancer Organizations	800/806-2226
National Breast Cancer Coalition	800/622-2838
National Breast Cancer Foundation	nationalbreastcancer.org

National Cancer Institute	800/4-CANCER
National Coalition for Cancer Survivorship	877/622-7937
OncoLink	oncolink.upenn.edu
SHARE	212/719-1204
Sharsheret	866/474-2774
Sisters Network	866/781-1808
Susan G. Komen Breast Cancer Foundation	800/462-9273
Y-ME	800/221-2141
Young Survival Coalition	212/916-7667

Cancers of an Unknown Primary Site (CUPS)

American Cancer Society	800/ACS-2345
American Society of Clinical Oncology	703/797-1914
Anderson Network	800/345-6324
Association of Cancer Online Resources	acor.org
Bloch Cancer Foundation	800/433-0464
Cancer Control PLANET	cancercontrolplanet.cancer.gov
Centerwatch	centerwatch.com
Coalition of National Cancer Cooperative Groups	877/520-4457
FindCancerExperts	findcancerexperts.com
International Cancer Alliance	800/422-7361
National Cancer Institute	800/4-CANCER
National Coalition for Cancer Survivorship	877/622-7937
OncoLink	oncolink.upenn.edu

Carcinoid

American Cancer Society	800/ACS-2345
American Society of Clinical Oncology	703/797-1914
Anderson Network	800/345-6324
Association of Cancer Online Resources	acor.org
Bloch Cancer Foundation	800/433-0464
Cancer Control PLANET	cancercontrolplanet.cancer.gov
Carcinoid Cancer Foundation	888/722-3132
Centerwatch	centerwatch.com
Coalition of National Cancer Cooperative Groups	877/520-4457
Life Raft Group	liferaftgroup.org
National Cancer Institute	800/4-CANCER
National Carcinoid Support Group	members.aol.com/thencg
National Coalition for Cancer Survivorship	877/622-7937
OncoLink	oncolink.upenn.edu

Cervix

American Cancer Society	800/ACS-2345
American Society of Clinical Oncology	703/797-1914
Anderson Network	800/345-6324
Association of Cancer Online Resources	acor.org
Bloch Cancer Foundation	800/433-0464
Cancer Control PLANET	cancercontrolplanet.cancer.gov
Centerwatch	centerwatch.com
Coalition of National Cancer Cooperative Groups	877/520-4457
National Cervical Cancer Coalition	800/685-5531
National Coalition for Cancer Survivorship	877/622-7937
OncoLink	oncolink.upenn.edu
Society of Gynecological Oncologists	312/644-6610
Society of Gynecologic Nurse Oncologists	312/434-8639

Also see Gynecologic

Chat Rooms

Note: Many more chat rooms appear on the Web sites of other listings.

Cancer Survivors Gathering Place	geocities.com/cancer_survivors
The Group Room *(Sundays, 4–6 P.M. EST)*	vitaloptions.org

Chemotherapy

American Cancer Society	800/ACS-2345
ChemoCare	800/55-CHEMO
Chemotherapy Foundation	212/213-9292
National Cancer Institute	800/4-CANCER

Children

Note: Many other cancer programs have divisions for children.

American Cancer Society	800/ACS-2345
American Society of Clinical Oncology	703/797-1914
Anderson Network	800/345-6324
Association of Cancer Online Resources	acor.org
Beyond the Cure	314/446-5215
Cancer Control PLANET	cancercontrolplanet.cancer.gov
Candlelighters Childhood Cancer Foundation	800/366-2223
Centerwatch	centerwatch.com
Children's Brain Tumor Foundation	866/228-4673
Children's Cause	301/562-2765
Children's Hospice International	800/242-4453

Children's Oncology Camps of America	803/434-3533
Coalition of National Cancer Cooperative Groups	877/520-4457
Friends Network (*The Funletter*)	805/565-7031
Hole in the Wall Camps	holeinthewallcamps.org
Hope Street Kids	800/227-2732
Intergroup Rhabdomyosarcoma Study	804/786-9602
Kids Cope	404/892-1437
Kids Konnected	800/899-2866
Leukemia and Lymphoma Society	800/955-4572
Make-a-Wish Foundation of America	602/279-9474
Melanoma Center	melanomacenter.org
Mercy Medical Airlift	888/675-1405
National Cancer Institute	800/4-CANCER
National Childhood Cancer Foundation	800/458-6223
National Children's Cancer Society	800/532-6459
National Coalition for Cancer Survivorship	877/622-7937
National Foundation for Facial Reconstruction	212/263-6656
NeedyMeds	needymeds.com
Neuroblastoma Children's Cancer Society	800/532-5162
OncoLink	oncolink.upenn.edu
Ronald McDonald House	630/623-7048
STARBRIGHT Foundation	800/315-2580
Starlight Foundation	323/634-0080
State Children's Health Insurance Program	877/543-7669
St. Jude Children's Research Hospital	866/278-5833
Sunshine Foundation	800/767-1976
SuperSibs!	866/444-7427
Teens Living With Cancer	585/334-0858

Clinical Trial

American Cancer Society	800/ACS-2345
American Society of Clinical Oncology	703/797-1914
Anderson Network	800/345-6324
Brain Tumor Cooperative Group	301/680-9770
Cancer411.org	877/226-2741
Cancer Care	800/813-4673
Center for Information and Study on Clinical Research Participation	ciscrp.org
Centerwatch	centerwatch.com
Children's Cancer Study Group	213/681-3032
Coalition of National Cancer Cooperative Groups	877/520-4457
Eastern Cooperative Oncology Group	608/263-6650
Gynecologic Oncology Group	215/854-0770

Intergroup Rhabdomyosarcoma Study	804/786-9602
National Cancer Institute	800/4-CANCER
National Surgical Adjuvant Project: Breast and Bowel Cancers	412/648-9720
National Wilms' Tumor Study Group	215/387-5518
North Central Cancer Treatment Group	507/284-4972
Pediatric Oncology Group	314/367-3446
Radiation Therapy Oncology Group	215/574-3195
Sarcoma Foundation	301/520-7648
Southwest Oncology Group	512/366-9300
Steve Dunn's Kidney Cancer Guide	cancerguide.org

Clinical Trial Results

Amedeo.com	amedeo.com
Center for Clinical Trials. . .	trialscentral.org
Drugs.com	drugs.com
Federal Drug Administration	fda.gov/medwatch
National Cancer Institute's registry of clinical trials	cancer.gov
National Institutes of Health register of clinical research	clinicaltrials.gov
National Library of Medicine	medlineplus.gov
NMT Weekly Trial Results	centerwatch.com

Colorectal

American Cancer Society	800/ACS-2345
American College of Gastroenterology	703/820-7400
American Gastroenterological Association	301/654-2055
American Society for Gastrointestinal Endoscopy	978/526-8330
American Society of Clinical Oncology	703/797-1914
American Society of Colon and Rectal Surgeons	847/290-9184
Anderson Network	800/345-6324
Association of Cancer Online Resources	acor.org
Bloch Cancer Foundation	800/433-0464
Cancer Control PLANET	cancercontrolplanet.cancer.gov
Centerwatch	centerwatch.com
Coalition of National Cancer Cooperative Groups	877/520-4457
Colon Cancer Alliance	877/422-2030
Colon Cancer Support Group	415/885-7546
Colorectal Cancer Network	301/879-1500
Crohn's and Colitis Foundation of America	914/328-1313
National Cancer Institute	800/4-CANCER
National Coalition for Cancer Survivorship	877/622-7937
National Colorectal Cancer Research Alliance	800/872-3000
OncoLink	oncolink.upenn.edu
United Ostomy Association	800/826-0826

Counseling

Note: Most disease-specific listings provide telephone counseling.

American Amputee Foundation	501/666-2523
American Cancer Society	800/ACS-2345
Bloch Cancer Foundation	800/433-0464
Bone Marrow Transplant Family Support Network	800/826-9376
Brain Tumor Society	800/770-8287
Burger King Cancer Caring Center	412/622-1212
Cancer Care, Inc.	800/813-4673
Cancer Conquerors Foundation	800/238-6479
Cancer Hope Network	877/HOPENET
Cancer Information and Counseling Line	800/525-3777
Cancer Support Network	412/361-8600
Cancer Survivors Network	877/333-HOPE
Cancervive	310/203-9232
Catholic Charities USA	703/549-1390
ChemoCare	800/55-CHEMO
Encore Plus	202/628-3636
Exceptional Cancer Patients	814/337-8192
Gilda's Club	888/GILDA-4-U
International Association of Laryngectomees	800/227-2345
Kids Konnected	800/899-2866
Leukemia and Lymphoma Society	800/955-4572
Look Good. . .Feel Better	lookgoodfeel better.org
Make Today Count	800/432-2273
Mautner Project for Lesbians With Cancer	202/332-5536
National Asian Women's Health Organization	415/989-9747
National Bone Marrow Transplant Link	800/546-5268
People Living With Cancer	703/797-1914
Sisters Network	713/781-0255
United Ostomy Association	800/826-0826
Wellness Community	888/793-WELL
Y-ME	800/221-2141

CUPS

See Cancers of an Unknown Primary Site

Death/Dying

Children's Hospice International	800/242-4453
Foundation for Hospice and Home Care	202/547-7424
Hospice Foundation of America	800/854-3402
Hospice Education Foundation	800/331-1620
Make-a-Wish Foundation of America	602/279-9474

Make Today Count	800/432-2273
National Cancer Institute	800/4-CANCER
National Hospice and Palliative Care Organization	800/658-8898
National Institute for Jewish Hospice	800/446-4448
Partnership for Caring	800/989-9455

Donor-Patient Matching Programs

Anderson Network	800/345-6324
Association of Cancer Online Resources	212/226-5525
Bloch Cancer Foundation	800/433-0464
Caitlin Raymond International Registry	800/726-2824
Cancer Hope Network	877/467-3638
National Cancer Institute	800/4-CANCER
National Foundation for Transplants	800/489-3863
National Marrow Donor Program	888/999-6743

Esophagus

American Cancer Society	800/ACS-2345
American Society of Clinical Oncology	703/797-1914
Anderson Network	800/345-6324
Association of Cancer Online Resources	acor.org
Bloch Cancer Foundation	800/433-0464
Cancer Control PLANET	cancercontrolplanet.cancer.gov
Carcinoid Cancer Foundation	888/722-3132
Centerwatch	centerwatch.com
Coalition of National Cancer Cooperative Groups	877/520-4457
National Cancer Institute	800/4-CANCER
National Coalition for Cancer Survivorship	877/622-7937
OncoLink	oncolink.upenn.edu

Eye

Eye Cancer Network	212/832-8170

Face

AboutFace	800/225-3223
American Cancer Society	800/ACS-2345
American Society of Clinical Oncology	703/797-1914
Anderson Network	800/345-6324
Association of Cancer Online Resources	acor.org
Bloch Cancer Foundation	800/433-0464
Cancer Control PLANET	cancercontrolplanet.cancer.gov
Centerwatch	centerwatch.com
Coalition of National Cancer Cooperative Groups	877/520-4457

Let's Face It	508/371-3186
National Cancer Institute	800/4-CANCER
National Coalition for Cancer Survivorship	877/622-7937
National Foundation for Facial Reconstruction	212/263-6656
OncoLink	oncolink.upenn.edu
Support for People with Oral and Head and Neck Cancer	800/377-0928

Fertility

American Cancer Society	800/ACS-2345
Fertile HOPE	888/994-HOPE
Impotence Institute of America	800/669-1603
National Cancer Institute	800/4-CANCER
National Infertility Association	617/623-1156

Financial Assistance (many types)

American Amputee Foundation	501/666-2523
American Cancer Society	800/ACS-2345
Amgen Safety Net	800/272-9376
AstraZeneca Foundation Patient Assistance Program	800/424-3727
Aventis Oncology	800/996-6626
AVONCares Program for Medically Underserved Women	800/813-4673
Bone Marrow Foundation	800/365-1336
Caitlin Raymond International Registry	800/726-2824
CHAMPUS (military veterans)	800/733-8387
Departments of Social Services (see your local white pages)	
Eli Lilly's Patient Assistance Programs	800/545-6962
Fertile HOPE	888/994-HOPE
GlaxoSmithKline's Commitment to Access	866/265-6491
Helping Patients.org	800/762-4636
Hill-Burton Program	800/638-0742
Leukemia and Lymphoma Society	800/955-4572
Medicaid	877/267-2323
Medicare	877/267-2323
Merck Patient Assistance Program	800/994-2111
National Association of Community Action Agencies	202/265-7546
National Council on Aging	benefitscheckup.org
National Foundation for Facial Reconstruction	212/263-6656
National Foundation for Transplants	800/489-3863
National Marrow Donor Program	888/999-6743
National Transplant Assistance Fund	800/642-8399
NeedyMeds	needymeds.com
ONCOLINE Roche Reimbursement/Patient Assistance Program	800/443-6676

Ortho Biotech Procrit Line   800/553-3851

PACT Plus   *See* Aventis

Partnership for Prescription Assistance   888/477-2669

Patient Advocate Foundation's Co-Pay Relief Patient
    Assistance Program   866/512-3861

Pfizer's Patient Assistance Programs   800/707-8990

Pharmaceutical Research and Manufacturers of America   202/835-3400

RxAssist and Rx Outreach Patient Assistance Programs   800/332-2056

Schering-Plough Pharmaceuticals Commitment to
    Care Program   800/521-7157

Social Security Administration   800/772-1213

South-Eastern Organ Procurement Foundation   800/543-6399

State Children's Health Insurance Program   877/543-7669

Together Rx Access   800/444-4106

Ulman Cancer Fund for Young Adults   888/393-FUND

Y-ME   800/221-2141

Financial Planners

Institute of Certified Financial Planners   800/282-7526

International Association of Personal Financial Planners   800/945-4237

National Association of Personal Financial Planners   888/333-6659

Personal Financial Planning Division, AICPA   888/777-7077

Society of Financial Service Professionals   888/243-2258

Food, Feeding
See Meals; Nutrition and Food Supplements

Gall Bladder

American Cancer Society   800/ACS-2345

American Society of Clinical Oncology   703/797-1914

Anderson Network   800/345-6324

Association of Cancer Online Resources   acor.org

Bloch Cancer Foundation   800/433-0464

Cancer Control PLANET   cancercontrolplanet
                                                                      .cancer.gov

Centerwatch   centerwatch.com

Coalition of National Cancer Cooperative Groups   877/520-4457

National Cancer Institute   800/4-CANCER

National Coalition for Cancer Survivorship   877/622-7937

National Organization for Rare Disorders   800/999-6673

OncoLink   oncolink.upenn.edu

Gastrointestinal

American Society of Clinical Oncology   703/797-1914

Association of Cancer Online Resources   acor.org

Centerwatch   centerwatch.com
Coalition of National Cancer Cooperative Groups   877/520-4457
Life Raft Group, The   liferaftgroup.org
National Coalition for Cancer Survivorship   877/622-7937
OncoLink   oncolink.upenn.edu
Also see Carcinoid

Genetics
Cancer Genetics Network   epi.grants.cancer
                                                     .gov/CGN

Gynecologic
American Cancer Society   800/ACS-2345
American Society of Clinical Oncology   703/797-1914
Anderson Network   800/345-6324
Association of Cancer Online Resources   acor.org
Bloch Cancer Foundation   800/433-0464
Cancer Control PLANET   cancercontrolplanet
                                                     .cancer.gov

Centerwatch   centerwatch.com
Coalition of National Cancer Cooperative Groups   877/520-4457
Gynecologic Cancer Foundation   800/444-4441
National Cancer Institute   800/4-CANCER
National Coalition for Cancer Survivorship   877/622-7937
OncoLink   oncolink.upenn.edu
Society of Gynecological Oncologists   312/644-6610
Society of Gynecologic Nurse Oncologists   312/434-8639
Also see Ovarian

Head
AboutFace   800/225-3223
American Cancer Society   800/ACS-2345
American Society of Clinical Oncology   703/797-1914
Anderson Network   800/345-6324
Association of Cancer Online Resources   acor.org
Bloch Cancer Foundation   800/433-0464
Cancer Control PLANET   cancercontrolplanet
                                                     .cancer.gov

Centerwatch   centerwatch.com
Coalition of National Cancer Cooperative Groups   877/520-4457
Let's Face It   508/371-3186
National Cancer Institute   800/4-CANCER
National Coalition for Cancer Survivorship   877/622-7937
National Foundation for Facial Reconstruction   212/263-6656
OncoLink   oncolink.upenn.edu

	Oral Cancer Foundation	949/646-8000
	Support for People with Oral and Head and Neck Cancer	800/377-0928

Herbs and Botanicals

About Herbs, Botanicals & Other Products	mskcc.org/ html/11570.cfm
Biological Therapy Institute Foundation	615/790-7535

Housing (near treatment centers)

American Cancer Society (Hope Lodges)	800/ACS-2345
National Association of Hospital Hospitality Houses	800/542-9730
Ronald McDonald Houses	708/575-7418

Impotence

American Cancer Society	800/ACS-2345
Impotence Institute of America	800/669-1603
National Cancer Institute	800/4-CANCER

Incontinence

American Cancer Society	800/ACS-2345
National Association for Continence	800/252-3337
National Cancer Institute	800/4-CANCER

Kidney

American Cancer Society	800/ACS-2345
American Foundation for Urologic Disease	800/242-2383
American Society of Clinical Oncology	703/797-1914
Association of Cancer Online Resources	acor.org
Cancer Control PLANET	cancercontrolplanet .cancer.gov
Centerwatch	centerwatch.com
Coalition of National Cancer Cooperative Groups	877/520-4457
Kidney Cancer Association	800/850-9132
National Cancer Institute	800/4-CANCER
National Coalition for Cancer Survivorship	877/622-7937
OncoLink	oncolink.upenn.edu
Steve Dunn's Kidney Cancer Guide	cancerguide.org

Larynx

American Cancer Society	800/ACS-2345
American Society of Clinical Oncology	703/797-1914
Association of Cancer Online Resources	acor.org
Cancer Control PLANET	cancercontrolplanet .cancer.gov
Centerwatch	centerwatch.com
Coalition of National Cancer Cooperative Groups	877/520-4457

International Association of Laryngectomees	800/227-2345
National Cancer Institute	800/4-CANCER
National Coalition for Cancer Survivorship	877/622-7937
OncoLink	oncolink.upenn.edu
Support for People with Oral and Head and Neck Cancer	800/377-0928

Legal and Procedural Counsel

Alliance for Lung Cancer Advocacy, Support and Education	800/298-2436
American Cancer Society	800/ACS-2345
Cancer Legal Resource Center	213/736-1455
Center for Patient Advocacy	800/846-7444
Kidney Cancer Association	800/850-9132
Lance Armstrong Foundation	512/236-8820
National Asian Women's Health Organization	415/989-9747
National Coalition for Cancer Survivorship	877/622-7937
Patient Advocate Foundation	800/532-5274

Leukemia

American Cancer Society	800/ACS-2345
American Society of Clinical Oncology	703/797-1914
Anderson Network	800/345-6324
Association of Cancer Online Resources	acor.org
Bloch Cancer Foundation	800/433-0464
Cancer Control PLANET	cancercontrolplanet.cancer.gov
Cancer Hope Network	877/467-3638
Centerwatch	centerwatch.com
Coalition of National Cancer Cooperative Groups	877/520-4457
Leukemia and Lymphoma Society	800/955-4572
Moving Forward Foundation	713/669-0908
National Cancer Institute	800/4-CANCER
National Coalition for Cancer Survivorship	877/622-7937
OncoLink	oncolink.upenn.edu

Also see Blood

Liver

American Cancer Society	800/ACS-2345
American Society of Clinical Oncology	703/797-1914
Association of Cancer Online Resources	acor.org
Cancer Control PLANET	cancercontrolplanet.cancer.gov
Centerwatch	centerwatch.com
Coalition of National Cancer Cooperative Groups	877/520-4457
Liver Cancer Network, Allegheny General Hospital	412/359-6738
LiverTumor.org	877/306-3114

National Cancer Institute ... 800/422-6237
National Coalition for Cancer Survivorship ... 877/622-7937
National Institutes of Health ... clinicaltrials.gov
OncoLink ... oncolink.upenn.edu

Lung

Alliance for Lung Cancer Advocacy, Support and Education	800/298-2436
American Association for Respiratory Care	972/243-2272
American Cancer Society	800/ACS-2345
American Lung Association	800/LUNG USA
American Society of Clinical Oncology	703/797-1914
American Thoracic Society	212/315-8700
Anderson Network	800/345-6324
Association of Cancer Online Resources	acor.org
Bloch Cancer Foundation	800/433-0464
Cancer Control PLANET	cancercontrolplanet.cancer.gov
Centerwatch	centerwatch.com
Coalition of National Cancer Cooperative Groups	877/520-4457
Its Time to Focus on Lung Cancer	877/646-5864
Lung Cancer Awareness Campaign (same org. as It's Time to Focus on Lung Cancer)	877/646-5864
National Cancer Institute	800/4-CANCER
National Coalition for Cancer Survivorship	877/622-7937
National Familial Lung Cancer Registry	410/614-1910
OncoLink	oncolink.upenn.edu
Pulmonary Hypertension Association	800/748-7274
Society of Surgical Oncology	847/427-1400

Lymph System / Lymphoma

American Cancer Society	800/ACS-2345
American Society of Clinical Oncology	703/797-1914
Anderson Network	800/345-6324
Association of Cancer Online Resources	acor.org
Cancer Control PLANET	cancercontrolplanet.cancer.gov
Centerwatch	centerwatch.com
Coalition of National Cancer Cooperative Groups	877/520-4457
Cure for Lymphoma Foundation	800/235-6848
Cutaneous Lymphoma Network	513/584-6805
Leukemia and Lymphoma Society	800/955-4572
Lymphoma Information Network	lymphomainfo.net
Lymphoma Research Foundation	800/500-9976
Moving Forward Foundation	713/669-0908
Mycosis Fungoides Foundation	248/644-9014

National Cancer Institute	800/4-CANCER
National Coalition for Cancer Survivorship	877/622-7937
National Lymphedema Network	800/541-3259
OncoLink	oncolink.upenn.edu

Magazines
Coping with Cancer	615/791-3859
CURE	800/210-CURE
Heal	214/820-7152

Marrow
See Bone Marrow

Meals (for the poor and disabled)
Catholic Charities USA	703/549-1390
National Meals on Wheels Foundation	616/531-9909
Ronald McDonald House	630/623-7048
Oley Foundation (meals by tube or IV)	800/776-OLEY

Melanoma
American Academy of Dermatology	847/330-0230
American Cancer Society	800/ACS-2345
American Society of Clinical Oncology	703/797-1914
Anderson Network	800/345-6324
Association of Cancer Online Resources	acor.org
Billy Foundation	510/264-9078
Cancer Control PLANET	cancercontrolplanet.cancer.gov
Centerwatch	centerwatch.com
Coalition of National Cancer Cooperative Groups	877/520-4457
Melanoma Center	melanomcenter.org
Melanoma Patients' Information Page	mpip.org
National Cancer Institute	800/4-CANCER
National Coalition for Cancer Survivorship	877/622-7937
OncoLink	oncolink.upenn.edu
Skin Cancer Foundation	800/754-6490
Also see Skin

Mesothelioma
American Cancer Society	800/ACS-2345
American Society of Clinical Oncology	703/797-1914
American Thoracic Society	212/315-8700
Association of Cancer Online Resources	acor.org
Cancer Control PLANET	cancercontrolplanet.cancer.gov

Centerwatch	centerwatch.com
Coalition of National Cancer Cooperative Groups	877/520-4457
Mesothelioma Applied Research Foundation	805/560-8942
National Cancer Institute	800/4-CANCER
National Coalition for Cancer Survivorship	877/622-7937
OncoLink	oncolink.upenn.edu

Military Programs (active duty, dependents, and retired)

Tricare, formerly CHAMPUS (eligibility line)	800/538-9552

Multiple Myeloma

American Cancer Society	800/ACS-2345
American Society for Blood and Marrow Transplantation	847/427-0224
American Society of Clinical Oncology	703/797-1914
Association of Cancer Online Resources	acor.org
Cancer Control PLANET	cancercontrolplanet.cancer.gov
Centerwatch	centerwatch.com
Coalition of National Cancer Cooperative Groups	877/520-4457
Institute for Myeloma and Bone Cancer Research	310/623-1210
International Myeloma Foundation	800/452-2873
Multiple Myeloma Research Foundation	203/972-1250
National Cancer Institute	800/4-CANCER
National Coalition for Cancer Survivorship	877/622-7937
OncoLink	oncolink.upenn.edu

Also see Blood

Neck

AboutFace	800/225-3223
American Cancer Society	800/ACS-2345
American Society of Clinical Oncology	703/797-1914
Association of Cancer Online Resources	acor.org
Cancer Control PLANET	cancercontrolplanet.cancer.gov
Centerwatch	centerwatch.com
Coalition of National Cancer Cooperative Groups	877/520-4457
National Cancer Institute	800/4-CANCER
National Coalition for Cancer Survivorship	877/622-7937
OncoLink	oncolink.upenn.edu
Support for People with Oral and Head and Neck Cancer	800/377-0928

Nursing at Home

Area Agencies on Aging	800/677-1116
Catholic Charities USA	703/549-1390
Hospicelink	800/331-1620
National Association for Home Care (and hospice)	202/547-7424

National Family Caregivers Association	800/896-3650
Visiting Nurse Associations of America	888/866-8773

Nutrition and Food Supplements

American Cancer Society	800/ACS-2345
American Institute for Cancer Research	800/843-8114
National Cancer Institute	800/4-CANCER
Oley Foundation	800/776-OLEY

Oncologists

American Society of Clinical Oncology	703/797-1914

Oral

American Cancer Society	800/ACS-2345
American Society of Clinical Oncology	703/797-1914
Association of Cancer Online Resources	acor.org
Cancer Control PLANET	cancercontrolplanet.cancer.gov
Centerwatch	centerwatch.com
Coalition of National Cancer Cooperative Groups	877/520-4457
National Cancer Institute	800/4-CANCER
National Coalition for Cancer Survivorship	877/622-7937
OncoLink	oncolink.upenn.edu
Support for People with Oral and Head and Neck Cancer	800/377-0928

Ostomy

American Cancer Society	800/ACS-2345
National Cancer Institute	800/4-CANCER
United Ostomy Association	800/826-0826

Ovary

American Cancer Society	800/ACS-2345
American Society of Clinical Oncology	703/797-1914
Association of Cancer Online Resources	acor.org
Cancer Control PLANET	cancercontrolplanet.cancer.gov
Centerwatch	centerwatch.com
Coalition of National Cancer Cooperative Groups	877/520-4457
CONVERSATIONS! Magazine	806/355-2565
Encore Plus	202/628-3636
Facing Our Risk of Cancer Empowered (FORCE)	866/824-7475
Gilda Radner Familial Ovarian Cancer Registry	800/OVARIAN
Gilda's Club	888/GILDA-4-U
National Cancer Institute	800/4-CANCER
National Coalition for Cancer Survivorship	877/622-7937
National Ovarian Cancer Association	416/971-9800 X1320

National Ovarian Cancer Coalition	888/OVARIAN
OncoLink	oncolink.upenn.edu
Ovarian Cancer National Alliance	202/331-1332
Ovarian Cancer Research Fund	800/873-9569
Ovarian Plus International	703/715-6075
Ovarian Problems Discussion List	acor.org
SHARE	866/891-2392

Pain, Nausea, Anxiety Relief

American Academy of Medical Acupuncture	800/521-2262
American Academy of Pain Medicine	708/966-9510
American Alliance of Cancer Pain Initiatives	608/265-4013
American Association of Oriental Medicine	888/500-7999
American Cancer Society	800/ACS-2345
American Pain Foundation	888/615-7246
American Pain Society	847/375-4715
American Society of Anesthesiologists	847/825-5586
Association for Applied Psychophysiology and Biofeedback	aapb.org
National Cancer Institute	800/4-CANCER
National Certification Commission for Acupuncture and Oriental Medicine	703/548-9004
Partners Against Pain	partnersagainstpain.com

Pancreas

American Cancer Society	800/ACS-2345
American Society of Clinical Oncology	703/797-1914
Association of Cancer Online Resources	acor.org
Cancer Control PLANET	cancercontrolplanet.cancer.gov
Centerwatch	centerwatch.com
Coalition of National Cancer Cooperative Groups	877/520-4457
Hirshberg Foundation for Pancreatic Cancer Research	310/472-6310
Lustgarten Foundation	866/789-1000
National Cancer Institute	800/4-CANCER
National Coalition for Cancer Survivorship	877/622-7937
National Pancreas Foundation	866/726-2737
OncoLink	oncolink.upenn.edu
Pancreatic Cancer Action Network	877/272-6226

Parathyroid

American Cancer Society	800/ACS-2345
American Society of Clinical Oncology	703/797-1914
Association of Cancer Online Resources	acor.org
Cancer Control PLANET	cancercontrolplanet.cancer.gov

Centerwatch   centerwatch.com
Coalition of National Cancer Cooperative Groups   877/520-4457
National Cancer Institute   800/4-CANCER
National Coalition for Cancer Survivorship   877/622-7937
Norman Endocrine Surgery Clinic   813/991-6922
OncoLink   oncolink.upenn.edu

Prayer and Spiritual Counseling
   Christian

      Coming Home Network (Catholic and Protestant)   800/664-5110
      700 Club (Evangelical)   800/759-0700
      Upper Room Living Prayer Center   800/251-2468

Jewish
National Center for Jewish Healing   212/399-2320

Muslim
CARE (Council on American-Islamic Relations)   714/776-1847 or
                                                     202/488-8787
Islamic Education Center   909/594-1310

Nonspecific
Dave Dravecky's Outreach of Hope   719/481-3528
World Prayer Team   800/990-6150

Products and Supplies
Abledata   800/227-0216
American Amputee Foundation   501/666-2523
American Cancer Society   800/ACS-2345
Cancer Aid and Research Foundation   623/561-5893
Helping Patients.org   800/762-4636
Look Good. . .Feel Better   lookgoodfeelbetter
                                                     .org
Simon Foundation for Continence   800/237-4666

Prostate
American Cancer Society   800/ACS-2345
American Foundation for Urologic Disease   800/242-2383
American Society of Clinical Oncology   703/797-1914
Association of Cancer Online Resources   acor.org
Cancer Control PLANET   cancercontrolplanet
                                                     .cancer.gov
CaP Cure   800/757-2873
Centerwatch   centerwatch.com
Coalition of National Cancer Cooperative Groups   877/520-4457
Malecare   212/844-8369

National Cancer Institute	800/4-CANCER
National Coalition for Cancer Survivorship	877/622-7937
National Prostate Cancer Coalition	888/245-9455
OncoLink	oncolink.upenn.edu
Patient Advocates for Advanced Cancer Treatments	616/453-1477
Phoenix5	phoenix5.org
Prostate Cancer Education Council	303/316-4685
Prostate Cancer Foundation	*See* CaP CURE
Prostate Net	888/477-6763
Us Too! International	800/808-7866

Quackery and Fraud

National Coalition for Cancer Research	202/663-9125
National Council for Reliable Health Information	909/824-4690
Quackwatch	610/437-1795

Radiation Therapy

American Cancer Society	800/ACS-2345
American Society for Therapeutic Radiology and Oncology	800/962-7876
National Cancer Institute	800/4-CANCER

Rare Cancers

Adenoid Cystic Carcinoma Resource Center	home.paonline.com/knippd/acc/
Adrenocortical Carcinoma	pages.zdnet.com/beverlin/adrenocorticalcarcinoma/
American Cancer Society	800/ACS-2345
American Society of Clinical Oncology	703/797-1914
Anderson Network	800/345-6324
Association of Cancer Online Resources	acor.org
Cancer Control PLANET	cancercontrolplanet.cancer.gov
Centerwatch	centerwatch.com
Coalition of National Cancer Cooperative Groups	877/520-4457
National Cancer Institute	800/4-CANCER
National Coalition for Cancer Survivorship	877/622-7937
National Organization for Rare Disorders	800/999-6673
Neuroblastoma Children's Cancer Society	800/532-5162
OncoLink	oncolink.upenn.edu
VHL Family Alliance	800/767-4845

References (quick-lookup databases)

American College of Surgeons	facs.org
American Society of Clinical Oncology	asco.org
Association of Cancer Online Resources	acor.org

Cancer.com	cancer.com
Cancer Control PLANET	cancercontrolplanet .cancer.gov
Cancer Genetics Network	epi.grants.cancer .gov/CGN
Cancer Info Net	cancerinfonet.org
CancerSource	cancersource.com
Centerwatch	centerwatch.com
Clinical trials consortium	cancertrialshelp.org
Lung Cancer Online	lungcancer.org
National Breast Cancer Foundation	nationalbreastcan cer.org
National Cancer Institute	cancer.gov
OncoLink	oncolink.upenn.edu
Partners Against Pain	partnersagainstpain .com
People Living With Cancer	plwc.org
Phoenix5	phoenix5.org
Physician Data Query (or Protocol Data Query)	cancer.gov
Planet Cancer	planetcancer.org
Women's Cancer Network	wcn.org

Research Services (fee charged)

Doctor Evidence	310/650-8657
Health Resource	800/949-0090
Schine On-line Services	800/346-3287

Sarcoma

American Cancer Society	800/ACS-2345
American Society of Clinical Oncology	703/797-1914
Amschwand Sarcoma Cancer Foundation	713/838-1615
Association of Cancer Online Resources	acor.org
Bloch Cancer Foundation (and hotline)	800/433-0464
Cancer Control PLANET	cancercontrolplanet .cancer.gov
Centerwatch	centerwatch.com
Coalition of National Cancer Cooperative Groups	877/520-4457
GIST Support International	gistsupport.org
Institute for Myeloma and Bone Cancer Research	310/623-1210
Intergroup Rhabdomyosarcoma Study	804/786-9602
Liddy Shriver Sarcoma Initiative	liddyshriversarco mainitiative.org
Life Raft Group	973/837-9095
National Cancer Institute	800/4-CANCER
National Coalition for Cancer Survivorship	877/622-7937
OncoLink	oncolink.upenn.edu

Rare Cancer Alliance	206/600-5327
Sarcoma Alliance	415/381-7236
Sarcoma Foundation of America	301/520-7648

Second-Opinion Locators

American Society of Clinical Oncology	703/797-1914
Anderson Network	800/345-6324
Bloch Cancer Foundation	800/433-0464
FindCancerExperts	findcancerexperts.com

International Cancer Alliance	800/422-7361
National Coalition for Cancer Survivorship	877/622-7937

Skin

American Cancer Society	800/ACS-2345
American Society of Clinical Oncology	703/797-1914
Association of Cancer Online Resources	acor.org
Bloch Cancer Foundation (and hot line)	800/433-0464
Cancer Control PLANET	cancercontrolplanet.cancer.gov
Centerwatch	centerwatch.com
Coalition of National Cancer Cooperative Groups	877/520-4457
Melanoma Patients' Information Page	mpip.org
National Cancer Institute	800/4-CANCER
National Coalition for Cancer Survivorship	877/622-7937
National Council on Skin Cancer Prevention	skincancerprevention.org
OncoLink	oncolink.upenn.edu
Skin Cancer Foundation	800/SKIN-490
SunWise School Program	epa.gov/sunwise
Also see Melanoma	

Small Intestine

American Cancer Society	800/ACS-2345
American College of Gastroenterology	703/820-7400
American Gastroenterological Association	301/654-2055
American Society for Gastrointestinal Endoscopy	978/526-8330
American Society of Clinical Oncology	703/797-1914
Association of Cancer Online Resources	acor.org
Cancer Control PLANET	cancercontrolplanet.cancer.gov
Centerwatch	centerwatch.com
Coalition of National Cancer Cooperative Groups	877/520-4457
Colorectal Cancer Network	301/879-1500
Crohn's and Colitis Foundation of America	914/328-1313
Life Raft Group	liferaftgroup.org

National Cancer Institute   800/4-CANCER
National Coalition for Cancer Survivorship   877/622-7937
OncoLink   oncolink.upenn.edu
United Ostomy Association   800/826-0826

Speech
See Larynx

Stomach
American Cancer Society   800/ACS-2345
American Society for Gastrointestinal Endoscopy   978/526-8330
American Society of Clinical Oncology   703/797-1914
Association of Cancer Online Resources   acor.org
Cancer Control PLANET   cancercontrolplanet
                                                           .cancer.gov
Centerwatch   centerwatch.com
Coalition of National Cancer Cooperative Groups   877/520-4457
GIST Support International   gistsupport.org
Life Raft Group   liferaftgroup.org
National Cancer Institute   800/4-CANCER
National Coalition for Cancer Survivorship   877/622-7937
OncoLink   oncolink.upenn.edu

Support Groups
AboutFace   800/225-3223
American Amputee Foundation   501/666-2523
Bloch Cancer Foundation   800/433-0464
Blood & Marrow Transplant Information Network   888/597-7674
Brain Tumor Foundation   212/265-2401
Brain Tumor Society   800/770-8287
Cancer Care   800/813-4673
Cancer Support Network   412/361-8600
Cancervive   800/486-2873
Carcinoid Cancer Foundation   888/722-3132
Colorectal Cancer Network   301/879-1500
Gilda's Club   888/445-3248
Impotence Institute of America   800/669-1603
International Association of Laryngectomees   800/227-2345
Its Time to Focus on Lung Cancer   877/646-5864
Kidney Cancer Association   800/850-9132
Let's Face It   360/676-7325
Leukemia and Lymphoma Society   800/955-4572
Make Today Count   800/432-2273
Mautner Project for Lesbians With Cancer   202/332-5536
National Adrenal Disease Foundation   516/487-4992

National Infertility Association	617/623-1156
Pancreatic Cancer Action Network	877/272-6226
Partners Against Pain	partnersagainstpain.com
Rare Cancer Alliance	206/600-5327
Wellness Community	888/793-9355

Testicle

American Cancer Society	800/ACS-2345
American Foundation for Urologic Disease	800/242-2383
American Society of Clinical Oncology	703/797-1914
Association of Cancer Online Resources	acor.org
Cancer Control PLANET	cancercontrolplanet.cancer.gov
Centerwatch	centerwatch.com
Coalition of National Cancer Cooperative Groups	877/520-4457
Lance Armstrong Foundation	512/236-8820
Malecare	212/844-8369
National Cancer Institute	800/4-CANCER
National Coalition for Cancer Survivorship	877/622-7937
OncoLink	oncolink.upenn.edu
Testicular Cancer Resource Center	tcrc.acor.org

Thymus

American Cancer Society	800/ACS-2345
American Society of Clinical Oncology	703/797-1914
Anderson Network	800/345-6324
Association of Cancer Online Resources	acor.org
Cancer Control PLANET	cancercontrolplanet.cancer.gov
Centerwatch	centerwatch.com
Coalition of National Cancer Cooperative Groups	877/520-4457
National Cancer Institute	800/4-CANCER
National Coalition for Cancer Survivorship	877/622-7937
National Organization for Rare Disorders	800/999-6673
OncoLink	oncolink.upenn.edu

Thyroid

American Cancer Society	800/ACS-2345
American Society of Clinical Oncology	703/797-1914
American Thyroid Association	718/920-4321
Anderson Network	800/345-6324
Association of Cancer Online Resources	acor.org
Cancer Control PLANET	cancercontrolplanet.cancer.gov

Centerwatch	centerwatch.com
Coalition of National Cancer Cooperative Groups	877/520-4457
Light of Life Foundation	732/972-0461
National Cancer Institute	800/4-CANCER
National Coalition for Cancer Survivorship	877/622-7937
OncoLink	oncolink.upenn.edu
ThyCa: Thyroid Cancer Survivors' Association	877/588-7904
Thyroid Foundation of America	800/832-8321

Transplants (includes marrow and stem cell)

American Cancer Society	800/ACS-2345
American Society for Blood and Marrow Transplantation	847/427-0224
Coalition of National Cancer Cooperative Groups	877/520-4457
National Cancer Institute	800/4-CANCER
National Foundation for Transplants	800/489-3863
National Transplant Assistance Fund	800/642-8399
South-Eastern Organ Procurement Foundation	800/543-6399

Transportation

Note: Many other listings offer free or low-cost local transportation as part of their services.

AirLifeLine	877/247-5433
American Cancer Society	800/ACS-2345
Angel Flight America	800/446-1231
Area Agencies on Aging	800/677-1116
Catholic Charities USA	703/549-1390
Corporate Angel Network	866/328-1313
Mercy Medical Airlift	888/675-1405
National Patient Travel Helpline	800/296-1217

Urology

American Cancer Society	800/ACS-2345
American Foundation for Urologic Disease	800/242-2383
American Society of Clinical Oncology	703/797-1914
Association of Cancer Online Resources	acor.org
Cancer Control PLANET	cancercontrolplanet.cancer.gov
Centerwatch	centerwatch.com
Coalition of National Cancer Cooperative Groups	877/520-4457
National Cancer Institute	800/4-CANCER
National Coalition for Cancer Survivorship	877/622-7937
OncoLink	oncolink.upenn.edu

Uterus

American Cancer Society	800/ACS-2345
American Foundation for Urologic Disease	800/242-2383
American Society of Clinical Oncology	703/797-1914
Association of Cancer Online Resources	acor.org
Anderson Network	800/345-6324
Bloch Cancer Foundation	800/433-0464
Centerwatch	centerwatch.com
Coalition of National Cancer Cooperative Groups	877/520-4457
Gynecologic Cancer Center	800/444-4441
National Cancer Institute	800/4-CANCER
National Coalition for Cancer Survivorship	877/622-7937
OncoLink	oncolink.upenn.edu

Vagina

Gynecologic Cancer Foundation	800/444-4441

Voice / Voice Box
See Larynx

Welfare and Charitable Services

Area Agencies on Aging	800/677-1116
Catholic Charities USA	703/549-1390
Departments of Social Services (see your local white pages)	
Medicaid	877/267-2323
YWCA	202/467-0801

Young Adults

Planet Cancer	planetcancer.org
Ulman Cancer Fund for Young Adults	888/393-FUND

Index

About the Author

Dave Visel has written for newspapers, magazines, radio, and television since the early 1960s, including a fourteen-month stint in Thailand and Vietnam. There, he wrote stories and took combat photographs for most of the world's major newsgathering organizations.

When the digital age began to flower in the late 1970s, Visel cofounded an advertising agency that specialized in high-tech marketing. The emergence of micro- and minitechnology for business applications, the development of computer software and the many scientific advancements of that era were major multiclient marketing focuses of the agency.

Since he sold his advertising agency in 1990, Visel has participated in a number of startup enterprises through initial public offering, merger, or acquisition.

Visel now gives first priority to support of the cancer struggle of his lady. Second precedence is to a careful consideration, by both the author and his wife, of how they can help others through the lessons they have learned over the past six years.